Dec 2001

To: Jeannie
+
Nick,

wishing you good
health as you read
through these pages.

Sueanne
Langdon

David
Rourke

THE FOOD CONNECTION

THE RIGHT FOOD AT THE RIGHT TIME

THE FOOD CONNECTION

THE RIGHT FOOD AT THE RIGHT TIME

Sam Graci

Macmillan Canada
Toronto

First published in Canada in 2001 by
Macmillan Canada, an imprint of CDG Books Canada

National Library of Canada Cataloguing in Publication Data
Graci, Sam, 1946–
   The food connection: the right food at the right time
Includes bibliographical references and index.
ISBN 1-55335-008-1
1. Nutrition.   2. Diet.   3. Hormones.   I. Title.
RA784.G72 2001   613.2   C2001-901530-5

1 2 3 4 5   FP   05 04 03 02 01

Cover design by Tania Craan
Cover photograph by Ralph Ferri
Text design and typesetting by Heidy Lawrance Associates

A portion of the proceeds of the sale of this book will be donated to Scouts Canada for their tree planting program.

Macmillan Canada
An imprint of CDG Books Canada Inc.
Toronto

Printed in Canada

Text pages printed on New Leaf Eco (100% Post Consumer Waste)

This book is available at special discounts for bulk purchases by your group or organization for sales promotions, premiums, fundraising, and seminars. For details, contact: **CDG Books Canada Inc.**, 99 Yorkville Avenue, Suite 400, Toronto, ON, M5R 3K5. Tel: (416)-963-8830. Toll Free: 1 (877)-963-8830. Fax: (416)-923-4821. Web site:cdgbooks.com

DEDICATION

I owe a great debt to so many people who have encouraged my personal growth and helped to bring this book to fruition.

There are three people I would like to dedicate this book to. They are listed in alphabetical order.

STEWART BROWN is my most trusted and valued best friend. He has been sensitive and progressive at one and the same time. This book is only possible because of him. He stands for high ideals and ethics that I continually admire. As the initiative behind this book, it is he who is helping, encouraging and motivating you to optimum health.

JOE GRACI, JR., is my brother. It is hard to express the enormous love I have for him and the total belief I have in him! He never stops trying to bring happiness, joy, love, goodwill and health to everyone he encounters. Bravo Joe! Job well done.

SHANTA MA is Mrs. Hilda Densmore, my adopted mother. "Shanta Ma" means Peaceful Mother. Ah! This is one truly beautiful human being who prays for me, her children and so many others, with conviction and earnestness. We are so very fortunate to bathe in her love. I need her and I know she is and will always be there. "Thank You" eternally, Ma!

CONTENTS

FOREWORD

Over the past 25 years, I have treated thousands of patients using diet, exercise and nutritional supplements as my primary treatment modalities. The power of these simple, inexpensive therapies is completely overlooked by most physicians, who may give lip service to lifestyle changes but rarely spend the time to underscore their importance or help their patients implement them.

As a result, people are looking for guidance elsewhere, as the glut of health-related books on the market attests. Unfortunately, the conflicting advice offered in these books leaves many people confused and frustrated.

This is why I highly endorse Sam Graci's new book, *The Food Connection*. Eschewing the trendy high-fat and high-protein approach, Sam clearly and concisely presents the rationale for a diet centered around vegetables, fruits, whole grains, lean protein and essential fats. He not only provides recipes and easy-to-follow tips for getting started, but he also explains exactly how food can improve—or worsen—your mood, energy level, mental acuity, competent immune surveillance and your health and spontaneous healing.

One of my favorite sections of *The Food Connection* is the discussion of hormonal balance. I have long felt that consideration of hormone levels is a crucial, yet overlooked aspect of health, particularly as we age and levels of certain hormones decline. Sam's explanation of hormonal interactions and his recommendations for optimizing hormone function are unparalleled.

Whether your goal is to stay healthy, age gracefully and avoid the diseases that plague our culture, such as heart disease, diabetes, arthritis, and osteoporosis, or you are looking to reverse these or other chronic, degenerative conditions, I urge you to embrace the principles outlined in *The Food Connection*. Sam's thoughtful, readable book—written in his inimitable and enthusiastic style—deserves a place in the library of anyone seeking optimal health.

The Food Connection is one wake-up call you cannot afford to miss.

Julian Whitaker, M.D.
Author, *Health & Healing* newsletter

ACKNOWLEDGMENTS

To Robert Harris, vice-president and publisher of CDG Books, who from the very beginning inspired my confidence as a writer.

I would especially like to extend my utter gratitude to Susan Girvan who single-handedly contributed not only an enormous number of hours, but her literary acumen to ensure that the material and presentation in this book are both accurate and up-to-date. My great appreciation to both Rebecca Conolly and Anita Castaldi and the team at CDG Books, whose patience and awesome editing brought clarity to my thinking and helped to improve every chapter of this book. They encouraged my personal growth and brought this volume to fruition.

To Patricia Deauville of Vero Beach, Florida, Brad King and Carolyn Lightbourn for their valuable advice, input and insightful comments. The ever-exuberant Brad King always was available to help me translate cutting-edge science into easily understood terms for the general public.

Many thanks to Dianne Fidler for her typing, patience and good will. Special thanks to Karen Corley for her drawing at the end of the Epilogue and to Sallie Stanley-Adams for her supportive encouragement.

Dr. Julian Whitaker, M.D., is a wonderful person whose efficacy, dedication, clarity and brilliance I greatly admire. I am most fortunate to count him as a friend and contributor to this book.

And especially to Abigail Pearpoint, Elvira Graci and Karen Corley—our deep friendships, the inspiring insights we shared together, and their literary guidance were all evolutionary experiences for me. They each did an outstanding job of fine-tuning this book and always remained patient and enthusiastic. They believe in this message. In the process they are helping to improve the lives of hundreds of thousands of people. Bravo! I owe each of you a great deal of gratitude.

And thank you, the reader, for using the dietary strategies in this book to achieve optimum health.

My one dream is to relieve suffering and allow humanity optimum mental, emotional and physical good health for a potentially better world.

Consequently, I have never charged money for lecture series, radio interviews, television interviews, magazine articles or newspaper articles. The author's royalties from my first book, *The Power of Superfoods,* was 100 percent given to non-profit groups that feed children in Canada. *The Power of Superfoods* became the number one best-selling book on health and nutrition in the history of Canada.

To be consistent with my ideals, 100 percent of all profits or author royalties that I receive from the sale of this book will go to support environmental issues across Canada. I will receive no money from the sale of this book.

The book is written on 100 percent recycled paper; set with biodegradable vegetable inks; and a portion of the proceeds will be donated to the tree planting program of Scouts Canada.

INTRODUCTION: UNDERSTANDING THE CONNECTION

WORLDS APART

In a small village in the Chinese countryside, outside the seaport city of Shanghai, 12-year-old Lin Chen arrives home from school to a cup of green tea. Soon after, Lin sits down with her family to enjoy dinner.

The Chens' main dish is a miso-type soup full of garlic, onions and sea vegetables, with slices of tofu and slivers of fish. There is also a separate small bowl of steamed rice topped with chopped scallions. A plate of stir-fried bok choy accompanies a platter of sliced raw tomatoes, green peppers and carrots drizzled with borage oil. After cleaning up, each member of the Chen family enjoys a handful of ripe, local blackberries that are just in season.

In a small town somewhere in British Columbia—or perhaps California, Florida or Nova Scotia—12-year-old Lynn Kristen conveniently rendezvous with her mom and dad, who are both just coming from work. They meet at a busy hamburger chain for dinner.

Lynn orders a burger with mayo, ketchup and mustard, as well as a large order of French fries she covers with table salt and vinegar. She completes her meal with a frosty cola. When Lynn reaches home, she has two scoops of creamy, fudge-brownie chocolate ice cream.

THE BAD NEWS

Statistics show that the Canadian Lynn has already begun to make herself 50 percent more eligible for PMS, a difficult menopause, osteoporosis, high blood pressure, high cholesterol, a poor complexion, weight gain and steadily declining energy than the Asian Lin. Lynn is reaching her "total load" of cumulative toxic damage quickly and is making herself 85 percent more eligible for cancer and heart-related degenerative diseases than Lin, her Chinese counterpart.

After 25 years of nutritional research, I have concluded that lifestyle is a significant factor in this increased risk of disease and certainly the body's diminished ability to spontaneously heal itself. The addition or omission of a single nutrient in your diet can make or break your attention span, learning capability, mood and energy.

In the 1990s there were great hopes, fueled by intensive medical research, that many of our diseases and ailments would prove to be genetic in origin and would, in the foreseeable future, be curable through sophisticated gene therapy. This has yet to be realized and does not appear possible for a long time to come. It is becoming more and more apparent that lifestyle and diet are far more important to your health than your genetic makeup is. It is now very clear that at least 80 to 85 percent of your ailments are caused by your diet, lifestyle or environment, while less than 15 to 20 percent are genetically ordained: your genetics are not your destiny. Here are just a few of the most recent findings:

- Researchers at the U.S. Centers for Disease Control report that both women and men can reduce their risk of dying from stroke or heart disease by 15 percent simply by supplementing with antioxidants and multivitamins daily.
- Harvard Medical School researchers estimate that 85 percent of all deaths from heart disease among women could have been avoided with regular exercise, a healthy diet and avoidance of smoking.
- A large study completed at the U.S. National Heart, Lung and Blood Institute concluded that an adequate vitamin C intake can reduce the risk of dying from cancer by 62 percent.
- Researchers at the Karolinska Institute in Stockholm, Sweden, undertook a major study to determine the most important causes of cancer. They concluded that diet, lifestyle and the environment account for 85 to 90 percent of all cancers. Even among identical twins, the genetically determined cancer risk is less than 15 percent. Robert M. Hoover, M.D., of the National Cancer Institute, wrote an editorial in the July 2000 issue of the *New England Journal of Medicine* to accompany this Scandinavian study. In clarifying the genetic versus environmental contribution to cancer, he writes, "genes and environment interact to produce a risk greater than the sum of their independent effects, which can be reduced by advances in either area."

Our Nutritional Downfall

The Asian Lin ate a satisfying dinner comprised of a variety of unprocessed, unadulterated whole foods. The Western Lynn described *her* dinner as "delicious" because it looked good, smelled good and tasted good. Unfortunately, however, modern technology had refined her food and taken out the nutrients necessary for good health, while leaving behind a variety of chemical compounds that lead to cell damage, resulting in such ailments as fatigue, cloudy thinking, lowered self-esteem, leaky-gut syndrome, poor complexion, weight gain, irritability and poor digestion. These processed foods also contain foreign and toxic compounds called preservatives, taste enhancers, moisturizers, coloring agents, artificial flavors, fungus retardants, hydrogenated oils or fats, lots of empty calories and few nutrients. Researchers call these foreign chemicals xenobiotics because residue from them slowly builds up in your 100 trillion cells causing unnecessary rust and decay. In research, we generally call these accelerated aging factors and health deterrents.

The cause-and-effect relationship between the wrong food choices and negative moods or impaired mental faculties can become a vicious cycle. If poor eating habits are the initial problem, then mood swings, poor concentration, depression and fatigue develop because of dietary deficiencies or excesses, which in turn result in further poor food choices. If, for example, Lynn experiences a mid-afternoon energy sag, she may find herself reaching for a candy bar. From this, she would gain an almost immediate sugar boost. But when her body recovers from this an hour later, she'll find her energy stores even further depleted and perhaps she'll be feeling a bit irritable. She'll likely go looking for another sugar spike, maybe in the form of some high-carbohydrate potato chips. And on and on the declining spiral goes.

Lin's body is regenerative and using its infinite capacity to self-diagnose and self-heal. Lynn's body, on the other hand, is losing its natural ability to self-diagnose and self-heal as she continues to eat this type of synthetic food. Her body is "falling out of its natural rhythm" and into a state of accelerated aging, pain, discomfort, disease and possibly premature death. Lynn needs to readjust her physiology to a regenerative mode and beware of the burger as "King" and the dairy as "Queen."

THE GOOD NEWS

There is plenty of time for Lynn (and you) to take evasive action from chronic disease by readjusting her (and your) physiology to a regenerative mode—if you know how. Much of it depends on the lifestyle choices you make. Those concerning food and water are particularly important because we have control over those choices. There is general agreement that we are what we eat, digest and absorb, whether our food sources are synthetic or from natural, whole food sources.

Each one of your 100 trillion cells is a little molecular motor designed to run at peak efficiency if you fuel it properly. Cells need water, vitamins, minerals, fats, carbohydrates and protein to produce the energy to sustain your body's many and varied functions. The nutrients in natural, unrefined, whole foods— which I call high-octane fuel—keep your cells operating at peak performance and give you the reserve for healing. If the deliveries of necessary nutrients don't arrive, the cells slow their work down—and so do you!

Most of this is not news. Neither is the fact that we need regular exercise. But, did you know that to guard your health and survival you require at least 8.25 hours of sleep a night in a totally dark environment?

The Divine Blueprint—Bioenergetic Whole Foods

The earth naturally produces all sorts of healing bioenergetic foods. Bioenergetic foods are plant-based foods grown under the direct energy pathway of the sun and equally infused with the energies of the soil and rain. They convert their energy (energetic) to the efficient and effective biological (bio) rejuvenation and revitalization of every cell in your body. They promote "high-fidelity" hormone communication in supersymmetry, so they can instantaneously turn any chemical relay system "on" or "off."

Each of the bioenergetic foods contains a variety of nutrients that help ensure your optimum health and healing. You may also consume them indirectly by eating the fish, chickens, animals or wild game that initially ate these bioenergetic whole foods.

Each of these foods, as found in nature, is called a "whole" food because it has all of its naturally occurring parts intact. Lin ate whole foods; Lynn unfortunately ate processed foods that are no longer whole foods. Many of their necessary parts are missing because of refining and processing.

With this book, you'll gain a solid understanding of all the natural foods—such as colorful vegetables, herbs, fruits, berries, grains, lean proteins, beans, nuts, seeds, pollens, grasses and sea vegetables—that will ensure your optimum health and healing and extend your life. These real foods sustain hormone synthesis in the daily tug of war to survive well, and both monitor and adapt you to your internal and external environments.

You'll also learn about how these foods promote "high-fidelity" communication within your hormone system—the control of which is key to your sustained health and longevity. It's critical to understand that hormones left to run at random create senseless chemical reactions that, over time, put your system at high risk.

Finally, you'll learn how to assess your current health, how to apply the principles of eating right, which foods are nutritional powerhouses and why, and which choices will help you control the healthfulness of your personal environment.

Your Most Intimate Experience Ever

Eating food is the most intimate experience you will ever be involved in. Every mouthful of food becomes your skin, hair, body weight, muscles, bones, heart, organs, nervous system, brains, immune system, energy, enzymes and hormones. More importantly, food can be used to enhance your lifelong hormonal control program.

From this point forward, every time you go to eat any food, look at it carefully. Ask yourself, "Do I want this food to become my face, hair, energy, thinking, moods, bones, muscles, organs or immune system?" Remember, modern technology has now made foods look good, smell good and taste good, but they carry a deadly price tag. Don't pay that painful price.

Every minute 200 million new cells are renewed, revitalized or reformed in your body. This is a total of 300 billion new cells a day. The quality of the food you eat daily directly influences the high-quality or low-quality development and functioning of each and every cell.

The Food Connection is not a diet—it is a lifelong hormonal control program. So eat as if your life depends upon it. Embark on a lifelong path of choosing bioenergetic whole foods and accelerate your health and healing. You will never feel sorry you did!

Part I

WHAT HAS FOOD GOT TO DO WITH IT?

1

THE LOSS OF OUR SURVIVAL EDGE

CIRCADIAN RHYTHMS—ON NATURE'S TERMS

Our hunter-gatherer ancestors of the Paleolithic Era ate what we refer to as the "Paleolithic Diet." It was comprised of a lot of wild game, fish, seasonal wild fruits and berries, nuts, leaves, tender green grasses, wild vegetables, herbs, tubers, edible roots, bark, wild whole grains, ocean algae (referred to as sea vegetables)—anything they could hunt or gather—with clean water as their only beverage.

Perhaps it is even more important to note what they did not eat: sugar or artificial sweeteners, salt, cultivated grains (since agriculture had not yet begun) and vegetable oils—in other words, they ate absolutely no processed food. They also did not smoke or consume alcoholic beverages.

Our common ancestors lived off the land and took their cues from nature and the circadian rhythms of night and day (dark and light), as well as cyclical seasons, in order to prepare for different times of the day and different seasons' variations. They followed the 24-hour circadian rhythm of night and day, and so stopped eating and went to sleep when it was dark, and arose when it was light. For eight months of the year—during spring, summer and autumn—they lived primarily on wild game and colorful vegetation. They migrated whenever they needed to. In winter, they slept and rested more, thereby slowing their metabolic processes and slowing the aging of their hormones, neurotransmitters, glands, organs and bodies. Seasonal variations in the circadian rhythms of plants and animals are easily noticed in their adapting to the amount and intensity of heat and light during sprouting, budding, growth, flowering and dormancy. Seasonal changes were the traditional cue for our hunter-gatherer ancestors to migrate, hibernate and breed.

Procreation, for the survival of our human species, was also cyclical and followed the seasons. Children were generally conceived in late August or September (at the end of the "feasting" of summer), lay protectively incubated and developing within their mothers—who could survive the "famine" of winter and nourish their offspring—and were born in May or June, as the "feasting" would begin again.

Our ancestors and the genes they developed were based on the cycles of "feast or famine," within the seasons and balances of nature. Those who had great storage capabilities lived and thrived; those who did not died and their genes became extinct. Today, we are the direct descendants of those who survived, of those who had great potential to store carbohydrates as fat and survive the "famine" of winter until the earth made an orbital shift and the warmth of spring returned.

For over 100,000 years, our ancestors thrived on a diet comprising 60 to 70 percent lean protein (100 to 200 grams of protein daily) in the form of lean, wild game. This meat, due to the organic vegetation the animals ate, contained exceptional amounts of long-chain Omega-3 essential fatty acids. These Omega-3 fatty acids provided humans with DHA (docosahexaenoic acid) and EPA (eicosapentaenoic acid), referred to as EFAs (essential fatty acids). Dietary intake of EFAs both supported and boosted their central nervous system, learning ability, basic moods, superior intelligence and a host of critical mental functions. The remaining 30 to 40 percent of their diet was various, colorful vegetation rich in complex carbohydrates, vitamins, minerals, fiber and phytonutrients.

It is known that our ancestors were lean and strong. In 1988, a group of anthropologists and physicians (Boyd Eaton, M.D., Marjorie Shostak and Melvin Konner, M.D., Ph.D.) from Emory University in Georgia examined skeletal remains of our ancestors and considered their lifestyle and diet in their book *The Paleolithic Prescription*. They conclude that Paleolithic man, who averaged 6' 2", "was easily as strong as today's superior male and female athletes. They worked many fewer hours than the coming Agriculturists, but were significantly more robust."

THE END OF OUR COEXISTENCE WITH NATURE

The dawning of agriculture, just 10,000 years ago, ended the Paleolithic period and eliminated 95 percent of the hunter-gatherer lifestyle worldwide forever. This was the end of our existence on this earth on nature's terms. We began to cultivate the food and domesticate the animals we needed for our survival. Since the arrival of the industrial age, most of society has moved out of agriculture and into industry. So now we buy the foods we need, and the physical labor required is left to others. We live in heated and air-conditioned dwellings that insulate us from the weather. We eat food, far from its natural state, that has been refined and tampered with in one way or another. With the invention of artificial light, we have grown oblivious to the circadian rhythms of day and night and of seasons, and work and play around the clock and calendar, constantly shortening the dark (night) circadian cycle of the day, which is the critical time to revitalize our delicate hormonal and biological systems.

Our move from agriculture has had further detrimental effects on us, as T.S. Wiley and Bent Formby, Ph.D., point out in their book *Lights Out*: "If we were in trouble before, from that moment on, we were in serious danger." Brad J. King and Dr. Michael A. Schmidt, in their ground-breaking book *Bio-Age*, write:

> Things have changed in the last 100 centuries. In this time we seemed to reverse the fundamental law that shaped our physiology and have gone against the principles that got us this far to begin with. Now instead of eating like our ancestors, we have become carbohydrate addicts, consuming carbohydrates as our main source of food with protein as the supplemental food. So what does this have to do with healthy longevity, you ask? A lot!

So while our genetic makeup for digesting, absorbing, distributing and eliminating bioenergetic whole foods has remained largely unchanged in the last 10,000 years, our lifestyle certainly has not. Our hunter-gatherer ancestors were tall, lean, strong and aerobically fit. Although accidents, the trauma of birth and infectious diseases brought them down, they were free of the chronic "diseases of civilization" that cause 85 percent of all deaths in North America today.

Our shifts from hunting and gathering to agriculture, and then to industry, have drastically changed human nutrition and, in turn, have promoted stroke, heart disease, diabetes, obesity, depression and cancer. Modern medicine and infection prevention may have conquered many microbes, but we suffer chronically from diseases caused by our modern lifestyle—diseases that our ancestors effectively avoided. Change the environment—knowingly or unknowingly—and the environment is guaranteed to change us!

THE CHALLENGE OF SURVIVAL—MODERN-DAY ADAPTABILITY

Life has now become an interesting paradox. Our ability to function well, to stay alive, has been possible through some change and adaptability in response to our environment, but more to our ability to influence our environment. Since Paleolithic times, by controlling the weather's seasonal influences by living in protective dwellings, and by ensuring a constant and stable food supply, we have managed to change our environment, or at least mitigate its impact on us. But those changes have now started to hurt our chances of survival instead of helping them. Physically we haven't been able to adapt to the changes that we have made to our environment.

What have we been failing to adapt to? For one thing, a lack of sleep or a lack of deep sleep. We are now trying to run ourselves, with our foot down on the accelerator, 24 hours a day, seven days a week, 365 days a year. We work longer and harder than our ancestors did. We no longer get sufficient sleep, especially the deep sleep that they enjoyed and that our bodies need. For another, we now unsuccessfully try to adapt to synthetic foods made by marketing-driven companies, which have little or no protein, are dangerously devoid of the Omega-3 EFAs essential to human mental health, and are super-saturated with sugars, high-fructose corn syrup or artificial sweeteners. These processed or refined foods contain harmful hydrogenated vegetable oils, processed flour, preservatives, coloring agents and taste enhancers.

There is now a marked decrease in our consumption of high-quality protein, low-density or complex carbohydrates such as vegetables, and moderate-density carbohydrates such as fruits, berries and minimally processed grains that contain a little natural sugar and a lot of fiber, water, vitamins, minerals and phytonutrients. These bioenergetic whole foods are digested slowly and give off their sugar in small doses to ensure steady and productive insulin flow and hormonal balances. Instead, our consumption—or **"eating dumb"**—of processed or high-density carbohydrates with few fibers, vitamins, minerals, water or phytonutrients has skyrocketed, giving us huge amounts of simple sugars and subsequent detrimental "big hits" of insulin and hormonal imbalances. (See Part II, "Hormonal Balance: The Key to Our Well-Being.")

THE FALLOUT

The disruption of the natural circadian rhythm and lifestyle our ancestors had so beautifully adapted to has led to serious consequences for modern humans. Through natural selection, our species, Homo Sapiens, managed to evolve to meet the challenges of hungry predators and a hostile environment. We were and are the most complex physiological species and consequently we are also the most vulnerable.

The same physiological ability that allowed our Paleolithic ancestors to store calories during times of "feasting" for those times of "famine," as well as our shift to large amounts of sugar and fat from processed high-density carbohydrates, is causing us to store unnecessary amounts of fat. After all, we rarely experience times of "famine"—except when we diet.

Paleolithic people slept when the sun went down, reinvigorating, revitalizing and renewing their bodies' metabolic processes. We now stay up late at night under artificial lights, often glued to our television or computer, eating late dinners or high-carbohydrate snacks, accelerating aging and inviting weight gain and degenerative diseases.

We try to correct our resulting weight gain with miracle diets. But, as most of us now know, dieting has never worked and never will. An estimated 95 percent of dieters put the weight back on—if not more—because the Paleolithic ancestor within us recognizes a "famine mode," slows down our metabolism and conserves its portable energy stores from fat. We lose mainly critical water, muscle and bone. Once we begin eating again, our bodies store fat at an even greater capacity than before because we have been physiologically reminded that "famine" does still exist.

All of this is affecting our appetite and eating patterns, our mood, our ability to get a good night's rest, our ability to ward off degenerative diseases, our powers of thought and memory, and our very personality. Both our eating habits and lifestyle are so "out of whack" that our natural synchronicity for balancing internal survival switches that turn hormones "on" or "off" quickly and accurately, are being destroyed. We are accelerating our rate of aging and falling victim more frequently to pain, disease and an early extinction—death!

Improvements in modern life—such as cleaner water, better basic hygiene techniques, proper ventilation, rapid fluid replacement and more protein in the average diet—have reduced the basic killers of the 1940s, but, as the table below shows, poor nutrition, convenient processed foods, excess "empty calories," stress and a mounting "sleep debt" have given rise to modern-day lifestyle-related killers.

LEADING CAUSES OF DEATH IN NORTH AMERICA

1940	2000
1. Pneumonia and flu	1. Heart disease
2. Tuberculosis	2. Cancer
3. Diarrhea and intestinal ills	3. Stroke
4. Heart disease	4. Lung disease
5. Stroke	5. Accidents
6. Kidney failure	6. Pneumonia and flu
7. Accidents	7. Diabetes
8. Cancer	8. Suicide
9. Senility	9. Kidney failure
10. Diphtheria	10. Liver disease

RECOGNIZING THE ERROR OF OUR WAYS

We need modern-day adaptability to start working with the remarkable body evolution has given us. This means restoring its ability to spontaneously self-diagnose and self-heal. Once we understand in detail how our body, mind and emotions function, we can give all our cells, our 100 trillion little molecular motors, what they need to function optimally. We can largely avoid our modern-day "diseases of civilization" and live healthfully in our senior years. We can do this by learning to eat in harmony with our longstanding genetic predisposition to food. I like to call this **"eating smart."** Dr. David Jenkins of St. Michael's Hospital and professor of nutrition of the University of Toronto uses this

Paleolithic diet, which he calls the "Garden of Eden Diet," to lower cholesterol levels a staggering 30 percent in a mere two weeks with no medication.

WE ARE BUILT FOR WELLNESS—NOT ILLNESS

Will help, to keep us adaptable to the natural food chain, be coming soon to a drug store or doctor's office near you? In the "Divine Blueprint," the molecular architecture has given us everyday foods to keep the activities of our cellular, sub-cellular, molecular and even atomic levels running with accuracy and precision. Where are they? My goodness, they're right in our gardens, whole food stores, farmers' markets and produce sections of grocery stores as fruits, vegetables, herbs and sea vegetables. We can also find them in nutritional food stores in bins of grains, legumes, nuts, seeds, beans and peas. Right now, as you read these very words, they are probably right in your refrigerator, vegetable garden or cupboard.

Look for them vigilantly and use them wisely because—if you haven't noticed—you're running out of time!

Part II

HORMONAL BALANCE: THE KEY TO OUR WELL-BEING

GREAT CONDUCTORS IN THE SYMPHONY OF HUMAN LIFE

2

OPTIMIZING HORMONE FUNCTION

Anabolic capacity and anabolic drive—our cellular repair system—are both at their maximum levels when all of our body's hormones and neurotransmitters are in balance and at their peak levels.

All hormones and neurotransmitters were designed to be in supersymmetry with one another and in harmony with the natural circadian rhythms of nature's light, dark and seasonal variations.

All of your hormones—growth hormone, melatonin, testosterone, cortisol, DHEA, dopamine, insulin and others—interface between your environment and the thoughts and reactions it produces in your central nervous system. All of your information gathering that dictates a hormonal response comes from seeing, hearing, touching, tasting, smelling and thinking:

- Insulin levels dictate sex hormones like estrogen and testosterone.
- Light hitting your skin prevents melatonin secretion in the dark cycle.
- Melatonin cascades into prolactin, which triggers cortisol secretion and further cascades into dopamine, which are synergistic with your mood and food preferences.

Biologically, all this happens in the HPA axis (hypothalamus-pituitary-adrenal gland axis). This interaction between your hormones and the environment allows you to continually adapt and survive.

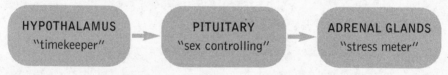

HYPOTHALAMUS
"timekeeper"

PITUITARY
"sex controlling"

ADRENAL GLANDS
"stress meter"

THE ROLE OF HORMONES

The word hormone is derived from the Greek word *hormao*, which means "arise to action." A hormone is a biochemical messenger that is a molecular call to action that can work with incredible speed, accuracy and complexity to communicate information from the brain to "target tissues" anywhere in the body. Any breakdown in the fidelity of your hormonal communication system will have negative consequences on your mental acuity, robust energy, sleeping, immune system, appearance and longevity.

Your ancestors survived by adapting to their food supply and environment. To survive well today, you require a superior biological communication system of hormones that can send accurate signals effortlessly, over discrete channels, at any time, anywhere in your body. You need a secure information network so that the right information gets to the right place at the right time without choking your system with contradictory input. If you don't—trouble!

Hormones are biochemical messengers that have the ability to modify the biological response of a cell, or complex network of cells, with which they are interacting "in real time." All hormones have positive feedback and negative feedback loops so their complex communication networks are not haphazard but efficient and specific. Positive feedback loops are wireless communications that "turn on" a biochemical reaction, and negative feedback loops can instantaneously "turn off" any reaction.

This complex feedback communication system is your hormonal lifeline.

Neurotransmitters: Our Hormones' Chemical Messengers

The human brain is made up of 100 billion nerve cells or neurons. Between each neuron is a tiny space called a synaptic gap. Since neurons don't touch the ends of one another, a "sending" neuron must send an electrical message to a "receiving" neuron. This message must find a way to "jump" across the synaptic gap so it can relay the message within the brain along millions of sending and receiving neurons, through the nervous system to the rest of the body.

Nature has developed nerve chemicals, called neurotransmitters, which are stored at the end of each neuron. When an electrical message (such as a thought) travels along a neuron, it arrives at the end and triggers neurotransmitters to be released. The neurotransmitters carry the electrical message across the synaptic gap to the receiving neuron. Once the neurotransmitter has completed its job, it is either recycled back to the end of the sending neuron or broken down.

This elaborate communication system between our brain and body is responsible for the orders that our glands secrete necessary hormones, that our muscles contract, and for every response, thought, accepting or repulsing emotion, and every mood. If messages from the brain could not be successfully transmitted, all processes dependent on the central nervous system would come to a grinding halt.

The imbalance deficiency of just one neurotransmitter alters neuron-reception quality or neuron-sending quality. This causes a "cascading" effect on other neurotransmitters that alters our peak physical, emotional and mental performance.

The brain may send an electrical message along a neuron, but if there is an insufficient supply of a neurotransmitter, the message is not communicated and thus causes an imbalance in the symphony of mind–body processes. For example, if there is a depleted amount of the neurotransmitter acetylcholine, we experience memory loss. Some neurotransmitters are affected by food additives in processed food, such as monosodium glutamate (MSG). In 1994, a dash of MSG in an airline salad put me in the airport hospital in San Francisco with symptoms mimicking a heart attack.

THE 11 CRITICAL HORMONES AND NEUROTRANSMITTERS

There are certain hormones and neurotransmitters that we should be aware of and take into consideration when making lifestyle and food choices. Some of these contribute to our anabolic drive or cellular repair, while others contribute to our catabolic drive or cellular "wear and tear."

All hormones and neurotransmitters were designed to be in harmony with one another and with the natural circadian rhythms of light, dark and seasonal variations.

> Well over 75 different neurotransmitters have been identified so far and there are many more yet to be discovered. The three main neurotransmitters are acetylcholine, dopamine and serotonin.

The Anabolic Hormones and Neurotransmitters

Insulin: This hormone is necessary for energy storage and protein synthesis. It promotes the synthesis and storage of glucose as glycogen, an on-demand energy source that is stored in the liver and muscles for short-term energy, and as fat for long-term energy. Insulin also helps to build protein from the building blocks you get from eating protein, called amino acids. It is secreted from the pancreas immediately following a meal and during periods of elevated blood sugar.

When there is not enough insulin you become "wasted" because the cells do not receive sufficient glucose, their primary fuel mix. When there is too much, insulin receptors stop working and glucose is stored long-term as body fat. Your brain uses 120 grams of glucose daily and the rest of your body about 240 grams of glucose daily. (Our brain is only 2 percent of our body mass, but utilizes 50 percent of the body's energy to function optimally.) The brain does not require insulin to pump glucose into its interior cells. Your brain absorbs glucose independently of insulin, which gives it first priority for bloodstream glucose over any other cells in the body.

Testosterone: This hormone is equally critical for men and women. It increases lean muscle mass, strong bones and red blood cell mass. It initiates protein synthesis and gives the ergogenic drive. Testosterone promotes growth hormone (GH) release and increases the metabolic rate, which burns fat.

Growth Hormone (GH): GH is released by the pituitary gland, in spurts, during deep sleep. It promotes a sense of well-being, increases lean muscle mass, strengthens bones, decreases body fat and boosts the immune system. It's our youth hormone. Growth hormone releasing hormone (GHRH) increases GH in the bloodstream, and another hormone, somatostatin, halts its production.

Serotonin: Our appetite, obsessive behavior and cravings are influenced by the neurotransmitter serotonin. It is also responsible for our peace of mind, tranquility and comfort. Serotonin "filters out" negative impulses and behaviors. Too much serotonin leads to nausea and diarrhea. Too little serotonin causes a person to be anxious, restless, depressed, impulsive and aggressive.

Serotonin needs to be balanced with melatonin (see below). An imbalance increases cortisol (see below) levels and stress, and can lead to poor impulse control, depression, and behaviors of overdrinking, overeating or a need to "get stoned." No other neurotransmitter is associated so strongly with our diet.

It is made in our brain from the amino acid tryptophan. As bloodstream levels of tryptophan rise or fall, so do levels of serotonin.

Melatonin: Melatonin operates our body's "biological clock." It influences a wide range of functions from fertility to insulin production to immunity—melatonin is our strongest anti-cancer hormone. Production of melatonin decreases dramatically with age from about 25.

It is produced by serotonin, in a two-step process, in the pineal gland of the brain. It is the second messenger, cyclic AMP, which carries the message to synthesize melatonin from serotonin. Once made, melatonin decreases cyclic AMP levels, thereby reducing all other hormones that require cyclic AMP to carry their message. Once this is accomplished, the body and mind can go into a deep sleep, since the body is less active. To further promote deep sleep and less activity, melatonin also reduces body temperature.

Melatonin production and release are governed mainly by cycles of light, dark and seasonal variations. It is turned "off" by daylight and turned "on" by darkness. Serotonin is made in your brain during the day as you eat carbohydrates and the amino acid tryptophan; then it rapidly converts to melatonin at sundown.

Dopamine: This neurotransmitter keeps us alert and vigilant. It is released just before we awake, but if we go to sleep too late in the dark cycle, it will not be released. Without it, we feel dull and out of sync.

It controls the "fight or flight" mechanism by controlling the release of adrenaline, which automatically alerts us in an emergency. It is also responsible for involuntary movements such as blinking and for emotional drive and spontaneity.

Dopamine also declines with age, but it can be "burned out" earlier by the continual use of drugs such as marijuana, ecstasy, speed, crack and cocaine. The "high" from drugs comes from the sudden release and surge of dopamine.

Ten million dopamine cells are located deep in the brain. As our brain uses dopamine, a toxic free radical is produced that contributes to the destruction of the dopamine neuron. Full-blown dopamine deficiency is known as Parkinson's disease.

Dopamine is oxidized (degraded) in the brain by the enzyme monoamine oxidase B (MAO-B), which increases progressively in activity from about the age of 30. It appears to be responsible for many of the physical and mental symptoms of aging: increasing lethargy, negativity and depression.

Dehydroepiandrosterone (DHEA): DHEA is the most abundant hormone in our bodies. It is produced by the adrenal glands and influences more than 150 different biochemical interactions throughout the body and brain. DHEA is called "the mother hormone" because it is the precursor for other adrenal hormones like estrogen, progesterone, testosterone and cortisol.

Properly elevated levels of DHEA sulfate in the bloodstream send anabolic instructions to each of our 100 trillion cells to repair, rebuild, restore and revitalize. This boosts our memory, mood, immune response and longevity. DHEA is classified as a youth hormone and typically declines about 2 percent a year after the age of 30; the average 70-year-old's DHEA levels will be only 10 to 20 percent of what they were at age 30.

DHEA can be supplemented. According to Dr. Sam Yen, a leading DHEA researcher at the University of California at San Diego, "DHEA in appropriate replacement doses has remedial effects with respect to its ability to induce an anabolic growth factor, increase muscle strength and lean body mass, activate immune function and enhance quality of life in aging men and women."

The Catabolic Hormones

Each of these hormones serves a specific beneficial purpose. However, when imbalanced or in excess they become detrimental to our well-being.

Cortisol: This hormone is secreted by the adrenal glands and takes control of metabolic networks in extreme stress. Cortisol becomes a problem when its temporary job becomes permanent in chronic stress. In excess, it increases insulin levels and blood sugar levels, decreases immune functions, increases blood pressure and causes brain damage. It is the second most abundant hormone in your body after DHEA.

Glucagon: Glucagon is concerned with processing glucose, the primary source of fuel for all our cells. It is the ratio between the hormones insulin and glucagon that determines whether there is storage or depletion of energy stores. Secreted by the pancreas, its action increases the blood glucose level between meals by stimulating the breakdown of glycogen in the liver. Glucagon increases with aging after 25 and promotes elevated glucose levels.

Epinephrine and Norepinephrine: These two hormones work with cortisol in times of danger, stimulating the nervous system, increasing heart rate and making us more alert. Too much can produce pronounced anxiety attacks, and if prolonged, can upset the insulin-glucagon ratio. Epinephrine is also called adrenaline.

Thyroid Hormone: The thyroid hormone regulates our resting metabolic rate and the effects of epinephrine and norepinephrine. Our bodies are hypersensitive to any imbalance. Too much thyroid hormone increases metabolism and accelerates aging; too little leads to depression and inertia. Too much thyroid hormone makes you agitated or jumpy; too little makes you unresponsive. It also magnifies cortisol's actions. Too much or too little accelerates aging.

A Delicate Balance

Both our hormones and neurotransmitters decline steadily with age. For most people, hormones and neurotransmitters will peak at about age 25, ride a plateau until 40, and then begin a steep decline. By the age of 75, most of us have only 20 percent of the vital hormones we had at 20. For example, growth hormone (GH)—our revitalizing and rejuvenating hormone that secretes primarily in small bursts while we are in a deep sleep phase—diminishes to only 10 to 15 percent of peak levels by the time we reach 75. The number of hormonal cell receptors also declines radically with aging. **Even one hormone out of balance with the others will throw the entire symphony out of tune.**

All of our hormones and neurotransmitters are working together with incredible speed, accuracy and complexity to communicate information from the brain to target tissues throughout the body.

Hormonal feedback loops operate on a hormonal axis that keeps all biochemical and biological functions within a "safe zone" because opposing hormones play a physiological tug-of-war to maintain balance.

For example, the control of blood glucose, our cells' primary fuel mix, is critical for optimal brain function. The primary hormonal axis that controls blood glucose is the insulin-glucagon axis. Insulin drives blood glucose down; glucagon raises blood glucose. As long as these two hormones are balanced in their opposing physiological actions, blood glucose levels are stabilized and brain function is optimal. This is an example of how our brain and body work hard every second to maintain efficient symmetry, balance and harmony in all our body's complex biochemical reactions.

Any breakdown in this system will have negative consequences on our mental acuity, energy, sleep patterns, immune system, appearance and longevity.

Let's look at an everyday example of how destructive a disruption in this insulin-glucagon axis can be: the consumption of a highly processed carbohydrate. If we eat a large plate of pasta at lunch, most of us will hardly be able to stay awake at 3:30 p.m. There is a reason this time of day has been dubbed "the afternoon doldrums."

The carbohydrates in the pasta have triggered a rapid release of insulin into the bloodstream, which drives blood glucose levels down. The pasta contains only a smidgen of the protein that is required to trigger the release of the hormone glucagon, which raises blood glucose. The long-and-short of it is that the carbohydrate-rich pasta lunch has temporarily disrupted the insulin-glucagon axis. We are sleepy three hours later because of a significant drop in brain function that resulted from a diminished supply of blood glucose (our brain's primary fuel).

FOODS, MOODS AND FEEDBACK LOOPS
Eating a 100% Processed Carbohydrate-Rich Snack or Meal Anytime

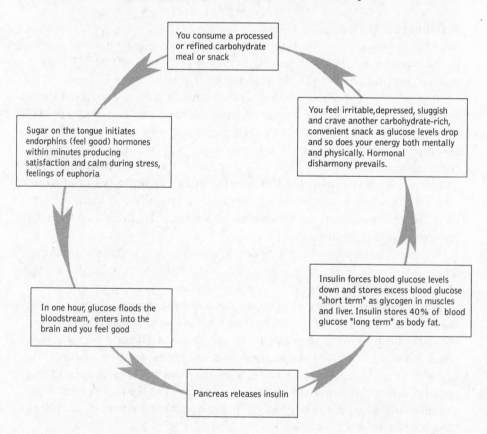

You consume a processed or refined carbohydrate meal or snack

You feel irritable, depressed, sluggish and crave another carbohydrate-rich, convenient snack as glucose levels drop and so does your energy both mentally and physically. Hormonal disharmony prevails.

Sugar on the tongue initiates endorphins (feel good) hormones within minutes producing satisfaction and calm during stress, feelings of euphoria

Insulin forces blood glucose levels down and stores excess blood glucose "short term" as glycogen in muscles and liver. Insulin stores 40% of blood glucose "long term" as body fat.

In one hour, glucose floods the bloodstream, enters into the brain and you feel good

Pancreas releases insulin

Our "Feel-Good" Hormones

The endorphins are your body's natural, morphine-like chemicals that boost mood and produce feelings of euphoria and satisfaction. They are released during intense exercise and referred to as "the runner's high." Meditation, Tai Chi, calming music, prayer, laughter, flowing dancing and pleasurable experiences raise endorphin levels. These endorphins increase your desire for "sweet treats." Satisfying sweet treat cravings is self-perpetuating since these foods further raise endorphin levels in the brain. This is why we cannot stop at one piece of chocolate, but eat the whole bar.

Fortunately, the 11 key players in our hormonal symphony can be positively influenced by what we eat.

TYPES OF HORMONES AND NEUROTRANSMITTERS

Amino Acid-Based

Endocrine hormones:	Insulin
	Glucagon
	Growth hormone (GH)
	Insulin-like growth factor (IGF)
	Thyroid hormone
Paracrine (pineal) hormones and neurotransmitters:	Melatonin
	Acetylcholine
	Dopamine
	Serotonin

Cholesterol-Based

Steroid endocrine hormones:	Cortisol
	Estrogen
	Progesterone
	Testosterone
	DHEA

Fat-Based

Autocrine hormones:	Eicosanoids
	Prostaglandins (PGE1, PGE2, PGE3)

Any general deterioration in your diet causes a system-wide information breakdown in your hormonal communication.

Polypeptide hormones and neurotransmitters are made from amino acids, which are the building blocks of protein. These include the endocrine hormones such as insulin, glucagon, growth hormone, insulin-like growth factor and thyroid hormone. They also include paracrine or pineal hormones and neurotransmitters such as serotonin, melatonin, acetylcholine and dopamine.

Steroid hormones are derived from unoxidized high-density lipoprotein (HDL) cholesterol or more accurately from the proper balance of HDL to low-density lipoprotein (LDL) cholesterol. These include cortisol, estrogen, progesterone, testosterone and DHEA.

Autocrine hormones like prostaglandins and eicosanoids are generated from fat and are lipid- or fat-soluble, allowing them to easily diffuse between fluid-filled cell hormone receptor sites.

OUR GLANDS

Each of the glands that make hormones are powerful manufacturing sites—in spite of their small size—that require precise nutrients daily. The pancreas that secretes insulin is only three ounces and the size of a clothespin. The pineal gland, which secretes serotonin and melatonin, is about the size of a grape seed.

These extremely sophisticated and precise communication systems require clean water, vitamins, minerals, protein, essential fatty acids (EFAs) like long-chain Omega-3 fish or algae oils and unsaturated fat—daily—or their performance declines—and so does ours.

What hormone-producing glands don't want are system-wide contaminants like sweeteners, excess fat, salt, fried foods, man-made chemical food additives and refined processed carbohydrates that clutter and clog these small factories. This raises havoc with hormone production and disrupts the generation of a biological message. Therefore, information transfer is reduced and everything declines.

The hypothalamus secretes what is known as hormone-releasing hormones that travel a short distance to the pituitary gland. The pituitary gland is a tiny gland, about the size of a kidney bean, that makes ten different hormones that are released directly into the bloodstream.

OUR HORMONES' EFFORTS TO COMMUNICATE

Our hormones must travel from our bloodstream to the cells they are targeting. But there are certain things that can impair this. For one, elevated insulin levels influence the production of inflammatory prostaglandins (PGE2) that cause artery and vascular walls to become severely inflamed; this decreased diameter impairs circulation that leads to reduced oxygen transfer. All high-quality hormonal production requires constant oxygen. Furthermore, as the vascular system swells up and the inside passageway diameter closes, veins and arteries lose their elasticity, become brittle and begin to become permeable. The resulting lesions cause our bloodstream nutrients to ooze out prematurely, and less nutritious blood circulates to the small periphery capillaries, the tiniest bloodstream channels.

Another hurdle for hormones is the fact that most cells of the brain, heart tissue, lungs and muscles are protected from the bloodstream by a group of cells called endothelial cells. These cells act as a persistent barrier to prevent harmful elements from passing from the circulating bloodstream into the interstitial space. Endothelial cells actually "feel" the blood flowing through them. They change shape and move around in response to velocity, blood pressure and hormones they detect in the blood. They spread out the forces to avoid dangerous extremes and are the sole control of the fluid dynamics of blood flow.

Between the endothelial cells and the actual target site tissues the hormones are trying to reach is the interstitial space, separating hormones from target tissue (see diagram on the following page).

TEN MAJOR HORMONE-PRODUCING GLANDS

Site	Gland	Biological Functions
Brain	Hypothalamus	Controls pituitary secretions, hunger, thirst, body temperature, sex drive
Brain	Pituitary gland	Regulates other endocrine glands that produce insulin, cortisol, growth hormone, thyroid hormones, estrogen and testosterone
Brain	Pineal gland	Main "biological clock" for sleep-wake circadian cycles
Throat	Thyroid gland	Controls all metabolism
Throat	Parathyroid gland	Controls calcium regulation
Lower throat	Thymus gland	Controls immune function
Abdominal region	Adrenal gland	Controls stress response above both kidneys
Abdominal region	Pancreas	Controls blood glucose levels
Female gonads	Ovaries	Control sexual development and release of eggs
Male gonads	Testes	Control sexual development and production of sperm

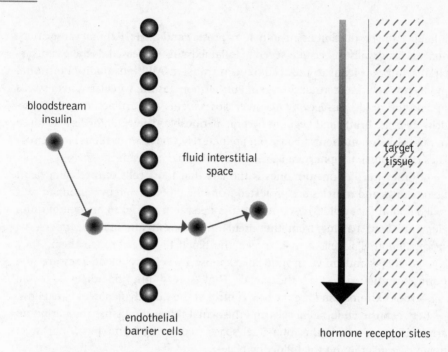

bloodstream
insulin

fluid interstitial
space

target
tissue

endothelial
barrier cells

hormone receptor sites

If the endothelial cell barrier is functioning well, hormone molecules move unimpeded through this line of protection to the target site tissues. If the endothelial cell barrier is dysfunctional, due to the lack of fortifying nutrients, fewer hormones get through intact and the concentration of active hormones in the interstitial space is severely decreased. Unable to reach their target site tissues, the hormones in the bloodstream are unable to communicate or transfer their commands. The inability to reach target cells is known as resistance.

The most common form of hormone resistance in humans is insulin resistance. Insulin resistance is the biological dysfunction leading to Type 2 diabetes, which affects more than 20 million North Americans according to the Centers for Disease Control and Prevention. They suggest the number will likely jump to 26 million by 2025, with the largest increase appearing in the 25 to 50 age group.

Even if the hormone, in adequate levels, reaches the interstitial space, it must still find its appropriate discrete receptors on the cell surface. This is a "lock and key" mechanism. The hormone key must precisely fit the lock on the receptor sites, to allow the hormone to release its biochemical message in the target tissue.

All of this intriguing biological action must do its "lock and key" process in a totally fluid environment. The fluidity of the cell membrane houses the locking mechanism. The more fluid the plasma (or outer membrane) of a receptor cell, the easier it is for the hormonal key to fit and unlock the receptor-site-locking mechanism. The less fluid the membrane environment is at the receptor site, the more difficult it is for the hormone key to quickly and efficiently flow unrestricted to the target cell lock.

Water consumption is critical for fluid content of blood and to carry the electrical charge, just like your telephone line or electric line, for hormone and neurotransmitter conduction. Water also cleanses all your organs and tissues like a giant bath. Drink a minimum of six to twelve glasses of pure water a day for superior well-being.

Endothelial cells require protein, vitamins and essential fatty acids (EFAs) to be strong, selectively permeable and vigilant and to maintain their fluidity. Saturated fats in full-fat dairy or in animal protein sources, such as red meat, significantly reduce membrane fluidity. EFAs rich in DHA and EPA are good sources of friendly Type-1 and Type-3 prostaglandin hormones, PGE1 and PGE3, that:

- thin the blood, preventing blood clots so hormones like insulin, which are not bound to a protein carrier, can move more quickly in the bloodstream to a target site tissue;
- act as anti-inflammatories, reducing the narrowing of the vascular system of veins and arteries, thereby facilitating the efficient flow of the bloodstream uninhibited, so hormones reach target sites intact;
- significantly increase healthy membrane fluidity of hormone receptor sites and in endothelial cells so hormone unlocking mechanisms work.

Many hormones do not travel beyond this external contact with the receptor site on the fluid membrane. They interact with the receptor site but do not enter the target tissue. They "download" or release their message through molecules known as second messengers. Second messengers are formed within the target tissue cell in response to the hormone unlocking the receptor site locking mechanism. This begins an unraveling chain of events referred to as a hormonal cascade.

The most researched second messenger is cyclic AMP (cAMP). cAMP is the most abundant second messenger that cells require high threshold levels of, especially endocrine hormones such as thyroid and growth hormone, to ensure transmission of their biological information. The enzyme adenylate cyclase initiates the synthesis of cAMP from the energy molecules ATP (adenosine triphosphate) that our cells make in their mitochondria (cellular energy factories). Mitochondria produce 90 percent of all free radical formations in our body from the burning of glucose, its fuel mix, to produce ATP from the food we eat.

Therefore, what we eat is vitally important. ATP is our body's energy for every function conceivable. Bioenergetic whole foods such as salads, colorful vegetables, ripe organic fruit, herbs, sea vegetables and "green drinks" supply us with enormous amounts of antioxidants to quench the destructive free radicals—smoke fumes—given off by our energy factories.

Some hormones, like insulin, do enter the target tissue cell and once inside connect with a second messenger. Second messengers represent the final "downloading" phase of hormonal communication.

Insulin uses two second messengers, DAG and IP3. Hormones such as insulin, in chronic high levels, are antagonistic to the availability of cAMP and decrease cAMP as they try to dominate. This is why high insulin levels are counterproductive to high-fidelity hormonal communication anywhere in the body.

Avoiding packaged snack foods and processed foods, laden with additional chemicals, can quickly reduce rising fluctuations in blood sugar and reduce the need for excess insulin. Good nutrition can quickly raise levels of second messengers, especially cAMP. So even though hormone levels decrease after the age of 25, if we produce enough cAMP, then hormonal communication is preserved, and we can function at our optimum—mentally, emotionally, physically and spiritually—well into our senior years.

Examples of Hormonal Miscommunication: Cortisol and Insulin Overload

The hormones insulin and cortisol are the only two hormones to increase continually after 25, accelerating aging and hormone communication havoc.

Cortisol, the hormone produced in the adrenal glands, was designed to be a short-term coping mechanism to deal with episodic stress. Today, we live in heightened stress continually. Dr. Hans Selye of Montreal, the author of *Stress Without Disease*, did exhaustive, pioneering studies on stress, the results of which were first published in 1937. He determined that seemingly small stressors can have devastating physiological consequences.

Excess cortisol not only inhibits the formation of good PGE1 and PGE3 hormones but also kills cortisol-sensitive cells in the brain and thymus. The immediate result is decreased brain and immune functions. Too little stress can be as detrimental to our health, however, as too much stress, as the adrenal glands tend to atrophy if not used daily.

Furthermore, poor diets punctuated with convenient processed foods create biochemical stresses and cause big hits of cortisol. Cortisol levels can get "out-of-whack" and eat away at muscle tissue and our central nervous system. In today's Western societies, elevated amounts of cortisol accelerate aging of our nerves and mechanical operations such as walking and fluid movements. Most worrisome, cortisol burns out the brain. As a result, we cannot deal with stress properly. Unmanaged stress causes agitation, pervasive panic and further emotional trauma.

Big hits of cortisol—all day long, all week long, all year long—kill our endothelial cells, wash over feedback loops and cause cortisol resistance. A little cortisol bath keeps the brain, heart and blood vessels slightly "tightened" for alertness. A lot of cortisol does irreparable damage by drowning endothelial cells and kills them by causing unrelenting sheer stress in artery walls, the heart, the brain and the sympathetic nervous system. Don't do it.

Insulin is the reason our blood sugar can be used as a fuel mix by our cells. Without insulin, our tissues would starve to death. But too much of a good thing is bad, and chronically high insulin levels are the norm for many who carry excess weight. We produce insulin in a relationship of grams to body weight. High insulin levels, from eating processed carbohydrates and packaged snack foods, hit the "overdrive switch" and overpower the negative feedback loop that says "stop." Once receptor sites burn out, we are unable to curb our appetite for sugar or sweeteners. This leads us to "sweet treat" binges that escalate the problem even further. We now become insulin-resistant and crave an all-sugar, all-the-time diet. This is modern-day self-extinction. We are all witness to it!

If we lose excess weight properly, insulin production goes down and insulin receptor sites go "back on," so we can more efficiently deal with the occasional blood glucose rise.

Elevated insulin levels must be implicated in the rise of cancer. Consider that the prevalence of a high-density carbohydrate diet began escalating after 1945. We know that this diet is largely responsible for the rise in insulin levels. We also know that elevated insulin levels result in obesity and diabetes. And, we know there is a link between excess weight and cancer. Therefore, the rise of diabetes and cancer should correspond perfectly. It does.

> Did you know that animals in nature do not get cancer? Only domesticated animal pets or animals raised for human consumption do. The implication is that the diet we feed them and the change in their circadian rhythms — because they stay up late under electric lights to produce milk and eggs — are the cause of this. What are we doing to "man's best friend"? What kind of friend does that make us?

THE HORMONAL DOWNFALL OF OUR MODERN DIET

The low-fat, high-carbohydrate, low-protein diets of the 1970s, 1980s and 1990s have had wide-sweeping implications on our health. These diets have triggered high frequencies of degenerative diseases, unmanageable levels of stress and excessive weight gain. No attention was paid to the importance of hormonal balance or the nature of a functional hormonal axis.

Many nutritional researchers feel that accelerated aging, beginning from 35 to 50 years of age, is mainly due to hormonal dysfunction or hormonal miscommunication.

The following four factors are the primary markers of accelerated aging—all of which stem from poor food choices and excess stress.

Excess Blood Glucose Levels: Excess glucose, from eating refined or processed food that is high in calories and sweeteners, can combine with proteins in our body to make advanced glycated end products (AGEs). AGEs represent a serious problem for our body. They are very sticky and quickly adhere to places they shouldn't, causing accelerated biological damage to all cells. They accelerate the occlusion (opposing walls stick together) of blood vessels and capillaries that nurture the heart, eyes, kidneys and brain. This means we become more prone to heart attacks, blindness, kidney failure and stroke.

Excess sugar consumption (natural or synthetic sweeteners), from any source, elevates blood glucose levels. Part of the hypothalamus is responsible for sensing the amount of glucose in the blood and controlling the pancreas hormonally, to stabilize blood sugar levels using the hormone insulin. Chronic sugar consumption leads to constantly high blood glucose levels that wash over the hypothalamus in a glucose swell that causes glucose-induced toxicity in the hypothalamus that jams its switches on "off." In this situation, insulin cannot do its job well and we become insulin resistant, a primary marker of aging.

We can stabilize blood glucose levels by only eating bioenergetic whole foods.

Excess Insulin Levels: Insulin is secreted by the pancreas in response to incoming calories (primarily processed carbohydrates). The fewer the calories consumed, the less insulin is secreted. As insulin levels go down, we lose excess fat and support the synthesis of hormones such as testosterone, DHEA and growth hormone and hormonal communication. High levels of insulin inhibit the release of the important brain-feeding hormone called glucagon. The stress hormone cortisol acts as a back-up system to raise blood sugar levels for the brain. Cortisol is able to make more glucose by cannibalizing existing body structures such as muscle. The problem is that even though cortisol may be trying to help the brain by raising blood sugar levels, elevated cortisol levels destroy the hippocampus portion of the hypothalamus.

"Chronic high insulin racks up a 'clock time' of four years for every one you live," writes T.S. Wiley in his brilliant book *Lights Out*.

Excess Cortisol Levels: Too little stress in our body is just as bad as too much stress. To be alert, keen and observant, we require small amounts of the stress hormone cortisol. Cortisol is the body's molecular mediator of stress, for short periods of time.

Cortisol output is governed by circadian rhythms. Levels are highest in the bloodstream between 6:00 a.m. and 6:00 p.m., and then gradually decrease throughout the evening.

Excess cortisol has the capacity to kill at the cellular level. The thymus gland, the central control station of our immune system, is very sensitive to excess cortisol. This is why the thymus shrinks with age and we experience a loss of immune function. Excess cortisol also reduces brain longevity by directly destroying cortisol-sensitive neurons in our body's "control center"—the hypothalamus.

Engaging in low levels of prolonged moderate exercise (like walking) and simply learning to relax can dramatically help us to lower cortisol levels.

Excess Free Radicals: The mitochondria are the power generators, or furnaces, in each of our 100 trillion cells. A well-conditioned muscle cell may contain 1,000 to 3,000 mitochondria. They burn glucose to make adenosine triphosphate (ATP), or aerobic cellular energy. The constant biochemical functioning of mitochondria give off a "smoke" called a free radical. These free radicals are destructive to our cell walls and cellular processes.

In short, the fewer free radicals you make, the longer you can live.

Research shows that 90 percent of all free radicals are formed from the vast amounts of food we consume. Our body must do something with all of those incoming calories, after all. The bottom line is, the less food we take in and the fewer the calories we consume, the less energy is required to process incoming food, and hence, the fewer free radicals we make. The fewer the free radicals we make, the longer we live! In other words, unrestricted eating is the best way to accelerate aging.

There's no question. Most of us *are* overeating. The average North American woman requires only 1,400 to 2,000 calories a day, and the average man requires about 1,600 to 2,400 calories. And yet, most of us consume over 3,000 calories each day on average.

The goal, therefore, is to eat enough food—good food—to maintain optimum mental, emotional, physical and spiritual health, but never too many calories. Consider, for example, that a commercial cinnamon bun contains 670 calories and virtually no essential nutrients, while a power protein shake has only 130 calories with 35 grams of protein and adequate amounts of immune-supportive nutrients.

The process of calorie restriction is not starvation, extended fasting or malnutrition. If the average North American gradually and systematically reduced their calorie intake by 40 percent over one year, the results would be impressive from many perspectives.

LIVE A LONG, HEALTHY LIFE

If you practice voluntary and systematic calorie restriction, based on the work of Dr. Roy Walford, M.D., at UCLA Medical School, you can:
- reduce "corrosive" free radical proliferation;
- reduce excess blood glucose levels;
- reduce excess insulin levels; and
- reduce excess cortisol levels.

Dr. Walford and W. Windrich, Ph.D., of the University of Wisconsin, have extended longevity by 50 percent in all types of laboratory animals.

If you voluntarily reduce calorie consumption, conscientiously, while eating nutrient-rich bioenergetic whole foods, you will live a longer, healthier, happier life. You will then be eating in harmony with your longstanding genetic predisposition to the natural food chain.

We can also reduce gluttony, and then become more capable of being mentally clear, emotionally stable and physically robust.

With these three qualities maximized, we have the ability to compassionately help, love and support the mental, emotional, physical and ultimately the spiritual welfare of all humanity—one person at a time! Now we can develop into true selfless human beings, the quintessence of human evolution. The epitome of human excellence!

We are then in perfect supersymmetry with ourselves, with all other human beings, with all of nature, with our true self, with our divinity.

DAILY AVERAGE CALORIE CONSUMPTIONS BY COUNTRY

Country	Calories
USA	3,603
Germany	3,265
Mexico	3,100
Canada	3,093
Japan	2,880
England	2,800
Thailand	1,800

Unrestricted eating is the best way to accelerate aging!

BOOSTING OUR HORMONAL SYSTEM AND RESTORING BALANCE

As we've seen, hormonal imbalance can contribute to weight gain, depression, fatigue, mood swings, "out of whack" appetite controls, loss of motivation, poor sleep patterns and insomnia, and our cognitive abilities to hear, see, think, respond, remember, learn and be decisive.

But there are measures we can take to counter this. We can turn up, reinvigorate and balance our critical hormone systems.

One strategy is to target each diminishing hormone and make cellular receptor sites more sensitive to what is left. For example, exercise and diet management can shrink fat cells, which makes their receptor sites more receptive to insulin.

Another approach is to eat following the circadian rhythm, thereby releasing those hormones sensitive to a particular time of day or food. One such hormone is human growth hormone (GH), which is released by the pituitary gland in spurts, primarily during the later stages of deep sleep. GH is a powerful anabolic hormone that can renew a total sense of well-being. Unfortunately, if we eat a meal after 7:30 p.m., the digesting food and its conversion to blood-glucose will still be increasing our metabolism and insulin levels when we go to sleep, and this causes subnormal GH release. The unfortunate result is an accelerated-aging catabolic condition with no GH benefit for that night. We can correct this by eating our last meal of the day before 7:30 p.m. Likewise, certain foods can boost GH. Researchers have noted that GH secretion in seniors can be re-established to the active levels of their 30s by the appropriate nutritional stimulation of the pituitary gland. Seniors are still capable of making well over 80 percent of their youthful levels of GH. The only problem is that the critical switch on the receptor sites is stuck on "off" and must be activated.

Finally, we can critically review both our lifestyle and eating habits to determine if our habits are creating harmony or chaos with our hormonal symphony and, hence, our state of mind. There is an immediate food-mood connection. What we ate at our last meal or snack is having a profound and direct hormonal and neuro-transmitter effect on our present mood, energy, clarity of thinking and emotional stability. Our dinner and evening snack will determine if we sleep well tonight. Furthermore, how well we sleep tonight will have a direct effect on our appetite tomorrow, our ability to fend off colds, the flu and other illnesses, and our moti-vation, decisiveness, energy levels and overall mood. Our lifestyle and eating habits will also determine our ability to heal and grow radiant skin and vibrant hair.

Targeting Specific Hormones and Neurotransmitters

Serotonin: Your best dietary strategy is to optimize the natural cycle of sero-tonin production, which is during the day, from the foods you consume. Here's a summary of serotonin-boosting menu:

- Breakfast: a 30 percent lean protein, 60 percent low-density complex carbo-hydrates
- Mid-morning snack: raw, very low-density complex carbohydrates from carrots, celery, zucchini, etc.
- Lunch: high in lean protein with complex carbohydrates from veggies and salad
- Mid-afternoon snack: fresh fruit as a low-density complex carbohydrate
- Dinner: high in complex carbohydrates and low in protein to supply lots of tryptophan and ensure both sufficient serotonin for a calm evening and mela-tonin for a deep, regenerative sleep

Breakfast and lunch should have the greatest amount of protein in order to stockpile protein for the day ahead. Throughout the day, the amount of protein should be gradually decreased and complex carbohydrates such as fruit, whole grain pasta, vegetables, bread, salads, grains and legumes should be increased to produce serotonin. Too much protein at night and not enough complex carbo-hydrate promotes a restless night's sleep.

A potent serotonin-elevating compound, 5-hydroxytryptophan (5-HTP) is available and 10 times as potent as L-tryptophan. It converts to serotonin very quickly, but has the risk of dramatically elevating blood levels of serotonin. Too much serotonin in the blood stream may damage heart valves. If you use 5-HTP, take 50 mg once or twice a week only, one hour before going to sleep with one piece of plain bread (without any fat such as butter or protein such as cheese or almond butter) to produce lots of serotonin and melatonin for deep sleep. A piece of plain bread or three handfuls of plain popcorn is safer and can also work well on their own naturally.

Dopamine: Meditation can dramatically reduce the stress hormone cortisol and greatly enhance the synthesis—naturally—of both dopamine and DHEA. DHEA and cortisol are both steroid endocrine hormones manufactured from cholesterol in the two adrenal glands. DHEA levels and dopamine levels have been documented to rise by 25 to 30 percent in people who meditate or pray for one-half hour or more each day. This is the safe, natural way I highly recommend you use to raise your DHEA and dopamine levels after the age of 30. Furthermore, if you get 8.25 hours of deep sleep in a totally dark room each night, cortisol levels naturally decline during the night, growth hormone (GH) increases in the dark cycle of the night, and both DHEA levels and dopamine levels increase in the early morning.

Not only will you reduce cortisol levels and increase both DHEA and dopamine levels with meditation, but you will be calmer, more peaceful and experience greater physical, mental and emotional vitality. Believe in Nature, it always has a safe, natural means!

Meditation also revitalizes the pineal gland, which is located in the brain, just between the two eyebrows. According to Dr. Herbert Benson of Harvard Medical School, meditation is a practical method of extending brain longevity. The pineal gland becomes calcified (hardened) over time, beginning at about age 35 and it becomes difficult for the pineal gland to secrete the hormone melatonin, even though it still synthesizes melatonin when you are in your 80s or older. Therefore, "eating smart" means having a high-quality "green drink" each day with natural vitamin K, which recent research shows will decalcify and restore the pineal gland. Combined with meditation, this dietary strategy will naturally allow you to synthesize and excrete large amounts of the cancer protective and deep-sleep inducing hormone, melatonin.

Likewise, you will also decrease cortisol levels and increase DHEA levels by consuming daily 650 mg of DHA and 1,000 mg of EPA—the critical long-chain Omega-3 EFA derivatives—as well as 1 tablespoon of Omega-3 EFAs flax, perilla or hemp oil, and 1/2 teaspoon of borage oil, providing 500 mg of GLA, the critical Omega-6 EFA derivative.

You can increase dopamine levels by using a half teaspoon of the amino acid L-tyrosine mixed in 4 oz (125 mL) of water and swirling it in your mouth so it is absorbed sublingually. The L-tyrosine mix needs 500 mg of vitamin C, 40 mg of magnesium and 100 mg of vitamin B6 to be converted to dopamine.

Both dopamine and its close relative, the compound norepinephrine (also called noradrenaline), are manufactured from substances found in food: the amino acids tyrosine (TYR) and phenylalanine (PHE), folic acid, magnesium and vitamin B12.

Consuming tyrosine-rich foods naturally and quickly boosts levels of these neurotransmitters and keeps you vigilant, alert and in an elevated good mood with the ability to deal with stress from the day. I highly recommend you use the foods below to safely raise dopamine levels. Chocolate that is 70 to 75 percent cocoa, generally referred to as semisweet dark chocolate, is very rich in tyrosine. Use small amounts, if you choose, mid-afternoon, to raise endorphins and dopamine levels. It can really elevate your mood and increase alertness.

DOPAMINE-BOOSTING FOODS

Food	Calories	TYR*	PHE*	Fat	Carbo-hydrate	Protein
		(mg)	(mg)	(grams)	(grams)	(grams)
Alphapure whey protein isolate powder, 2 scoops	110	1,500	1,200	1.5	15.0	30.0
Fat-free cottage cheese, 1 cup	164	1,495	1,500	1.2	6.0	4.0
Soy protein isolate powder, 2 scoops	105	1,200	1,490	10.0	15.0	25.0
Soy beans, 1 cup	290	1,100	1,498	15.0	16.9	28.0
Chicken breast, no skin, 6 oz (170 g)	193	950	1,150	7.5	0.0	29.1
Salmon, broiled, 3 oz (85 g)	127	734	850	3.8	0.0	22.0
Fat-free yogurt, 1 cup	130	600	645	3.5	15.0	12.0
Legumes, baked, 1 cup	350	395	725	13.0	52.9	15.0
Peanuts, dry-roasted, 1 oz (28 g)	160	365	440	13.5	6.0	6.5
Brown rice, 1 cup	216	190	260	1.8	45.0	5.0
Almonds, 6	150	165	325	14.0	5.2	6.0
Egg white	17	135	205	0.0	0.3	3.5
Egg yolk	59	124	119	5.1	0.3	2.5
Banana	105	29	45	0.6	27.0	1.2
Raw apple	81	6.0	7.0	0.5	21.1	0.3

*TYR = tyrosine; PHE phenylalanine

DHEA: If you supplement with DHEA, have your physician run a DHEA sulfate blood test first, to determine whether it's necessary. If your physician feels you could benefit from DHEA supplementation, you can use 5 mg of pharmaceutical-grade 100 percent pure DHEA and 15 mg of 7-Keto with a small amount of fat (1/4 teaspoon of flax oil, hemp oil or fish oil) 20 minutes before breakfast. Use the most important DHEA analog of all, 3-acetyl-7-keto DHEA (generally called

7-Keto). It is "downstream" from sex steroid metabolism and therefore is not converted to testosterone or estrogen, which could be very dangerous. DHEA and growth hormone (GH) are very closely linked. And, in fact, increasing DHEA also makes your body produce more IGF-1, the actual messenger hormone for GH. DHEA may produce more GH receptor sites on our cells, which would make us more sensitive to the GH we normally produce. Maintaining youthful levels of DHEA is a counter-balance to rising cortisol levels and reduces destructive elevated cortisol levels.

Hormones: Under Our Direct Dietary Control

Usually, the role of nutrition as a factor impacting human evolution is over-looked. Likewise, the fact that food plays such a critical role in hormonal communication seems to be largely ignored by the medical and dietetic commu-nities of our society. However, it is a survival technique under our direct control.

The more well-nourished we are, the more likely we will pass on strong, resilient genes to the next generation. We now understand that all functions in the human organism decline with age. But nature gives us time to make a contribution to life and sufficient time to rear the next generation of our species, then wants us to make an exit.

From this point of view, organisms like ours that developed more sophisti-cated hormonal systems based on the food they ate had a better chance of survival to rear their offspring and were more likely to pass on their healthy genes. Therefore, the hormones that are directly regulated by our diet will have the greatest effect on survival, if we can optimize their performance.

Eating a Variety of Bioenergetic Foods

All of our hormones—growth hormone, melatonin, testosterone, cortisol, DHEA, dopamine, insulin and others—interface with our environment and all of the thoughts and reactions it produces in our central nervous system. All of our information gathering— seeing, hearing, touching, tasting, smelling and thinking—produces a hormonal response. And so does everything we eat. The more variety of fresh, seasonal foods you have in your diet, the greater chance of getting the nutrients your body needs. Surveys indicate that the average person has a very set and narrow pattern of eating, which becomes even more entrenched as they get older. As a result, you can develop deficiencies that may take years to accu-mulate and cause disease. By "eating smart" you can increase your anabolic capacity and drive. You can, with nutrients and food, rebalance the neurological messengers, the neurotransmit-ters, and return your hormone messengers and receptors to a fully operational level.

What You Eat Affects How You Feel

What you eat at each of your three meals and two snacks each day directly influences your moods, stress level, robust energy, food cravings and sleep habits.

The "mind-body" connection really is the "mind-body-diet" connection. A hormonally correct diet becomes your primary tool to improve emotional control. Conversely, a hormonally incorrect diet is your passport to emotional chaos.

Emotions cannot be isolated but hormones can. Far too often we let our emotions manipulate our diet. If you are stressed or depressed, you usually reach for comfort food that is typically carbohydrate rich. We are hardwired for the sweet taste. As soon as sugar touches your tongue, endorphins (feel good hormones) come gushing into your system. You instantly feel better. That is why it is easy to eat the whole package of cookies or container of ice cream. Your first food, mother's milk, is 50 to 60 percent glucose (sugar). We all acquire a "sweet tooth" at an early age. The acute influx of carbohydrates gives a temporary increase in blood glucose levels to the brain. You also trigger increased insulin secretion.

Chronically elevated insulin levels will promote the increased production of "bad" prostaglandins (PGE2), which generates more depression. You might solve the emotional problem temporarily with these comfort foods, but you have set in motion a cascade of hormonal events that leads to craving these foods, coupled with emotional trauma. On the other hand, fish or algae oil supplements rich in DHA and EPA, with the addition of more protein in the diet, will lead to better health and emotional stability.

This is why I recommend protein at all three meals and one of your two snacks each and every day. Look at a young child whose emotions are not as sophisticated as an adult's. Give them two chocolate bars and initially they are very happy and respond favorably. But within one to two hours they become uncooperative and are "bouncing off the walls." In comparison, feed them lean protein with bioenergetic vegetables and fruits and they are a pleasure to be with for the next four to six hours.

Meals and snacks should be eaten five times daily to avoid the peaks and valleys of moods that can accompany big meals. The idea is not to "graze" but rather to eat three planned and well-timed meals and two planned and well-timed snacks, never eating beyond 7:30 p.m. Avoid skipping meals or snacks as much as possible.

Always use food as your first line of remedy. Add supplements only when the bioenergetic food system is not enough for your individual biochemistry.

Returning to Our Ancestors' Protein-Carbohydrate Ratio

In 1992, researchers at *The New England Journal of Medicine* created a study based on a book by Dr. Boyd Eaton, M.D., et al, called *The Paleolithic Prescription*. Using anthropological data supplied and comparing a large number of existing hunter-gatherer tribes, these researchers estimated the average protein-to-carbohydrate ratio of ancestral man to be approximately 2 grams of protein for every 4 grams of carbohydrate.

A diet high in protein is anabolic. The rule of thumb for our daily protein requirements is 1/3 gram of protein per pound of body weight for ordinary daily activities, 1/2 gram of protein for moderate exercise training and 1 gram of protein for intensive tissue-building training.

Insulin drives nutrients into cells either for immediate use or future storage. Glucagon mobilizes stored energy (primarily carbohydrates) to circulate in the bloodstream as a source of energy, especially for the brain, between meals. These two hormones must work in close cooperation. This is why they form a hormonal axis that controls blood sugar levels with such precision.

To our hunter-gatherer ancestors, producing a strong insulin response to store incoming calories was a powerful survival mechanism. Today, that ancient survival mechanism has become a potent accelerator of aging because we are surrounded by excess calories from processed foods—day and night.

We can balance both our moods and our cravings by eating protein at the right time of day and in the proper proportions with carbohydrates. Reduce protein intake as the day goes on and increase bioenergetic complex carbohydrates. Use low-calorie, high-carbohydrate meals of five parts carbohydrate to one part protein when your mood is down or you're getting cravings and needing satisfaction. A small piece of tofu on a piece of whole grain bread, or 1 scoop of whey protein isolate powder in 8 oz (250 mL) of unsweetened rice milk or almond milk with 1/2 cup (125 mL) of blueberries, will give you some comfort and reduce your cravings within 45 minutes.

The Power of Physical Activity

Engaging in low levels of prolonged moderate exercise (like walking) and simply learning to relax, will dramatically help us lower cortisol levels.

But don't overdo it. Higher levels of exercise intensity generate significant, sheer stress, and cortisol levels dramatically rise. Our body instinctively knows high levels of stress means—emergency—"fight or flight." The more intense the exercise, the fewer benefits it has for our longevity. Free radical formation explodes with more intense exercise.

In his book *The Antioxidant Revolution*, Kenneth Cooper, the promoter of aerobic exercise, comes to a startling conclusion. Physically fit individuals who regularly engage in intense exercise may not be as healthy in the long term as a less physically fit person who follows a moderate, but consistent, exercise program. Moderate exercisers will also have fewer training-related injuries that prevent them from exercising.

"No pain, no gain" is not true, but "steady low-threshold pain can produce longevity gains" is true. The rule of thumb is never do more than 45 minutes of

EATING A 100% PROTEIN-RICH SNACK OR MEAL

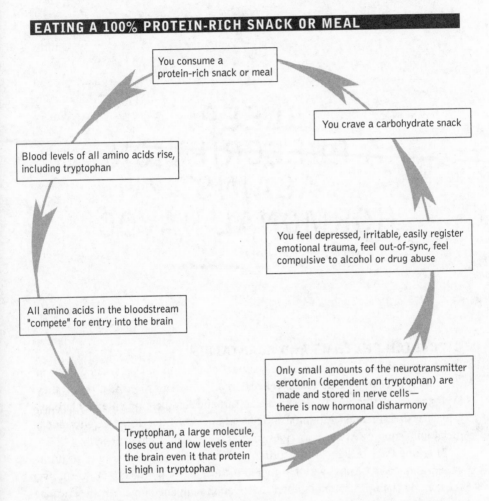

You consume a protein-rich snack or meal

You crave a carbohydrate snack

Blood levels of all amino acids rise, including tryptophan

You feel depressed, irritable, easily register emotional trauma, feel out-of-sync, feel compulsive to alcohol or drug abuse

All amino acids in the bloodstream "compete" for entry into the brain

Only small amounts of the neurotransmitter serotonin (dependent on tryptophan) are made and stored in nerve cells— there is now hormonal disharmony

Tryptophan, a large molecule, loses out and low levels enter the brain even it that protein is high in tryptophan

weight training. After 45 minutes, the levels of cortisol and free radicals rise to the point where recovery from exercise can be very difficult.

The Power of Mental Activity

There is a positive correlation between education and Alzheimer's disease. Lots of thinking produces lots of stimuli in the brain—and that produces a more active brain. A well-used brain develops more complex neurons and a thicker cortex. The functioning of an adult human brain can improve at any age when exposed to an environment rich in cognitive stimulation. We should read books, go to seminars, debate topics, take courses, try new hobbies—all these activities can keep our mind sharp well into our senior years.

3

SLEEP: A PRESCRIPTION AGAINST HORMONAL HAVOC

CIRCADIAN RHYTHMS AND ADAPTATION

Our hunter-gatherer ancestors were seasonal eaters and breeders. They went to sleep soon after it got dark and awoke soon after the sun rose. As a result, they averaged about 10 hours of sleep a night. This affected their appetite and fertility, as well as their mental, emotional and physical health. Their deep sleep hormone, melatonin, suppressed sex hormones such as testosterone and estrogen.

The long days of light, from spring to summer, meant ample time to hunt, gather and "feast." They were hardwired to store extra pounds of fat to survive the coming "famine" cycle of winter. Procreation happened instinctively, encouraged hormonally, in this circadian rhythm in late summer, allowing birthing to coincide with the return of the sun's light, heat and an abundant food supply the following spring. The excess light at night suppressed their deep sleep hormone, melatonin. The lack of melatonin increased their sex drive and fertility potential.

Late autumn began to be dominated by the longer, darker, colder days of winter. Instinctually, their perennial adaptation to long summer days was to "feast"—and for the ultimate survival of the species, mate during the "feasting" cycle. This ancient energy regulation system was the basis for their individual survival, as they knew summer comes before winter, and winter meant hibernation and a scarcity of food until the planet warmed up in spring. They instinctively observed the cues of nature, with their early detection cryptochrome light monitoring cells, and to avoid possible extinction, mated for the evolution of the human species.

In winter, when the days got longer, darker and colder, they adjusted once more. This was their "down" time and they slept during the 10 to 12 hours of dark. To conserve energy and to survive longer with the 20 pounds of portable energy or fat reserve they carried, their bodies lowered their thermostats by 1° Fahrenheit. This thermodynamic survival shift slowed and cooled down their resting metabolism rate (RMR). This is why we like a blanket while we sleep at night for most of the year.

In other words, our ancestors adjusted their sleep patterns to daily and seasonal changes as a basic survival mechanism.

Both our immune and metabolic energy systems are in direct communication with nature's light-and-dark cycles. Our skin contains thousands of photoelectric cryptochrome cells that receive and monitor the amount of direct light photons we are exposed to. These photons are carried in the bloodstream as blue light and inform our "systems control" center in the hypothalamus-pituitary axis of the brain of the light and dark phases of each day. In response, a myriad of hormones and neurotransmitters are switched "on" or "off." Daylight switches "on" dopamine and cortisol, as an example, and the dark of night turns dopamine and cortisol "off" but turns melatonin and growth hormone (GH) "on."

FALLING OUT OF SYNC—PARADISE LOST

Most North Americans don't want to say goodnight to fun and responsibility. Late-night television entices and family commitments beckon. The telephone, the Internet, e-mail, e-Bay and watching 100 channels, all rob us of sleep. We have extended our waking day and shortened the dark phase of the circadian cycle through artificial light.

Every night, we move farther and farther from the nine to ten hours of sleep a night the average adult got in 1920. Each weekday night we get an hour and thirty-six minutes less, on average, than the eight-and-a-half hours that sleep experts recommend. Each weekend night we receive one full hour less.

By the end of the year we are short 458 hours—almost three full weeks—of sleep. During an 80-year lifespan, we fall short a whopping 36,640 hours or 218 full weeks worth of lost sleep. We are the "great unslept," working our way through life on the verge of sleep bankruptcy.

Chronic inadequate sleep affects about 70 percent of adults. It is an intensifying collision between a non-stop society and human sleep physiology: "The 24-7-365 society is in direct opposition to how we're designed as humans," says Mark Rosekind, president of Alertness Solutions, which consults with businesses to reduce fatigue-related errors.

Not only are we not getting enough sleep, but how we're occupying ourselves during those waking hours has changed considerably. In the early 1970s, North Americans devoted 28 hours a week to leisure time and 40 hours a week to work. With the dawning of the new millennium, as of 2001, we're down to 15 hours a week of leisure time and have increased our work to 48 hours a week.

"Society is being victimized by not getting enough sleep," says Dr. David Dinges, director of experimental psychiatry at the University of Pennsylvania School of Medicine. He maintains, "Our productivity, our safety, our health are at risk."

Our combined sleep debt or sleep bankruptcy of 130 billion hours annually in North America has a direct annual cost of US$16.8 billion and an indirect cost, due to accidents and time lost to work required to correct fatigue-related errors, of more than US$100 billion.

A recent study showed that people who were awake for up to 19 hours scored worse on performance tests and alertness scales than those with a blood-alcohol level of 0.08 percent, which is considered legally drunk in most communities. If such individuals—surgeons, pilots, transport truck drivers, police, school teachers or the people responsible for overseeing your credit-card account—just pulled an all-nighter, they might as well be drunk.

The National Sleep Foundation attributes about 100,000 car crashes a year to sleep deprivation in the United States.

Dr. Thomas Wehr, chief of the section on biological rhythms at the National Institute of Mental Health (NIMH), believes few adults have the crystal-clear sensation of being completely rested. "Perhaps we modern humans have never really known what it is to be fully awake," says Wehr.

How Much Is Enough?

The NIMH's Wehr has found that in the absence of lights and alarm clocks, the length of the full sleep cycle is eight-and-a-quarter hours to eight-and-a-half hours of sleep a night. While Wehr thinks this is the physiological ideal, he points out that some individuals may require more—up to nine hours for some adults.

For every hour or fraction under eight hours, you need to double that and add it on to the next night's eight hours. Or take the time for a catnap. Rosekind of Alertness Solutions gives the rule of thumb on length. "There are two numbers to remember: 45 minutes and two hours," says Rosekind. "A short nap works best up to 45 minutes. After that, you'll be in deep sleep and may feel a groggy inertia upon awakening. If you need a longer nap, go for about two hours, allowing you to slumber through a full 90-minute sleep cycle and wake rested."

Sleep settles us emotionally, cognitively, immunologically and hormonally. Nothing else can do that. And yet inadequate sleep is a workaholic's badge of honor. But to brag about cheating sleep is equivalent to bragging about eating junk food and never getting off the couch; it is consciously undermining our own well-being and equilibrium.

And we're passing on our bad habits to our children who are rapidly becoming as sleep deprived as we are.

Our Kids: Overscheduled and Overtired

Surveys from the National Sleep Foundation reveal that only 15 percent of adolescents say they sleep eight-and-a-half hours or more on school nights. A quarter of adolescents usually sleep six-and-a-half hours or less.

Dr. Will Wilkoff, M.D., and author of *Is My Child Overtired?*, says the number of overtired patients has soared in the 25 years he has been in practice because families try "to squeeze 28 hours of living into 24."

Working parents, wanting to spend time with their children, let bedtimes slide. Homework and late-evening activities rev kids up just as they should be winding down. Teenagers may also be coping with jobs and relationships.

The effects are wide-sweeping. Tired students don't learn well. And too little sleep can contribute to depression. Dr. Wilkoff even suspects that some children who have been diagnosed with attention deficit disorder (ADD) or labeled hyperactive are that way simply because they are tired.

"Many sleep-starved kids are likely to go deepest into sleep debt when they hit the teen years," says Dr. Mary Carskadon of Brown University School of Medicine, who studies the sleep patterns of adolescents. She has found that their bodies' "biological clocks" reset themselves around puberty, ages 12 to 14, making their required length of sleep time about an hour longer than when they were children.

When a 10-year-old accustomed to going to sleep at 9:30 p.m., becomes a 13-year-old who goes to sleep at 10:30 p.m., the impact of that lost hour can be overwhelming, particularly on their attention span at school. Teenagers should feel wide awake, energetic and motivated after they wake up.

Sleep research indicates that most teens can manage well on eight-and-a-half hours of sleep, during the week, if they catch up with one extra hour on weekends. Younger children should get a full nine to 11 hours.

SLEEP IS NOT A WASTE OF TIME

The sleeping brain regulates gastrointestinal, cardiovascular and immune functions, and it energizes the body. Only the sleeping brain organizes and files all new information learned that day. It heightens cognitive processing, which includes reorganization of data already stored to mesh with the new data just filed.

As an example, if you study, read, hear or learn something new during the day, that night in your sleep your brain is actively processing that information. The more quality sleep you get nightly, the more you increase the likelihood of retaining that information and being able to access it easily.

If you have trouble sleeping, go to a sleep clinic at a local university. As an example, at the University of British Columbia (UBC), Dr. Jon Fleming runs the University Hospital's sleep clinic that saw 4,174 patients in 2000 and admitted 1,469 patients for overnight sleep studies, an average of 30 patients a week.

Dr. Fleming's advice is, "consistency—go to bed at the same time every night, up at the same time every morning."

It is interesting to note how long the average sleep cycle is for animals.

ANIMAL	HOURS OF SLEEP
Cat	15
Raccoon, rat, wolf	13
Gorilla	12
Fox, jaguar	11
Chimpanzee	10
Dog	10

The Sleep-Disease Connection

We have gone too far by turning night into day. We've crossed the line. Survival is all about equilibrium. But we have tipped the balance of homeostasis and created a declining catabolic spiral, encouraged accelerated aging and fostered an early extinction event.

Long-term sleep debt is a leading factor in the epidemics of diabetes, obesity, cardiovascular disease, depression, strokes and cancer. The advent of the light bulb—and our insistence on extending the light-cycle of each day and artificially reducing the dark cycle—is responsible for this increase in many modern-day diseases.

While limitless electricity has brought us the time to acquire more knowledge through watching television, reading books or surfing the Internet, and greater opportunities to attend theater or sporting events, it has also provided us with the accompanying hormonal imbalances that equate to metabolic havoc.

A ground-breaking study published in *Lancet* in 1999 clearly demonstrates the relationship between lack of sleep and the deterioration of health. Dr. Eve Van Cauter, a sleep researcher at the University of Chicago, studied a group of healthy young men for three weeks in a sleep lab. They were in bed eight hours per night the first week, four hours the second week, and 12 hours the third week. During the second week, when they were sleep-deprived, their blood samples showed impaired glucose tolerance. Without sleep, the central nervous system had become more active, which inhibited the pancreas from producing adequate insulin—the hormone the body needs to digest glucose. "In healthy young men with no risk factor, in one week, we had them in a pre-diabetic state," writes Van Cauter.

The study shows, says Van Cauter, that "sleep loss is partly involved in the epidemic of obesity." A lack of sleep drives down the secretion of growth hormone

(GH) and accelerates our excessive fat gain. Growth hormone burns fat and builds lean muscle mass when it is at normal levels of secretion. It drives childhood growth and controls an adult body's proportions of fat and muscle. We secrete growth hormone in spurts, with much of it secreted in the first round of deep, slow-wave sleep. As we age, we spend less and less time in deep sleep, which reduces growth hormone. Growth hormone triggers the release of insulin-like growth factor (IGF-1) from the liver. It is IGF-1 that carries out GH commands to burn fat and build lean muscle.

At a younger age, a lack of sleep could drive down growth hormone prematurely, accelerating weight gain and slowing the growth cycle, which ushers in a premature catabolic decline sooner. An ever-increasing number of our children will never experience their full potential because they never properly adapt to the light-dark cycles or the bioenergetic food chain.

The Van Cauter study also indicates that other hormones lose their balance and harmony when we accumulate sleep-debt. The hormone leptin, which tells the body when it should eat fat, for instance, is affected. When leptin levels drop, the body craves fats and carbohydrates, even if you've had sufficient calories. Satisfying that craving raises insulin levels, which further contributes to weight gain.

Another example is the stress hormone cortisol. It normally drops to low levels in the evening and adds to the melatonin-induced drowsiness that gets the body ready for sleep. Cortisol gradually rises overnight, reaching a peak about 6:00 a.m., just as the first rays of light appear. This cortisol surge helps to arouse and energize the body after a good night's sleep, getting us up and ready for the day's demands. But too little sleep, over as short a period as one week, leads to deterioration in overnight levels of cortisol, equal to the low levels typically seen in elderly people. This leaves us lacking any zest or energy when we arise.

The lack of sleep and its accompanying health problems are further aggravated by poor food choices. When we, or our children, eat processed or sweetened carbohydrates for supper or as an evening snack, we force insulin levels to rise. High insulin levels force growth hormone down.

THE POWER OF GROWTH HORMONE

Growth hormone (GH) declines in middle age from about 35 to 50, so that by the time we are 60, we have only a fraction of our peak levels.

There are a number of tests that screen for growth hormone deficiency, including the IGF-1 Somatomedin C blood test and the clonidine growth hormone stimulation test. Signs of adult growth hormone-deficiency include increased fat mass, especially around the belly; reduced energy and vitality; low self-esteem; poor general health; reduced exercise capacity; impaired cardiac function; and a decrease in "good" HDL cholesterol and an increase in "bad" LDL cholesterol.

Growth hormone is available only by prescription and can be administered only by injection. Physicians usually start patients, 50 and over, at 0.4 to 0.5 international units (IU) as a daily dose. Growth hormone therapy needs to be given for six months or longer to be effective. Most people over age 50 have enough growth hormone in storage in the pituitary gland. It just needs to be released.

L-glutamine Dr. Karlis Ullis, M.D., finds that the amino acid L-glutamine triggers the release of growth hormone better than any other amino acid such as arginine or lysine. Begin by taking 2 grams daily at bedtime. If there are no side effects such as diarrhea or upset stomach, increase to 5 grams after two weeks, and move slowly to 10 grams per day. A physician should measure IGF-1 levels before beginning, and again after two weeks, to quantify the results.

There is no guarantee that L-glutamine will release more growth hormone from the pituitary. L-glutamine is the most abundant amino acid in our body. At the very least, extra L-glutamine supplementation will repair the lining of the intestinal tract, build lean muscle tissue and greatly enhance the production of the important cellular antioxidant glutathione (see Chapter 10).

Nutritional Tips to Release Growth Hormone

1. Avoid sugary foods in the evening. The worst culprits are those foods with a very high ratio of sugar to fiber, such as ice cream, potato chips, cookies, candies, pies, chocolate bars, beer, liquor, wine, pretzels and gum. Growth hormone is mostly released while you sleep. Eating sweet or processed food elevates blood sugar levels, forcing a rise in insulin levels and turns the growth hormone releasing switch to "off."

2. Avoid eating before you exercise. Exercise releases GH and endorphins if it is energetic, but not totally exhausting. Combine 15 minutes of aerobic (treadmill or bicycle), with 30 minutes of anaerobic weight training, and then finish with 15 minutes of walking. Have a "green drink" in water before you exercise and a whey protein isolate power shake within one hour of finishing your exercise.

COMPROMISED IMMUNE DEFENSES—OUR HORMONAL REPORT CARD

There are several studies linking a lack of sleep to a decline in immune function. Research completed by James Krueger, Ph.D., a neurobiologist at Washington State University, showed that a rat not allowed to sleep dies of infection after about two weeks. This rat will also develop skin lesions—an indication of immune dysfunction.

Studies on humans show that inadequate sleep "down regulates" white blood cell counts and immune response modifiers, both of which are biological evidence that the body is having trouble fighting infection. When you have a severe flu you might be surprised that you can sleep for 15 or 18 hours a day.

Richard Stevens, Ph.D., a cancer researcher at the University of Connecticut Health Center, speculates that there is a connection between the epidemic of breast cancer and a woman's hormone cycles that are disrupted by late-night, artificial light.

The hormone melatonin is secreted about 90 minutes after we fall asleep. Melatonin triggers a reduction in a woman's production of estrogen. Light and high insulin levels interfere with and lower melatonin release, allowing estrogen levels to rise. Excess estrogen is known to promote the growth of breast cancer.

The light-melatonin-estrogen cancer theory is bolstered by a 1991 report released by the Centers for Disease Control and Prevention that determined blind women are only half as prone to breast cancer as fully sighted women. Two Scandinavian studies found a reduced incidence of breast cancer in blind people, as well as reductions in some other cancers. Blind women do not record late-night artificial light through their pupils. Therefore their melatonin secretion is not suppressed as often, and consequently their levels of estrogen are kept lower at night.

SLEEP AS NATURE INTENDED

Our hunter-gatherer ancestors probably did not get all their sleep at once. Historian A. Roger Ekirch, Ph.D., of Virginia Tech, has determined that they slept in two segments. References as far back as Virgil and Homer called it "first sleep" and "second sleep." In between is an hour of very quiet wakefulness that our ancestors called "the watch." It was a time to ponder, plan, meditate and think clearly.

NIMH's Dr. Thomas Wehr saw just that in his volunteers who were free to sleep and wake as their bodies willed. "They slept in two chunks with a period of wakefulness in between." Between the two sleep segments, or during the "watch," Wehr noted a rise in the hormone prolactin. Prolactin allows hens to sit contentedly for hours on their eggs. It also produces a similar meditative state in people.

It takes about three-and-a-half hours of melatonin secretion before prolactin is secreted. You need to go to sleep between 9:30 and 10:00 p.m. in the dark cycles of the winter and between 10:00 and 11:00 p.m. in the light-intensified summer to have melatonin secretion at peak levels and allow prolactin to be secreted at 3:00 a.m.

The bedroom must be fully dark for this to happen. Any light contamination from nightlights, clocks, televisions, VCRs—even blinking lights from electronic equipment—will interfere with this elegant process.

Stay Surcharged with Circadian Rhythms

Melatonin, prolactin and cortisol form the "biological clock" within us, an ancient sundial monitoring the dark and light cycles of each day. When we do not sleep in sync with both the daily and seasonal variations in light exposure, we fundamentally alter the internal "biological clock's" preprogrammed ability. This internal sundial, developed in our hunter-gatherer ancestors, was to be in circadian rhythm and hormonal balance with the "cosmic clock." The "cosmic clock" keeps us in tune with the cycles and rhythms of nature through our mind-body-planetary connection, in which we and nature, at every level, are in physical and biological sync.

The more we move out of tune with the "cosmic clock," a self-extinction process, the sooner we die.

Going to sleep with the sunset means a dark night's sleep with lots of melatonin and lots of prolactin. The red light or rose-yellow-orange light spectrum of the setting sun "turns on" melatonin production by striking the preoptic site connection in our eyes to the pineal gland in our brain. It is the green-spectrum light in bright morning that turns the melatonin switch "off" and turns the dopamine, cortisol and testosterone switches "on" in both males and females, so we awake energized and ready to go. These are ancient light-sensitive feedback loops.

In deep, dark sleep, melatonin surges shift our brain into superior immune maintenance. Melatonin is the most powerful antioxidant that prevents and quenches the corrosive free radical called the hydroxyl free radical. Our brain is 50 percent fat. Much of the fat in the brain is polyunsaturated, which makes it very prone to free radical attack and destruction. The pineal gland is in the center of the brain and the secretion of melatonin is ideally situated to quench hydroxyl free radicals.

Melatonin, as our most potent antioxidant, is our passport to remaining cancer free. If levels drop, we head into a catabolic nosedive and destroy proper hormone communication that leaves us prone to degenerative diseases.

Melatonin Supplements

In people 65 or older, peak night time melatonin levels are only 30 to 40 picograms per milliliter of blood, whereas a 25-year-old secretes 100 to 2,000 picograms per milliliter of blood at night. Melatonin is produced in the pineal gland. During normal aging, calcification of the pineal tissue is thought to cause the decline in melatonin synthesis. Vitamin K, in "green drinks" or green leafy vegetables prevents calcium from collecting and hardening in our arteries and glands.

A word of caution: if you choose to use melatonin for sleep or life extension, you may force the pineal gland to shrink and become less active. If you do choose to supplement with melatonin, the ideal amount to completely restore sleep cycles to normal is only 0.3 grams to 1 gram sublingually or up to 3 grams of time-released pharmaceutical pure melatonin every evening, once you reach the age of 40. This small dose keeps the serotonin-melatonin ratios favorable, even if you do not have a sleeping problem, and slows down the catabolic aging process.

Anything more is less effective according to Richard Wurtman, Ph.D., at the Massachusetts Institute of Technology's Brain and Cognitive Sciences Department.

Tips to Increase Melatonin and Stay Cancer-Free

1. Go to sleep early in the dark cycle of the evening and avoid the strong contamination of artificial light.
2. Eat no food beyond 7:30 p.m. (except your yogurt, garlic, flax seed oil recommendation), especially any sweetened or processed foods that raise insulin levels too high and "shut off" melatonin synthesis and secretion.
3. Restrict your daily calories by eating only bioenergetic, anabolic-supporting, whole foods—this increases melatonin levels by 50 percent.
4. Eat a bioenergetic, low-protein, complex-carbohydrate dinner to promote the absorption of the amino acid tryptophan and its conversion to serotonin, which cascades into melatonin.
5. Since melatonin protects the essential fatty acids in our body and brain from deterioration, be sure to consume Omega-3 EFAs from fish oils, eggs, sea algae, fresh fish, perilla oil, flax or hemp seeds and their oils, as well as Omega-6 EFAs from borage or primrose oils and animal fat in eggs or meat. This will also help ensure superior neurological processing.

As discussed in Chapter 2, serotonin is the precursor to melatonin. Serotonin levels are highest during the day and fall at night. Melatonin levels rise at night and fall during the day. The rise and fall of these two hormones in the pineal

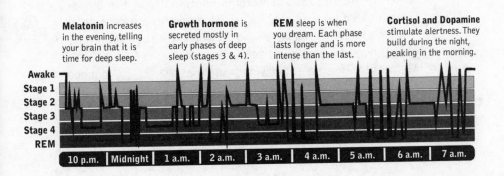

Melatonin increases in the evening, telling your brain that it is time for deep sleep.

Growth hormone is secreted mostly in early phases of deep sleep (stages 3 & 4).

REM sleep is when you dream. Each phase lasts longer and is more intense than the last.

Cortisol and Dopamine stimulate alertness. They build during the night, peaking in the morning.

Awake
Stage 1
Stage 2
Stage 3
Stage 4
REM

10 p.m. | Midnight | 1 a.m. | 2 a.m. | 3 a.m. | 4 a.m. | 5 a.m. | 6 a.m. | 7 a.m.

gland creates the circadian rhythms that bring balance and harmony to all hormonal synthesis and secretions. For example, growth hormone and prolactin are released primarily at night. Cortisol is released with the first "break of day." Dopamine, testosterone and estrogen peak just prior to waking and their levels drop throughout the day.

Ample melatonin will put you in a deep restorative sleep, trigger growth hormone and its active messenger, insulin-like growth factors (IGF-1, IGF-2 and IGF-3).

Natural Sleep Aids

1. **Herbs.** Passion flower, scullcap, griffonia, hops, lemon balm and kava kava, in combination, reduce anxiety and induce sleep. Have a cup or two of chamomile tea one hour before sleep to reduce anxiety.

2. **Bread.** Yes, you can eat one to two pieces of plain white bread, either toasted or not, one hour before sleep. Bread's glucose content will cause the resulting insulin to escort all the smaller amino acids from the bloodstream into cells, allowing tryptophan levels to rise in the bloodstream, find their way to the brain and convert to serotonin, which will synthesize melatonin and induce deep sleep. Put no butter, almond butter, peanut butter or cheese on the bread. This is the only time I recommend white bread or eating anything after 7:30 p.m.

3. **5-hydroxytryptophan (5-HTP).** 5-HTP supplementation is the immediate precursor for melatonin synthesis. Limited research indicates that 50 mg of 5-HTP, taken sublingually one hour before sleep, may do the trick. Only use 5-HTP one to two times a week, at the maximum, to keep serotonin levels from rising too high. It converts very quickly to serotonin and has the risk of dramatically elevating blood levels of serotonin. Too much serotonin continually in the bloodstream can damage heart valves. Use one 50 mg capsule of 5-HTP. Open the capsule and dissolve the powder under your tongue for two minutes.

4. **Melatonin.** If you absolutely must use it as a sleep aid, common doses range from 0.3 to 1 gram sublingually to 3 grams in a time-released form one hour before sleep.

The "Master-Switch" of Circadian Rhythms

Melatonin will also trigger the release of prolactin, which will calm your mind and nervous system and reduce the effects of accumulated stress.

Melatonin and prolactin are two powerful driving forces in controlling the "master-switch" in reproduction—for the regeneration of our human species. Melatonin also controls the production of estrogen and testosterone.

Prolactin: Prolactin makes milk and initiates both lactation and weight gain during pregnancy in humans and all mammals. It also enhances the production of immunological responses by producing both T cells and NK (natural killer) cells. Mother's milk builds a child's immune system with prolactin. As an adult, maintain your immune system with small amounts of prolactin while you sleep. Prolactin levels steadily increase with age and their eventual buildup causes the switch to be flooded and stuck in the "on" position. Excess prolactin causes weight gain and becomes an immune system suppressant.

No animals in nature experience cancer. Only humans and their domesticated pets or farm-raised animals experience cancer—because they are exposed to artificial light, robbed of diminishing dark cycles, and fed grains and synthetic, processed foods. Now you know how to reduce the likelihood of cancer in your lifetime. You control it hormonally through your own lifestyle.

Dr. Thomas Wehr, of the National Institute of Mental Health, also discovered that longer periods of melatonin secretion greatly increased bacteria and virus-fighting white cell macrophage and lymphocyte production. Longer periods in dark sleep also raised prolactin levels. This consistent elevation of prolactin fosters the same brain-waves observed during deep meditation.

Wehr's study goes on to stress that "prolactin in humans probably facilitates a switch to 'quiescent wakefulness,' just as it promotes brooding behavior in birds," such as hens, to sit on eggs calmly for six or more hours at a time. It is during this circadian rhythm of between 1:00 a.m. and 4:00 a.m. that we are in a meditative state with high endorphin (painkiller) levels and elevated prolactin levels.

Prolactin produced in the middle of the night gives us deep, rich, calm dreams to imagine, plan or foster better communication and artistic imagery. Prolactin is at its highest between the two periods of sleep—during the "watch"—and allows us to calmly plan, think and sort out life. Prolactin production shifted toward the morning means reduced cortisol, leading to less dopamine, leading to "hung-over" mornings with no zest and finally—we daydream during the daytime but are generally a little out of sync.

Mothers who breastfeed are calmer and more in tune with their babies, as the "mothering hormone," as prolactin is sometimes called, is elevated. Breastfed babies also develop stronger immune systems.

Following the Circadian Rhythm

Timing is everything. We cannot make melatonin in daylight or with the lights on. As far as melatonin synthesis goes, the darker the better. Our cytochrome light monitoring cells on our skin "turn off" cortisol—our ready-to-respond-or-adapt hormone, and dopamine—our alert, motivated-to-action hormone, and "turn on" the two-stage conversion of serotonin to melatonin.

Nature fosters superior hormone balance and harmony during the dark cycles of sleep in order to build immunity, cool our resting metabolism rate, and allow our brain to sort out and file information we learned that day. Nature accomplishes this by secreting the hormone leptin from fat tissues into our body. Leptin tells the brain we are "full." Melatonin enhances leptin's appetite-suppressing effect so we stay asleep all night instead of wandering sleeplessly looking for food.

Furthermore, as insulin levels drop and melatonin levels rise, glucagon rises. Glucagon is the hormone secreted by the pancreas to stimulate the breakdown of the "short-term" storage of glycogen, into blood glucose, in the liver, to feed the body and especially the brain while we sleep.

This is a feedback loop: melatonin surges enhance leptin to tell the brain it is well fed and suppresses appetite, while triggering the release of glucagon hormone to feed the brain and body with stored energy, as glycogen. This allows us to sleep deeply and to successfully restore, rejuvenate and reinvigorate our 100 trillion cells to boost our optimal anabolic capacity—to fuel an anabolic drive.

When we stay up late with artificial light, our brain says it is summer. Summer in our ancient, inherited feedback loops means we should load up on carbohydrates in order to create and store fat.

The saving grace is that the carbohydrates at least make serotonin, which makes melatonin, and puts us to sleep. This is a survival mechanism, in a topsy-turvy way, that puts us into a hibernation mode to sleep off the excess blood sugar blast. It is an instinctive adaptation trying to make something a little good out of something that is bad.

The drawback is, as long as it is light outside or the lights are on inside, cortisol levels rise and don't drop. High cortisol levels were meant to be episodic, not chronic. It geared our ancestors up for a quick "fight or flight" response. Chronically elevated cortisol levels from staying up too late literally kill the cells in the thymus gland and destroy the immune system. High cortisol levels eat lean muscle mass and destroy the hypothalamus-pituitary-adrenal axis—the "master hormonal switch" in the brain.

High cortisol levels cause depression. As the cortisol switch remains jammed in an "on" position, we feel the modern-day feeling of pervasive, sheer panic. If this happens day after day, week after week, month after month, real mental illness pushes us into severe depression and schizophrenia. At the very least, heightened stress causes high blood pressure and heart failure. Doctors can prescribe drugs for depression that help put our sleep cycles back in rhythm, but now we know we can reset our cycles without drugs.

It is all ultimately in our hands. The choice to follow the ancient circadian rhythm of sleeping and eating as means of achieving optimum energy and well-being is ours to make. Choose wisely for your own sake!

Natural Sleep

"The lamb and the lion shall lie down together. But the lamb will not be very sleepy."

—Woody Allen

Stress is the most common cause of restless sleep and insomnia. But there are measures we can take to ensure a good night's sleep.

1. Foster effective coping skills during the day.
2. Don't allow stress into the bedroom. Keep televisions, computers, calculators, arguing and so on, out of the bedroom. Do not pay bills or balance your bank account in your bed.
3. Eat your largest meal at breakfast or lunch and a light meal of 500 calories at supper.
4. At supper include salads, vegetables, whole grain pastas or breads and only a little protein, about 15 to 25 grams. This will promote serotonin synthesis.
5. Do not eat past 7:30 p.m. except for your yogurt, garlic, flax seed oil preparation or plain white bread to help induce sleep. Try the herbal sleep aid called sleep+.
6. Eat slowly and chew your food thoroughly at dinner.
7. Avoid caffeinated beverages after early morning, as caffeine can linger for up to 12 hours in your blood.
8. Avoid alcohol in the evening.
9. Go to sleep and rise at the same time each day.
10. Make sure your dietary intake of calcium, magnesium, manganese, copper, chlorophyll, B vitamins, vitamin C, vitamin E and vitamin D is adequate.

WE ARE THE "GREAT UNSLEPT"

Easily accessible calories from mostly processed carbohydrates—combined with the lights left on too long in the dark cycle of night—provide ancient mind-body-planetary cues that tell your body's systems that it's the endless summer of

August. Endless summer has always been followed by winter, so you instinctively store portable energy as a fat pad.

But the endless summer of late-night artificial light and the endless calorie-laden, synthetic carbohydrate "foods," alcohol and the exhausting "high" of drugs and stimulants—day after day, week after week, month after month, year after year—propel you out of circadian rhythm and out of sync with yourself, with other human beings and with nature. Furthermore, you gain an enormous sleep debt and your hormones are completely "out of whack."

Hormone havoc is defined as death. You are suddenly a threat to nature itself—you are unnatural, and you hasten your very own early extinction, by your very own hands.

One question I ask you to seriously ponder: Does this behavior pattern truly express my gratitude for the wondrous gift of life I have been given? It's your call now. Be wise!

4

WOMEN: YOUR HORMONAL HEALTH

Declining or imbalanced hormones, in both women and men, contribute to loss of lean muscle mass, thinning hair, decreased vision, fragile bones, diminishing skin quality, weight gain, food cravings and lack of good quality sleep.

For women, one of the chief culprits is estrogen. The estrogen decline in postmenopausal women is so severe that the average 55-year-old man has more estrogen than the average 55-year-old woman. Men's estrogen supplies, while much smaller than women's, do not decline with age, which may be the reason that twice as many women have Alzheimer's as do men.

BOOSTING HORMONES

Therapy to replace diminishing hormones such as estrogen became a well-accepted technique in the 1990s. Premarin, the synthetic version of the female sex hormone estrogen, is the most widely prescribed drug in North America, with about 50 million prescriptions written every year. Other hormones are being used in replacement therapy as well.

But estrogen replacement therapy is not for all women, and there is continuing debate as to whether it is advisable at all. There is a debatable association between estrogen replacement therapy and cancer in North American women, particularly breast cancer and, to a lesser degree, cancer of the ovaries and uterus. The risk of cancer can be mitigated by using the lowest effective dose possible. Estrogen users are less likely to get Alzheimer's disease, osteoporosis and heart disease.

There is mounting evidence that natural forms of hormones are safer over the long haul. Natural estrogen is not only safe, but it actually protects against breast cancer.

Three different estrogens are produced by the female body: estrone, estradiol and estriol. Estrone is the strongest, estradiol is somewhat weaker and estriol the weakest. Stronger estrogens are believed to be more apt to stimulate tumor growth; therefore, you should steer away from them.

If you use Premarin (**pre**gnant **ma**re's u**rine**), I highly recommend that your health care professional have a knowledgeable pharmacist replace it with a natural combination therapy blend of human estrogens comprised of estrone, estradiol and estriol, balanced with a natural progesterone cream and a touch of testosterone (for anabolic drive)—not synthetic estrogens from horses, or synthetic progesterone called Provera. Determining the appropriate hormone ratios among these five hormones in women over age 35 is a most effective strategy to diminish perimenopausal or menopausal effects, which can include hot flashes, night sweats, vaginal dryness, and dramatic mood swings.

Estrogen Alternatives

Premarin is a blend of 10 different types of estrogen found in the urine of pregnant mares and is stronger than the estrogen produced in a woman's body. The only estrogen replacement I believe women should use is a mix of two or three natural estrogens that are identical in chemical structure to the estrogen produced by a woman's own body.

I encourage you to talk to your physician about Bi-Estrogen, which is 80 percent estriol and 20 percent estradiol, or Tri-Estrogen, which is 80 percent estriol, 10 percent estradiol and 10 percent estrone. Studies show that estriol has a protective effect against breast cancer, and in contrast to stronger estrogens, it appears to inhibit tumor growth. Asian women and vegetarians, who have much lower risks of breast cancer than the average for North American women, have higher levels of estriol. There is no estriol in Premarin.

Jesse Hanley, M.D., a California family physician and personal friend, with 15 years of experience in natural hormone replacement therapy, recommends complete blood testing to determine if you should use Bi- or Tri-Estrogen plus however much progesterone, testosterone and DHEA you require. The mandatory blood tests are for total estrogens, progesterone, testosterone, DHEA sulfate, thyroid function, liver function, luteinizing hormone (LH) and follicle-stimulating hormone (FSH).

In either Bi- or Tri-Estrogen replacement, plant-derived estriol makes up 80 percent of the hormone replacement. Estriol is the dominant estrogenic hormone in women who do not have breast cancer and in women who are pregnant. Scientific evidence demonstrates that estriol is safer as a replacement than either estrone or estradiol. Please understand, however, that estriol is natural and therefore cannot be patented by a commercial company. Estriol has been slow to gain the attention of physicians since pharmaceutical companies do not promote it; there is no financial advantage to do so.

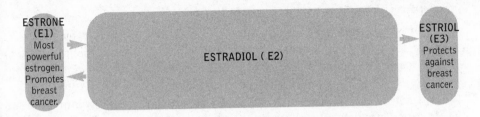

ESTRONE (E1) — Most powerful estrogen. Promotes breast cancer.

ESTRADIOL (E2)

ESTRIOL (E3) — Protects against breast cancer.

Estriol leaves a woman's body more quickly than estradiol and estrone, which is why it is referred to as the "weak" estrogen and why a higher dose is required: for a dose equivalent to 0.6 to 1.25 mg of Premarin, a woman would require 2 to 5 mg of estriol. But this so-called weakness is a benefit, because the more estriol a woman takes, the less likely she is to get breast cancer.

Furthermore, estriol supplementation increases friendly lactobacilli bacteria and near elimination of pathogenic or undesirable bacteria in the intestinal tract. Estriol also restores normal vaginal mucosa and promotes a return to normal low vaginal pH.

Adding Progesterone to the Mix

Any woman who takes estrogen must also take progesterone to protect against uterine cancer. The exception to this is a woman who has had a hysterectomy.

Progesterone is a precursor hormone that makes other hormones, such as estrogen, testosterone, DHEA and adrenal corticosteroids. It prevents osteoporosis and fibrocystic breasts, is a natural energizer and anti-depressant, and optimizes the libido.

Do not confuse natural progesterone with synthetic progesterone like Provera or with Mexican yam extract that, contrary to popular belief, is not a good source for progesterone.

Use about 1/4 teaspoon of natural progesterone creams twice a day, applied to the soft skin of the abdomen, inner thighs or inner arms. Use between 100 and 200 mg of oral capsule progesterone daily if you do not want to use the creams.

Use micronized progesterone creams for better absorption. The micronization process allows the transdermal delivery of a progesterone cream or gel to effectively be absorbed through the skin. Micronized progesterone is also less likely to be broken down by the liver.

Provera is the most popular synthetic progesterone. It is a synthesis of new progesterone analogs called progestins. These progestins have their own side effects and I do not recommend them. Progestins are not the same thing as natural progesterone. Your body knows how to handle progesterone, whereas progestins are unnatural drugs.

Recent research indicates that estrogen seems to play a role in governing the secretion of insulin. As total estrogen levels decrease, insulin resistance and insulin levels rise.

THE IMPACT OF LIFESTYLE AND FOOD

Estrogen is a good example of how hormone peaks and receptivity are influenced by lifestyle. The amount and degree of discomfort a woman goes through at menopause depend on many variables, such as smoking, drinking, diet and exercise, as well as her country of origin, her culture and genetics.

Japanese women, who outlive North American women by seven or eight years, experience only 50 percent of the incidence of osteoporosis, even though their intake of milk is low. Japanese women also have 75 percent fewer deaths from heart disease and 70 percent fewer deaths from breast cancer.

When I studied in China and Japan, I realized they have no word for "hot flashes." In Japan, China and other Asian countries, women experience fewer symptoms of menopause. Traditionally, women in Japan or Asia do not drink alcohol or smoke. Their traditional diets are filled with isoflavone phytonutrients, phytoestrogens and antioxidants from natural bioenergetic whole foods—especially from fermented soy products. The best source of dietary estrogen is soy beans and soy bean products such as extra-firm tofu, tempeh, miso, soy burgers, soy nuts and soy protein isolate powder.

Herbal combinations have enormous success balancing out-of-harmony female hormones with their estrogenic effect. Chaste berry, for example, has been found "highly effective in reducing PMS symptoms" in extensive German research according to *The British Medical Journal* (vol. 322, Jan. 20, 2001). Whenever using herbs, ensure that each is a standardized extract. Some herbs you might consider using to reduce the adverse side effects of menopause include black cohosh, chaste tree berry (vitex agnus castus), dandelion, don quai and red clover.

Some foods can be helpful as well. Cruciferous vegetables like broccoli, Brussels sprouts, kale, cauliflower and broccoli sprouts contain indole-3-carbinol (I3-C). This powerful phytonutrient forms into diindolylmethane (DIM) in the stomach, which, according to research, significantly reduces the level of 16-alpha-hydroxy-estrone—a known promoter of breast cancer. I3-C or DIM upregulates the tumor-suppressor gene BRCA-1, which blocks estrogen from sending the signals that enhance the growth of breast cancer.

A Long Island University Hospital study presented as a paper to the Society of Gynecologic Oncologists, in March, 2001 and funded by the National Cancer Institute, demonstrated that when indole-3-carbinol (I3-C) and diindolylmethane (DIM) were mixed in test tubes, ovarian cancer cells in those tubes died within days. Moreoever, both compounds also enhanced the effectiveness of the chemotherapy drug cisplatin, making it more deadly to the OVCAR-3 cell line, known to be resistant to cisplatin. One hundred percent of the malignant tissue died when cisplatin was combined with DIM.

Cruciferous vegetables also increase the protective estrogen metabolites 2-hydroxyestrone and 2-methoxyestrone and, therefore, may reduce the risk of hormone and estrogen replacement therapy-related cancer. If you do use hormone replacement therapy, do supplement with capsules of diindolyl-methane (DIM) to help protect you from possible cancer.

Estrogen and progesterone are the primary female sex hormones. But women also produce a small—but very important—amount of testosterone, which slowly dwindles after the age of 35. Testosterone keeps a woman's muscles and bones strong and gives her an anabolic boost. Women only require a tiny bit of testosterone, but experience a big feel-good boost, especially if they are on estrogen replacement therapy. Testosterone is not only necessary for a woman's emotional well-being, but it is vital for normal physical development.

Women's blood levels of testosterone range between 15 and 100 ng/dL, while for men the range is 300 ng/dL to 1,200 ng/dL. Women who take Bi-Estrogen hormone replacement therapy should speak with their physician about using a small testosterone dose of 2.5 mg three times a week. (This should be taken in the morning with a fat, to help absorption.) This small amount will not produce any masculine side effects such as a deepening of the voice or excess facial hair growth.

Testosterone comes as a pill, gel, cream or injections. Testosterone cream can be included in your estrogen or progesterone preparations by a knowledgeable pharmacist.

As hormones decline during perimenopause (generally 35 to 50 years of age), the ratio of estrogen to testosterone shifts and melatonin declines until post-menopause. At this point, progesterone, melatonin and estrogen are all but gone, with a little testosterone still lingering. After menopause, a woman's hormonal makeup is closer to a man's than to a premenopausal woman's. This is a phase shift that can initiate cancer.

PREMENSTRUAL SYNDROME

Premenstrual syndrome (PMS) is the name given to those symptoms many women experience seven to ten days before their periods. These can include mood fluctuations, depression, anxiety, food cravings and bloating. Many women experience heightened emotions and sensitivity for about a week before their periods. Despite its pervasiveness, PMS has been a challenge to isolate or define because of its complexity. A woman may experience breast tenderness one month; a combination of anxiety and food cravings the next; then headaches, backaches, fatigue and forgetfulness the next month; followed by mood swings and weight gain the next month.

PMS signals that a woman did not get pregnant during her last ovulation and her body is now preparing for a possible conception next month.

A large variety of lifestyle factors can aggravate symptoms of PMS. A diet high in sugar and refined carbohydrates, alcohol, caffeine, fat and saturated fat, stress and an inadequate amount of outdoor exercise or activity can all be factors. Normal levels of the female hormones estrogen and progesterone, as well as the hormone serotonin, are sensitive to fluctuations during PMS and may also be contributing factors.

A Food Supplement: It is beneficial to supplement with diindolylmethane (DIM) daily, if you experience PMS, since two capsules contain the equivalent to eating 2 pounds of raw or lightly cooked cruciferous vegetables. It is possible to reduce your PMS symptoms with your bioenergetic food choices. The following offer some suggestions.

Eat More Soy Products: Dr. Mark Messina, Ph.D., an associate professor at Loma Linda University and an expert on soy beans and soy products, recommends that women consume more soy products. Soy contains estrogen-like compounds called phytoestrogens, which help to offset the fluctuations in a woman's natural monthly estrogen. Phytoestrogens act very much like the female hormone estrogen by binding to the body's estrogen receptor sites, promoting natural estrogen "feedback loops."

Eat Enough Fiber: Estrogen levels swell during PMS and any excess estrogen is eliminated through the intestinal tract. It is fiber in the intestinal tract that soaks up estrogen and carries it out. If there is insufficient fiber, the estrogen gets reabsorbed into a woman's system, exacerbating further estrogen swells and promoting the symptoms of PMS. Asian women do not experience PMS to the degree North American women do. They consume 30 to 40 grams of fiber daily on average, while most Western women consume only 15 to 20 grams of fiber daily.

To meet a recommendation of at least 30 grams of fiber daily, consume two to three servings of colorful fruit, a large leafy salad with 1 tablespoon of olive oil, three servings of fresh vegetables steamed "crunchy-tender" and several servings of whole grains in the form of oatmeal, seven-grain cereal, or minimally processed whole grain breads.

Avoid Binges and High-Carb Treats: PMS typically triggers food cravings. Women who turn to chocolate, ice cream or cinnamon buns for satisfaction can quickly add 25 to 30 teaspoons of sugar daily to their diets.

Researchers at Massachusetts Institute of Technology compared PMS sufferers to women who did not experience PMS symptoms, and found that the former group increased their daily caloric intake from an average of 1,892 calories to 2,395 calories during this time. Their processed carbohydrate consumption increased 24 percent during meals and 43 percent during snacks. After consuming high-carbohydrate snacks, women experienced relief from tension, anger, fatigue, depression and felt more alert and calm. Researchers concluded that these women were trying to raise their serotonin hormone levels to negate declining moods.

Eating "sweet treats" gives short-term relief but actually aggravates PMS. Sugar-sensitive women can severely magnify their PMS symptoms by allowing a minor food craving to escalate into a binge.

Avoid Saturated Fats: The saturated fat in fatty dairy products and meat raise blood levels of estrogen. Switch to vegetables, salads, legumes, fruit, whole grains, fat-free dairy (but keep dairy to a minimum by using only fat-free plain white organic yogurt), tofu, fish and whey protein isolate or soy protein isolate powders.

Get Enough Omega-3 Essential Fatty Acids: One study on long-chain Omega-3 essential fatty acids from salmon, mackerel or tuna, suggests foods rich in DHA (docosahexaenoic acid) and EPA (eicosapentaenoic acid) or supplements of cod liver or other fish oils or algae oils reduce headaches, irritability and anxiety. One-half teaspoon of organic, cold-pressed borage oil on your salad or vegetables would do much the same. Borage oil contains a special fat called gamma linolenic acid (GLA) that regulates prostaglandins, which are hormone-like compounds that cause the abdominal bloating and tender breasts associated with PMS.

With the borage oil, I also recommend you take a supplement of evening primrose oil that is high in gamma linolenic acid (GLA), which also regulates the production of prostaglandins.

Try using all three of these essential fats along with a daily total of 1,200 IU of vitamin E in the dry powder form called a succinate.

Drink Plenty of Water: PMS sufferers should consume more clean water. University of Alberta researchers found that PMS sufferers drink much less water than other women do. Drinking water does not cause fluid retention but actually helps the body rid itself of excess fluid and reduce bloating.

Coffee and other caffeinated beverages appear to cause more acne, irritability, anxiety and fatigue in PMS sufferers.

Take Supplements: Supplements can greatly reduce or even eliminate PMS symptoms. Consider the following:
- Magnesium levels drop during the last two weeks of the menstrual cycle, which could contribute to water retention, cramping, headaches, tearfulness and an over-sensitized nervous system. Consume magnesium-rich foods such as leafy green vegetables, organic bananas, raw nuts and wheat germ, or take a 250 mg capsule of magnesium citrate with supper.
- Taking calcium supplements in a dose of between 1,300 and 1,600 mg reduces PMS symptoms by 48 percent. Researchers speculate that the mineral might increase serotonin activity.
- Researchers at the U.S.D.A. Forks Human Nutrition Research Center, in North Dakota, showed that mood swings, depression and poor concentration were associated with low intakes of vitamin A, B2, B6, folic acid, calcium, magnesium, copper and zinc. It would be wise to include for one week before and during menstruation, a multi-B vitamin with 50 mg of each B vitamin, two capsules of beta and alpha carotene soft gels from palm oil and a multi-mineral supplement. Many women successfully control PMS with transdermal progesterone cream and some have used it successfully to normalize irregular periods, according to Dr. John R. Lee, M.D, author of *Medical Letter.*

The birth control pill is not as widely recommended today as a treatment for PMS as it once was. It does block the surging of female hormones such as estrogen and progesterone, but the safety of long-term use is questionable.

HEALTHY BREASTS, NATURALLY

In 1960, one in 20 women developed breast cancer. In 1975, it was one in 17. In 1995, the number rose to one out of every nine women.

The incidence of breast cancer is 85 percent dependent upon your diet and lifestyle, and 15 percent dependent on your inherited genes. Even though breast cancer rates are constantly rising among North American women, there are exciting nutritional breakthroughs that can help women prevent breast cancer and have healthy breasts all their lives.

It is vitally important that you do everything within your power to reduce your risks by taking preventive action.

It is possible to get an idea of the influence of diet by looking at the effects of dietary change in large populations and through epidemiology, the study of the incidence and frequency of diseases in different populations. Japanese women on traditional diets have one of the lowest rates of breast cancer in the world, but when they move to North America and eat like North Americans, their breast cancer risk quickly rises. At this time, Japan and China are both in the midst of sweeping dietary changes, in which traditional patterns of eating are weakening in the shift to Western diets, with increased consumption of dairy products, beef and even North American fast food. Their breast cancer rates are rising quickly and dramatically. These countries are living laboratories. Studies also show that Seventh Day Adventists in North America, a vegetarian Christian group that also avoids tobacco and alcohol, have much lower rates of breast cancer than the North American average.

Diet has special significance among lifestyle factors in that you have total control. Dietary modification is a primary therapeutic intervention in Ayurvedic medicine and traditional Chinese medicine, and in both Indian and Chinese cooking, ingredients are valued for both their health-promoting properties and flavors. They have both produced healing cuisines.

Fats That Heal vs. Fats That Kill

The fats you eat impact the quality of your breast tissue and can be responsible for tenderness, cysts and inflammation. Inflammation is a mechanism of the body's healing system that increases circulation and immune activity at the site of slight injury or minor infection. When inflammation is unwarranted or excessive, it is generally a symptom of a hormonal imbalance. The major hormones, which are made from the fatty acids you eat, that can increase or decrease inflammation in breast tissue are called prostaglandins. Depending on which fatty acids are predominant in your diet, this synthesis can favor pro- or anti-inflammatory prostaglandins. This means there are therapeutic opportunities through immediate dietary change.

Both inflammation in your breast tissue and depression are highly correlated with elevated levels of pro-inflammatory hormone-like prostaglandins called PGE2. High levels of PGE2 also force serotonin levels down so you feel depressed, confused and indecisive, and you put your breast tissue at high risk. This is one major symptom of PMS.

By lowering the production of "bad" pro-inflammatory hormone-like prostaglandin PGE2, while simultaneously increasing the production of "good" anti-inflammatory prostaglandins PGE1 and PGE3, you are restoring your body to proper hormonal balance. This leads to healthy breast tissue, and boosts both your alertness and mood.

There are two ways you can increase the production of the "good" prostaglandins:

- Decrease insulin production by not eating sweetened or processed carbohydrates such as cakes, cookies, crackers, rice, white potatoes, simple white or dark wheat bread and "sweet treats."
- Increase your long-chain Omega-3 essential fatty acid consumption by eating broiled salmon, mackerel or tuna at least three times a week. You can also use a fish oil supplement, such as cod liver oil, supplying 1,000 mg of EPA and 650 mg of DHA per day. If you are vegetarian, use 1 tablespoon of flax seed or hemp seed oil or 2 tablespoons of their ground seeds daily and consume a "green drink" daily, rich in algae such as spirulina, chlorella and Nova Scotia dulse. Also take between 1 and 3 grams daily (which may be five to ten capsules) of EPA-rich vegetarian algae oil extract. EPA can make DHA in your body. When these fatty acids predominate in your diet, you produce lots of healthy anti-inflammatory PGE1 and PGE3 and your breast tissue will be in optimal health. Take 1/2 teaspoon of organic borage oil daily.

If you eat a lot of safflower, sunflower, corn, palm or sesame oils, or products made from them such as margarine, vegetable shortening, bottled salad dressings, commercial bread, buns or bakery items, or egg yolks, red meat or organ meats, or partially hydrogenated oils full of dangerous chemically altered trans-fatty acids, you are boosting dangerous PGE2 levels. All food sources of arachidonic acid (AA), a hormone-like fatty acid, boost the synthetic pathways that produce more of the depressing, pro-inflammatory prostaglandin PGE2.

Read labels carefully. You might be shocked to know how many unfriendly fats you are consuming daily. They are in many packaged, processed, restaurant and fast food products. When PGE2 predominates, your breast tissue is compromised and put at a heightened risk of inflammation, infection, cyst development and ultimately cancer.

There are also several other positive dietary and lifestyle strategies you should adopt to maintain healthy breast tissue:

- If you eat poultry, meat or dairy products, make an effort to purchase local organic products that are certified to be free of hormones which are estrogenic and add to the hormonal "total load" capacity of cells in your breasts.
- Be sure to avoid the use of artificial sweeteners and products containing them.
- Avoid fried foods and the saturated, unhealthy fats in red meat and full-fat dairy. Do use plain white, unsweetened, fat-free yogurt each day.
- Eat two to three pieces of ripe, colorful fruit each day. Make one serving fresh or frozen blueberries or any other berry.
- Eat a large salad each day with 1 tablespoon of extra-virgin olive oil, fresh lemon or apple cider vinegar, and salt-free herbal seasonings.
- Use carrot sticks, celery sticks, red pepper rounds and sunflower sprouts as a mid-day snack. Eat all the lightly steamed "crunchy tender" vegetables you can, especially broccoli, red beets, squash, yams, carrots, kale, Swiss chard, asparagus, red cabbage, garlic and ginger.
- Avoid the common "button" mushroom either raw or cooked.
- Reduce or eliminate your consumption of alcohol. There is growing concern that, because alcohol affects your body's production and use of estrogen, even moderate intake may significantly raise the risk of breast cancer in susceptible women.
- Quit smoking tobacco or marijuana. Not only is it damaging to your lungs and liver, it proliferates the production of free radicals and accelerates your aging.
- Increase your intake of lean protein. Researchers have concluded that eating more protein increases a breast cancer patient's chance of survival. The average woman should eat about 27 grams at each of her three meals.
- Learn to examine your breasts yourself each month, and get a baseline mammogram by age 50.
- Avoid the use of toxic household detergents, washing sodas and cleaners. Use biodegradable alternatives. Avoid pesticides, herbicides and chemical cleansers around your property and toxic agrichemicals in food. Pesticides and other environmental pollutants are now believed to be key factors in the worldwide epidemic of breast cancer. Protecting yourself wisely from toxins is a very crucial step in developing healthy breast tissue and a healthy lifestyle.
- Get 8.25 to 8.5 or even 9.0 hours of sleep each and every night in a totally dark room to put you in symmetry with the dark phase of the circadian rhythm. This is the time to restore and rejuvenate, as well as synthesize your hormones and neurotransmitters. Go to sleep as close to sundown as you are able to, so as to lower your body temperature to secrete cancer-protective melatonin and rejuvenating growth hormone, and rise with the morning sun.

Fibrocystic Breasts

Nothing gives a woman more relief than learning that a lump in her breast is harmless. Generally, these benign lumps get larger and more tender just before menstruation. This condition, called fibrocystic breasts, occurs when tiny, fluid-filled sacs form in the milk-producing glands. According to Dr. Bruce H. Drukker, M.D., professor of obstetrics and gynecology at Michigan State University in East Lansing, diet may help you eliminate these fibrous lumps entirely.

Here are some recommendations on making dietary, lifestyle and supplemental choices that will help.

Avoid Excess Bad Fat: Reduce fat, especially saturated fat, in your diet. Never consume more than 20 percent of your daily calories from good fats. A high-fat diet increases the amount of estrogen in the body, which fuels the growth of lumps in the breasts.

Increase Fiber Intake: Increase fiber to 40 grams a day because eating more fruit and vegetables not only reduces fat but provides the fiber that can reduce the swelling and tenderness in the breasts by absorbing excess estrogen and carrying it out of the body.

Supplement with Progesterone Cream: Dr. Norman Shealy, M.D., Ph.D., author of *Natural Progesterone Cream*, highly recommends using 1/4 teaspoon of natural progesterone cream twice a day for fibrocystic breasts. This is equivalent to about 100 to 120 mg of progesterone. He recommends using it only during the two weeks before the onset of the menstrual cycle. It takes two to four months for fibrocystic lumps to disappear. A majority of women have a very small to moderate amount of fibrocystic breast lumps.

NUTRITIONAL CONTENT OF VARIOUS CARBOHYDRATES

Carbo-hydrate	Amount	Vitamin A	Vitamin C	Calcium	Magnes-ium	Fiber
		(IU)	(mg)	(mg)	(mg)	(g)
Broccoli	3 cups	6,492	350	215	85	14
Kiwi	1 cup	135	60	20	15	2.5
Brown rice	1/2 cup	0	0	1.5	0.5	2
Apple	1 small	340	175	40	20	2.8
Black beans	1 cup	50	60	35	15	13
Avocado	1/2 cup	250	40	60	30	7
Oatmeal	1 cup	25	30	50	32	10
Sweet potato	1 cup	5,900	375	50	19	10
Croissant	1 pce.	1	5	6	4	1
Donut	1 pce.	2	3	4	1	2

Take Vitamin E-Complex: Vitamin E-complex helps stabilize fluctuations in a woman's hormones and can reduce the size and pain of fibrous cysts. Try using the dry white powder form of vitamin E called d-alpha succinate with other mixed tocopherols including 20 percent gamma-tocopherol. It is natural and better absorbed after 30 years of age and may be your best source of vitamin E. Use three 400 IU-size capsules daily, one at each meal. Vitamin E complex suppresses the level of inflammation-promoting cytokine called Interleukin-6 (IL-6) that triggers the secretion of C-reactive protein levels (CRP). Both IL-6 and CRP are directly implicated in the increased prevalence of heart attacks and strokes. Both IL-6 and CRP are sharply reduced by a vitamin E-complex.

Supplement with Calcium and Magnesium: Add 1,000 mg of calcium citrate and 1,000 mg of magnesium citrate, together at bedtime, preferably with 1/2 cup of non-fat plain, organic yogurt, two cloves of garlic finely minced, and 1/2 table-spoon of flax seed, hemp seed or perilla oil.

Exercise: Exercise five days a week, but avoid damaging your body by going too hard, too soon. Do a combination of aerobics and anaerobic weight training. Don't slight walking, as it may be your best form of exercise.

Ensure Your Personal Environment Is Toxin-Free: Avoid all toxic pesticides and herbicides. Do not use them in your garden or on your lawn. Xenoestrogens and petrochemical estrogens are potentially carcinogenic for women's breasts and men's prostates. Xenoestrogens, sometimes called organochlorides, are estrogenic compounds that encompass a wide variety of pesticides and other chemicals introduced into the environment. The increase in these compounds since 1960 is thought to be related to increased breast lumps, breast cancer and the increased incidence of male infertility.

Reduce Stress: Explore the wonderful spiritual current within yourself and consider meditation, prayer, pondering, spiritually elevating reading and nightly watching the stars as a star gazer.

5

MEN: YOUR HORMONAL HEALTH

Men experience the same dramatic decline in their sex hormones as women do. Male hormone decline begins at approximately 35 years of age, a process that is called andropause.

THE SIMILARITY OF ANDROPAUSE TO MENOPAUSE GENERALLY SEEN BETWEEN 35 AND 50 YEARS OF AGE

Andropause in Men	Menopause in Women
• Testosterone decreases	• Estrogen decreases
• Body fat increases	• Body fat increases
• Biological status decreases	• Biological status decreases
• Osteoporosis increases	• Osteoporosis increases
• Cardiovascular disease increases	• Cardiovascular disease increases
• Prostate cancer increases	• Breast cancer increases

Andropause occurs when testosterone, the hormone essential to maintaining a man's youthful vigor, dwindles. Researchers estimate that 20 percent of men and 15 percent of women in their forties are deficient in testosterone. (Sometimes low testosterone in men and women is caused by following a low-fat diet—we can starve our bodies of the cholesterol we need to make testosterone.) This hormone not only controls the sex drive, but also builds and maintains muscle mass, bone strength, fat content and distribution—making a man leaner, and boosting vitality, skin elasticity and, in an indirect way, the hair on a man's head. Athletes take it illegally to increase endurance and strength.

Testosterone is also responsible for the libido. It promotes the initial sexual urge, then facilitates performance. Sexual stimulation begins in the brain when neurotransmitters ignite neurotestosterone receptor sites, which start a hormonal cascade that ignites testosterone sites in the nerves, blood vessels and muscles.

THE ESTROGEN CONNECTION

Men need estrogen as well as testosterone throughout their lives. Testosterone is a "prohormone" responsible for making the male hormone dihydrotestosterone and estrogen. The overall effect associated with testosterone is really the result of the combined effects of testosterone plus dihydrotestosterone and estrogen.

As men reach 40, the ratio of testosterone to estrogen changes. This change is accompanied by an increase in fat and a decline in the male body's energy metabolic system. This increases central abdominal fat—what men call a "beer gut" and physicians call "central adiposity"—and is generally a sign of low testosterone levels.

Why the increase in fat? With the onset of andropause, men begin to lose their fat-burning muscle mass as testosterone diminishes, and excess glucose turns into abdominal fat. This "fat-pad" makes estradiol, a form of estrogen, and somewhere between the ages of 55 and 60, with low testosterone and high estradiol levels, hormonally, men become similar to women.

While women experience a decline in all of their sex hormones, men only experience a decline in testosterone. Their estrogen levels increase. The main source of estrogen in adult men is from the breakdown of testosterone. In boys, estrogen is responsible for bone growth and skeletal muscle, and in mature men it prevents bone loss and keeps the brain's neurotransmitters, especially acetylcholine, working at optimum. Thus the transformation at andropause is from one of he to he-female. Elderly men, for all intents and purposes, are more woman on the inside after andropause. After andropause, elderly men are more hormonally similar to women than to younger men. This phase is when men are more likely to develop cancer.

Aging can also lead to an increase in insulin production. The more insulin produced, the greater the accumulation of stored body fat. That stored body fat contains the enzyme that converts testosterone to estrogen. And so the cycle continues.

Balancing Estrogen

There are certain measures, however, that can be taken to safely reduce estrogen levels. I recommend the following options.

Lower Insulin Levels: The only way to reduce estrogen build-up is to reduce excess body fat. That can only be done by lowering insulin. Lowered insulin levels can quickly be achieved by removing processed and sweetened foods from your diet, and eating more bioenergetic whole foods instead.

Don't Gain Weight: Employ voluntary calorie restriction and eat only bioenergetic whole foods. There is no disagreement among nutritional researchers in the world of longevity research that voluntary calorie restriction works in every animal species tested. The elusive goal of living a longer, leaner, healthier life can now become a reality. To achieve such powerful benefits you must consciously understand the exact way you need to eat and live. Food and lifestyle are strong therapeutic drugs that you can control effectively—right now. With better hormonal control you will have more zest, clarity and sleep more soundly.

Work Out Regularly: Exercise daily with aerobics and anaerobic weight-resistance training to build fat-burning muscle.

Get a Good Night's Rest: Avoid the hormonal falloff that occurs during peri-andropause in men aged 35 to 55. Get 8.25 to 8.5 hours of sleep a night in total darkness. Go to sleep early, at sundown, so that your body temperature drops off and keeps you in "temperature rhythm." In this cool-down, critical phase of climate control, testosterone and estrogen levels will drop dramatically and melatonin levels will rise to help keep you cancer-free. If you stay up too late and in warm light, you will not cool down, and estradiol will soar. This is the catalyst of cancer. Both your melatonin and growth hormone levels will remain critically low because your climate control mechanism is stuck in the "off" position.

TESTOSTERONE THERAPY BENEFITS

Ensuring that testosterone is at optimal levels is crucial to a man's physical and emotional well-being. In the early 1960s, a physician named Tiberius Reiter published the results of 12 years of experience using testosterone replacement therapy in 240 men (aged 45 to 75) who complained of premature aging. The results showed that after two to four months of testosterone administration, significant improvements occurred in the areas of depression, impotence, urinary disturbances and other aging-related disturbances.

Dr. Malcolm Carruther, M.D., completed an 18-year study on 1,000 men, ranging in age from 31 to 80 years, administering synthetic testosterone with similar findings. He reports that all of the men experienced "an overall feeling of increased vitality and well-being," and they had "less depression and irritability and increased drive and assertiveness."

Time magazine ran an April 24, 2000, cover story on testosterone. It noted a UCLA study that revealed that men with low testosterone levels frequently exhibit signs of anger, irritability and aggression. When these men went on testosterone replacement therapy, their anger diminished and their sense of well-being increased.

If you want more ergogenic drive, better cardiovascular health and enhanced strength, as well as emotional stability, maintaining testosterone levels is the key.

Natural Testosterone Is Better

Today, men have access to natural testosterone therapies that restore youthful hormonal levels. Testosterone, like estrogen, is available only through a doctor's prescription. It is available in compounding gels, easy-to-use patches and oral tablets that are generally taken three times a day. In Canada, a physician can prescribe and have a knowledgeable pharmacist make a topical gel from 10 or 20 percent natural testosterone. In the U.S., the prescription hormone replacement gel, AndroGel®, is now available. Recent research by endocrinologists indicates that natural testosterone gels are very effective at raising testosterone levels for improved mood, increased lean muscle mass, ergogenic drive, libido, bone density and muscle strength.

In addition, there are other natural measures you can take to boost your testosterone levels.

Reduce Stress: To increase testosterone levels, you must reduce cortisol levels by reducing stress. As cortisol levels rise, testosterone levels drop, because the steroid hormone pregnenolone, which is required to make testosterone, is diverted to make more cortisol. Reduced cortisol levels indicates successful stress reduction.

Herbert Benson M.D., a cardiologist at Harvard Medical School, believes that the most effective way to reduce cortisol—which has been used successfully for thousands of years—is meditation. Meditation is a practical method of extending brain longevity and spiritual awakening.

Work Out: It is possible to stimulate testosterone production with early-morning, weight-resistance exercises when testosterone production is heightened. These exercises must be very intense, brief (from 15 to 30 minutes) and not exhausting. Try to alternate aerobic exercise, such as cycling or walking, with a weight-resistance program to really increase testosterone.

Testosterone peaks between 2 a.m. and 4 a.m. and stays elevated until about 9 a.m. Therefore, if you do any weight training, it is better to do strength training in the morning than at night. (Bill Pearl, the only man ever to defeat Arnold Schwarzenegger for the Mr. Universe title, does his strength training at 3 a.m. to take full advantage of his peak testosterone levels.)

Eat Soy Products: Soy beans and fermented soy bean by-products such as extra-firm tofu, tempeh, miso, soy burgers and soy protein isolate powder appear to regulate estrogen and modulate testosterone production.

Use Herbal Aromatase Inhibitors to Reduce Estrogen: In youth, low amounts of estrogen are used to "turn off" the powerful cell-stimulating effects of testosterone. As estrogen levels increase with age, testosterone cell stimulation may be locked in the "off" position and cause the loss of libido in older men. As more and

as you age

more testosterone is converted to estrogen, the estrogen is taken up by testosterone receptor sites in cells throughout the body. When an estrogen molecule occupies a testosterone receptor site on a cell membrane, it blocks the ability of serum testosterone to induce a healthy hormonal signal. It does not matter how much free testosterone is available if excess estrogen is competing for the same cellular receptor sites. For testosterone to function, it must be freely available to cell receptor sites in the brain, nerves, muscles and genitals.

As men and women age, testosterone becomes bound to serum globulin and is not available to cell receptor sites where it is needed to initiate stimulation centers in the brain. The component in the blood that renders free testosterone inactive is called sex hormone-binding globulin (SHBG) and is made in the liver. Excess estrogen can increase the production of SHBG and block testosterone receptor sites.

Testosterone must be kept in the "free" form in the bloodstream as "bound" testosterone cannot be picked up by testosterone receptors on cell membranes. For aging men, it is desirable to suppress excess levels of SHBG and estrogen while boosting free testosterone levels.

The safest and easiest way to increase free testosterone is to prevent it from being converted into excess estrogen (estradiol). While estrogen levels are necessary for men, high levels also trick the brain into thinking that enough testosterone is being produced, thereby slowing the natural production of testosterone. *what is the level?* If blood test results show estradiol levels greater than 30 pg/mL, men should consider radical lifestyle changes and use an aromatase-inhibiting nutrient.

In a study conducted by the Life Extension Foundation, in Hollywood, Florida, and reported in January 2000, herbal aromatase inhibitors reduced estradiol levels from 54 to 36 and increased free testosterone levels from 14.4 to 22.5 in 30 days. Herbs that increase testosterone and suppress estrogen are highly desirable for men over 40 who show the premature aging effect of a testosterone deficit.

Conversely, it is not advisable for prostate cancer patients to increase testosterone. *The New England Journal of Medicine* (1998, 339; 785–791) showed that an herbal preparation called PC Spes had the dual effect of suppressing testosterone and increasing estrogen and was, therefore, beneficial in the treatment of prostate cancer.

Chrysin *(Passiflora Coerulea)*, a bioflavonoid extracted from plants, is a natural aromatase inhibitor. Chrysin is not well absorbed. A study published in *Biochemical Pharmacology* (1999, vol. 58) identified the specific mechanisms of chrysin's absorption impairment and concluded that the addition of a black pepper extract called piperine significantly enhanced the bioavailability of chrysin. There are drugs such as Arimidex that inhibit stinging aromatase, but chrysin is natural.

A highly concentrated extract from the nettle root *(Urtica dioica)* provides a unique mechanism for increasing levels of free testosterone. The prostate gland also benefits from nettle root.

In Germany, for 30 years, nettle root has been used as a treatment for benign prostatic hyperplasia (BPH), enlargement of the prostate gland. A metabolite of testosterone called dihydrotestosterone (DHT) stimulates prostate growth, leading to enlargement. Nettle root inhibits the binding of DHT to attachment sites on the prostate membrane. Nettle root extracts also inhibit enzymes such as 5-alpha-reductase that cause testosterone to convert to DHT. It is the DHT metabolite of testosterone that is known to cause benign prostate enlargement, excess facial hair and hair loss at the top of the head.

About 90 percent of all testosterone is produced by the testes, the remainder by the adrenal glands. Testosterone functions as an aphrodisiac hormone in brain cells, and as an anabolic hormone in the development of bone and skeletal muscle. As men age past 40, sex hormone-binding globulin (SHBG), which is made in the liver, increases dramatically—by 40 percent. The associated decline in sexual interest is not due to the amount of testosterone produced, but rather to the increased binding of testosterone to globulin by SHBG.

But testosterone is more than a sex hormone. Protein synthesis for maintaining muscle mass, bone formation, improved oxygen uptake, cholesterol regulation, blood sugar balancing and competent immune surveillance requires testosterone, as do cardiac functioning and neurological functions.

Have a knowledgeable physician check your hormone levels from simple blood tests to review your hormonal report card and establish your specific dietary strategy.

The tests I recommend and the ideal ranges are:

Testosterone, total	241–827 mcg/dL
Free testosterone	7.2–24 mcg/dL
Progesterone	0.3–1.2 mcg/dL
Estradiol	0–54 mcg/dL
DHEA sulfate	70–310 mcg/dL
Prostate-specific Antigen (PSA)	0–4 mcg/dL

Women have successfully used natural hormone replacement therapy for 20 years. Natural hormone replacement therapy for men is the next step, as it becomes popular, accessible and socially acceptable.

YOUR PROSTATE

Prostate disease begins as the male hormones decline and estrogens rise, usually around age 40. Some medical researchers estimate that 70 to 75 percent of men in North America will experience some degree of prostate cancer by the age of 70.

As noted, it is not testosterone levels alone that are important to a man's hormonal health, but the ratio of testosterone to estrogen. When the ratio of estrogen to testosterone increases, prostate problems escalate. When estrogen breaks down it produces 4-hydroxy estradiol, which acts as destructive free radicals in the prostate.

Seventy-five percent of all prostate cancers are diagnosed in men over 60. But this is not a magical number, and it's probable that many of these cancers developed years before they were diagnosed. Prostate cancer is slow-growing. The five-year survival rate for localized cancer is good news—100 percent. However, after five years, the survival rate gradually declines to 52 percent at ten years. This argues for prevention.

Strategies to Reduce Prostate Cancer

Supplement: After the age of 40, use diindolylmethane (DIM) explained on page 58, on a daily basis to reduce conversion of testosterone to DHT and estrogen, while improving prostate function.

Avoid Animal Fat: While no single cause of prostate cancer has been determined, the single biggest risk factor for prostate cancer is eating products that contain animal fat. In one study involving over 6,000 men, those who routinely ate milk, cheese, eggs and meat had a 3.6 times greater risk of fatal prostate cancer than those who did not. Studies on vegetable fat do not show a relationship to prostate cancer. Studies on carcinogens formed when meat is cooked also don't show a strong association.

Prostate cancer is one of the few cancers where a strong link exists between it and eating one type of food—red meat from mature cattle that have accumulated a long lifetime of environmental chemicals in their fat. Eliminate full-fat dairy from your diet and eat lean red meat sparingly.

Load Up on Lycopene: The carotenoid lycopene gives tomatoes, watermelons, grapefruit and papaya their red color. Researchers are realizing that the cancer-preventive effects of the Mediterranean diet, which have been attributed to olive oil, may in fact be due to lycopene.

On April 12, 1999, at a meeting of the American Association of Cancer Research in Philadelphia, a study was presented that shows lycopene can shrink existing prostate tumors and slow their spread. The doctors found that men receiving lycopene were less likely to have cancer cells extend to the edge of the prostate gland and precancerous cells were less abnormal looking. They determined this by measuring the level of Prostate-Specific Antigen (PSA) (which indicates the volume of cancer cells in the prostate gland. PSA levels in men receiving lycopene, at 15 mg two times a day fell by 20 percent, indicating a decrease in prostate cancer cell volume.

Eat tomatoes in your salads, tomato sauces and cooked tomatoes in which tomatoes lycopene is especially concentrated. Lycopene requires a fat to be absorbed, so after your tomato sauce is cooked drizzle it with some olive oil or sprinkle flax seed oil over your salad.

Take Vitamin E Supplements: According to a study published in the *Journal of the National Cancer Institute* (Dec. 20, 2000), and conducted at the prestigious John Hopkins School of Public Health, that evaluated 10,456 men who were studied over a seven-year-period, higher levels of gamma tocopherol (vitamin E subfraction) significantly reduced prostate cancer risk, and both selenium and alpha tocopherol (vitamin E subfraction) also reduced prostate cancer incidence, but only when gamma tocopherol levels were high.

Scientists at the National Academy of Sciences suggest that alpha tocopherol (or tocopheryl) vitamin E supplements must contain at least 20 percent gamma tocopherol, ideally giving you 210 mg of the gamma portion daily. Commercial alpha tocopherol (vitamin E) without 20 percent gamma tocopherol can deprive cells of the gamma form and actually lower the levels of the critical gamma forms of vitamin E. Use the dry form of vitamin E called a succinate.

Take an Herbal Combination: The five powerful herbs listed below have been shown in numerous clinical settings to prevent and treat benign prostatic hypertrophy or BPH, a tendency for the prostate gland to enlarge and become inflamed. They work to reduce inflammation in the prostate gland, improving urinary flow and relieving urgency. They block the detrimental effects of testosterone and estrogen on the prostate. I personally use this herbal combination and highly recommend it to men 35 years of age and older. Please note that each herb must be an herbal extract for you to receive their therapeutic supportive benefit.

HERB	RECOMMENDED DAILY DOSAGE
Saw palmetto (serenoa repens)	450 mg
Chinese licorice	225 mg
Pygeum africanum	125 mg
Corn silk	480 mg
Stinging nettle root (urtica dioica)	300 mg

PROGESTERONE AND DHEA

Progesterone is one of the two most important hormones in your body. It is a natural energizer and anti-depressant, it optimizes your libido and is a precursor for estrogen, testosterone, cortisone, aldosterone and dehydroepiandrosterone or DHEA—the second most important hormone. Some men, when they enter andropause, may experience a decrease in their progesterone levels just as women do.

DHEA is your body's most abundant hormone responsible for health and longevity. After the age of 35, DHEA levels drop as well. Natural progesterone cream can help to replenish the loss of both progesterone and DHEA. Many physicians have noted that some men who use natural progesterone cream rubbed into the skin see a striking rise in depleted DHEA levels.

Some men, after the age of 50, can benefit from the overall health-enhancing benefits of natural, standardized USP progesterone cream rubbed into the skin. Natural progesterone is the only known replacement hormone that does not suppress or turn "off" the body's own production of that hormone. About 1/4 teaspoon of the cream should be applied to the scrotal skin twice a day.

Applying 1/4 teaspoon twice a day is equivalent to approximately 100 to 120 mg of natural progesterone. Many physicians have noted increases of DHEA levels ranging from 30 to 100 percent over their baseline, when men apply the cream to scrotal skin.

After using natural progesterone, you will notice that you have more energy and a better memory. You will also benefit from the reduced risk of heart disease, increased fat loss and improved immune function.

DHEA is the most abundant steroid hormone produced by a man's body in the adrenal glands. The average male synthesizes between 25 and 30 mg each day. The second most abundant steroid hormone is cortisol, which is synthesized at the rate of 10 to 20 mg every day. If stress is higher, then cortisol output is higher.

Your body makes more DHEA because it inhibits excessive cortisol action by binding it to its receptors. Therefore, if DHEA levels decline, which they do from age 35 on, there is no "braking mechanism" to "turn off" the excess cortisol, which literally destroys your brain, heart, arteries and muscle tissue.

Of interest to us is that men (and women) with higher DHEA levels do appear to have less heart disease and lower overall premature mortality than men and women with lower levels. Any decline in DHEA can have devastating consequences on the aging process.

As discussed, physicians have noticed that progesterone raises DHEA levels. And DHEA may increase testosterone production. Therefore, progesterone cream may increase testosterone. Men who use progesterone cream should take, daily, the herbal extract combination noted on page 74, to protect free testosterone levels.

After the age of 30, men should consider using two capsules of this herbal combination a day to achieve this amount of herbal extracts. Men who begin to go bald or have benign prostatic hypertrophy (BPH) before the age of 50, should consult with a knowledgeable physician or health professional and use two capsules of this formula three times a day for a total of six capsules daily.

Following a lifelong commitment to stress reduction, aerobic and anaerobic exercise, getting 8.25 to 8.5 hours of sleep a night, coupled with eating bioenergetic whole foods, helps men maintain their ergogenic drive and their anabolic reserve. This is the quickest, surest and best way known to achieve the goal of optimum physical, emotional and mental hormonal synthesis, output, balance and health.

Part III

THE POWER OF FOOD: THE DIVINE BLUEPRINT

6

BIOENERGETIC WHOLE FOODS

Astronomers generally agree that our Milky Way galaxy contains over 400 billion suns just like ours. There are 500 to 600 galaxies recognized beyond our own and if we imagine that each one has a similar number of suns, our universe would be home to about 40 trillion suns. That's a lot of light.

There is a saying that incorporates the phrase, "everything good under the sun." This sun of ours is 93 million miles from earth and it takes a pulse of the sun's energy, a sun beam, eight full minutes to reach the earth traveling at the speed of light (186,000 miles a second). This is all perfectly designed in the Divine Blueprint. For, if the sun were closer, we would have excessive heat and droughts—and if the sun were farther away, the earth would be too cold for us to survive or to grow food upon.

The explicit and dynamic passage from the Old Testament, "Let there be light," draws us closer to the infinite and awe-inspiring power of this first-created manifestation, light!

LIGHT IS ENERGY AND THERMODYNAMICS

The First Law of Thermodynamics is based on the conservation of energy. This law states that energy can neither be destroyed nor created. Albert Einstein made us aware that energy can constantly transform into matter, and matter can constantly transform into energy.

The sum total of energy and matter is always equal, although it could vary in proportion as being all energy at one time, or some other combination of the two at another time. Basically speaking, everything, then, is energy or can be converted into energy.

When you use plants for your food and energy source, you directly eat foods alive with energy. If you use animals as a food source, then you eat the energy of plants indirectly, since the plants are converted to the animals; and the animals then convert into the tissues, cells, atoms and sub-atomic particles of your body.

Energy cannot be created or destroyed, but it can be stored. This First Law of Thermodynamics reminds us that if we eat more food than our body's energy requirements for that particular day, then that excess energy must be stored. The body stores energy as fat. As a survival mechanism during our forefathers' and foremothers' hunting and gathering days, before our ancestors were agrarian or animal herders, the human body developed an almost infinite capacity to store fat. The physiology is that the body developed an enzyme called lipoprotein lipase to collect digested fat in the bloodstream and then to stuff it into cells. This was necessary then and remains today in affluent societies as an outdated survival mechanism that keeps 40 percent of North Americans overweight. This enzyme was originally designed to see us through times of famine or "down time" due to injury or illness, but today it keeps storing extra calories, especially fat calories, as excess body fat we do not need.

The Second Law of Thermodynamics states that any energy system left to its own will break down and fall apart. Entropy is the name of the force that makes all energy systems fall apart.

Entropy is the body's natural transformation from matter to energy. Everything in nature is subject to entropy. The matter that comprises your body experiences the natural state of entropy, so it eventually returns to the vast storehouse of universal energy—from which it originally came. This energy then is potentially capable of replenishing itself as matter once again … and so this perfectly balanced process of the recycling of energy and matter, of life and creation itself, goes on and on.

The human body was designed for wellness, not illness. Every single one of your 100 trillion cells is made to function extremely well and cohesively to give you dynamic mental and physical vitality and well-being. Nature, in the Divine Blueprint, has skillfully allowed the plant kingdom to continually capture the life force of the sun. This is the process of photosynthesis, which allows plants steeped in sunlight and infused with the energy of rain and rich soil to literally manufacture oxygen, protein, vitamins, minerals, phytonutrients, fiber, cell salts, essential fatty acids and energy.

THE ORIGIN OF BIOENERGETIC FOODS

Bioenergetic foods, as I mentioned earlier, are the natural high-octane fuels the human body requires to support an anabolic drive. They convert their energy fuel (energetic) to the efficient and effective biological (bio) rejuvenation and revitalization of every cell in your body.

Food is energy. This is a basic scientific principle. Your body is an energy system. Every single one of the 100 trillion cells (little molecular motors) in your body requires energy to work. Digestion, respiration, talking, seeing, hearing, circulation, thinking and metabolism all require energy. Every cell, every tissue, every muscle requires energy to function healthily. When your body's energy is low, it just does not have the resources to run well, and that is when illness begins to dominate. When your energy is high, your peak performance and health are optimal. Food is the source of energy your body needs most. With precision and deliberate measure, nature has designed high-octane fuels for your energy support and biological functions.

Food can either give you dynamic energy or rob you of it. Your body is an extremely efficient piece of machinery that can absorb virtually all the food you consume. What you eat on a daily basis either nourishes your anabolic state and health or it diminishes the healthy balance into a declining catabolic state. If your last meal or snack did not promote your anabolic drive, then it accelerated your aging.

Bioenergetic whole plant-based foods are pure life energy. Grown in sunlight and infused with the energy of the soil and water, they can increase your energy and improve your moods and motivation. They can bring you back to an energetic anabolic drive. You only have to eat them. It is that simple!

A Second Gift from Plants

During photosynthesis, plants create the oxygen that is fundamental to the very survival of the human race. Equally important is the fact that plant-based foods, during photosynthesis, take in and recycle our waste product, carbon dioxide. Without plants, sunlight, soil and water, we would have no oxygen and we would suffocate from our own accumulated carbon dioxide.

Five hundred million years ago, the atmosphere of the earth was 98 percent carbon dioxide plus a smidgen of methane and nitrogen. There was virtually no oxygen. Bacteria in the first stage began to "breathe in" the carbon dioxide and produce oxygen as a waste product, as plants still do today. In the more sophisticated second step of photosynthesis, which took place over millions of years, a blue-green phytoplankton called spirulina, along with other algae, learned to also "breathe in" carbon dioxide and produce oxygen as a waste product. Carbon dioxide began to dwindle to its present fraction of one percent, and the atmosphere on earth grew to its present oxygen-rich status of 21 percent.

This increase in oxygen made human life possible on earth but, ironically, it poisoned the atmosphere for the very same bacteria that made it. These bacteria had to take refuge in oxygen-free environments. Today, they live on in the darkest recesses of the human gastrointestinal tract and play an important role— along with some other 40 to 50 species of "friendly" bacteria—in destroying bacteria, viruses and toxins, in digesting foods, assimilating fats, preparing proteins for absorption and contributing to human biological wellness.

Your body is tightly interwoven with nature. The sulfur in proteins that comprise half the dry weight of your body is absorbed by plants from the soil. This sulfur is continually recycled by nature and plants for your well-being. The sulfur, left to its own, will be leeched from the soil by rain and run-off to our rivers, lakes and eventually oceans. A versatile small plant, a photoplankton called emiliana hyxleyi, which grows profusely in the oceans, produces tens of millions of tons of dimethyl sulfide, which evaporates from the oceans, forms into clouds and returns to the land, in rain, where once again plants can take it back up in photosynthesis. This is again nature's gift of a miraculous plant-giving life to all humankind.

All human cycles are part of the energy pathway. The sun is the principal controller of all life simply because of the nature of matter in our universe. The life force of the bio-ecosystem is all the energy of the sun captured in the food chain. In the food chain, all species and substances interact with one another in "feedback loops" that are interdependent on each other, yet independent on their own. For example, humans eat big fish, big fish eat small fish, small fish eat smaller fish, the smallest fish eat algae and algae derive their nutrients from rocks. These are positive "feedback loops" that intimately weave animals, plants, microbes and humans into parts of the entire bio-system.

The sun is the giver of life on this planet and indigenous cultures from every continent have instinctively worshipped or greatly honored the sun. Each day you should pause in awe and gratitude for your remarkable body and equally thank the plants, soil, rain and sun for their light, energy, nutrients and disease prevention.

Daily express your sincere gratitude, remain open, loving, appreciative, alert and calm. If you feel more comfortable, "thank" the Divine Blueprint. Whatever you do, reconsider the blind trust you have given to tasty donuts and other fast or processed foods and their brilliant, Porsche-driving marketing wizards.

For 3 billion years, there was only anaerobic life on earth that did not require oxygen. With the advent of photosynthetic organisms about 500 million years ago, oxygen began to accumulate in the atmosphere.

Energy generation during aerobic metabolism drives your 100 trillion cells. That energy is stored in a molecule known as adenosine triphosphate (ATP). ATP is essential to sustain the physiological and biological reactions of human life.

Your body has a limited ability to store ATP. ATP is constantly generated by the quality of foods you eat daily. Bioenergetic whole foods are the preferred fuel to sustain life energy and prevent you from reaching your "total load" of cumulative toxic damage too early in life.

REFINED FOODS: INTERRUPTING THE CYCLE

Plants, with all of their naturally occurring parts intact—whole foods—are critical to our health and vitality. Researchers refer to these foods as energy-rich or bioenergetic.

On the other hand, foods that have been refined—which have many of their essential nutritional elements and components removed or damaged through

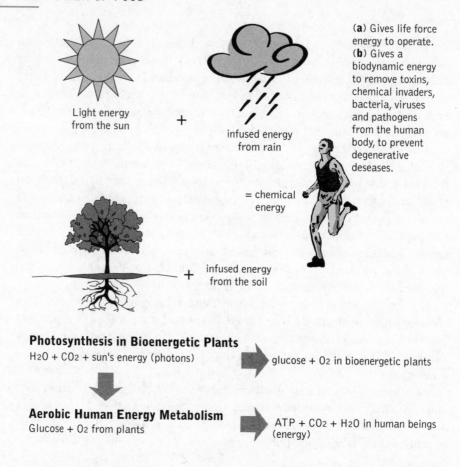

(a) Gives life force energy to operate.
(b) Gives a biodynamic energy to remove toxins, chemical invaders, bacteria, viruses and pathogens from the human body, to prevent degenerative deseases.

Light energy from the sun

+

infused energy from rain

= chemical energy

+

infused energy from the soil

Photosynthesis in Bioenergetic Plants
$H_2O + CO_2$ + sun's energy (photons) → glucose + O_2 in bioenergetic plants

Aerobic Human Energy Metabolism
Glucose + O_2 from plants → ATP + CO_2 + H_2O in human beings (energy)

processing—contribute little or nothing to our well-being. In fact, most contribute to our negative moods, weight gain, accelerated aging and ill health.

The dilemma is that most of these refined or processed foods are attractive to us because they are convenient and tasty. But through processing, many of their necessary parts have been removed and they have gained foreign and toxic compounds in the form of preservatives, taste enhancers, moisturizers, coloring agents, artificial flavors, fungus retardants, hydrogenated oils or fats.

Fast Foods: Hazardous Waste?

The convenience of fast foods that Lynn ate, or maybe they are foods you eat quite often, are attractive because they are convenient, predictable, tantalizing, palatable and delectable. We must acknowledge the fact that fast-food production has become an art, and manufacturers have made these foods very tasty and appealing. The fast-food industry world-wide now tops well over US$300 billion a year in sales and is growing at a rapid pace. We'd better be careful!

Fast food is the most unhealthy dietary development in human history. In

North America, we have perfected fast foods, especially their extremely attractive packaging, and have exported them quickly through seductive advertising, all over the world. People now love fast food, especially children. For children, and for most adults, fast food is compellingly attractive because it caters to our inherited tastes for sugar, fat, animal protein, and our learned taste for salt. Fast-food chains have worked tirelessly to perfect the texture, flavor and aroma of their foods.

As I travel the world doing nutritional research, I am amazed at the enormous success and appeal French fries, cinnamon rolls, burgers, milk shakes, cola, pizza, potato chips and onion rings have to people in China, Japan, Morocco, India, Latin America, the Caribbean and even more remote indigenous cultures. I witness the clever marketing, powerful advertising, attractive and colorful packaging and the appealing taste that fast-food chains utilize to turn people from healthy dietary choices to readily available, unhealthy fast foods—very quickly.

In our 24-7-365 fast-paced societies, people no longer appear to have the time to shop for fresh produce, wash, cut and cook vegetables or prepare entire, balanced meals. Furthermore, many families have both parents working, and likewise in single-parent families, time is in short supply, so fast foods become a very tasty and convenient option.

In our hectic mobile cultures, convenience and predictability of fast food appear to reassure and offer comfort to work-weary, shopping-exhausted, late-night-carousing, or hungry road travelers who recognize the logo of a fast-food restaurant in malls, shopping centers and strategically located roadsides. This warm familiarity invites you because the food always looks the same, tastes the same, is prepared the same, costs the same and you and your kids know there will be no surprises.

The Science Behind the Appeal

Nothing draws us to food like its aroma. Fast-food chains have employed psychologists, sociologists and marketing wizards to make the smell of their offerings irresistible. They know that if something smells good, we are most likely to eat it. Fat is one of the best carriers of aroma. We are drawn to the smell of buttery buns baking, rich chocolate melting, fries and onion rings frying, and tofu and burgers sizzling.

From a taste standpoint, we have an inherent love of sweetened fat, according to research done by Adam Drewnowski, Ph.D., director of the Nutritional Sciences Program at the University of Washington. It leads us to cookies, cakes, croissants, chocolate and ice cream.

Fat alone is unpalatable. But sugar can mask the taste of pure fat. When people are asked to taste foods containing various amounts of sugar and fat, their perception of the fat content decreases as the sugar content increases. On the other hand, fat can make foods taste less sweet. Chocolate icing, as an example, contains

70 percent sugar and 15 to 20 percent fat, which is too sweet for most of us. However, this icing gains in appeal if the fat content is increased to 25 percent or more. So fat makes fast foods desirable, and sugar makes the fat taste invisible.

Through fast, processed foods, we consume a whopping number of excess calories in the form of saturated fats, sugar, salt and dangerous trans-fatty acids. The fat clogs our arteries and makes our metabolic processes sluggish, while the sugar is just excess calories that will add unwanted weight and hurl us into a catabolic nosedive.

Fast-food manufacturers spend an enormous amount of money to ensure their foods are highly appealing. They want us to crave their fast foods, in spite of the fact that they are unhealthful. Feel duped and used? You should.

Why Are We So Susceptible?

Stress, for one thing, magnifies our cravings for fast food. The stress hormone cortisol, secreted from the adrenal gland during stress, triggers the release of other hormones, which increase food cravings and overeating.

Our reproductive system may also trigger cravings and overeating. There are nerve cells in our brain that control eating as part of ensuring both energy and hormonal balance. Dr. Sarah Leibowitz at Rockefeller University notes that this appetite-control center in the brain is immediately next to the reproductive center. She believes that the cycle of sugar and fat craving coincides with reproductive needs. "Nature is seeking reassurance that we have enough energy and body fat for survival of the species," says Dr. Leibowitz. For example, men have a species-survival need for greater muscle mass and prefer protein fats such as double-patty hamburgers and roast beef sandwiches. Women, on the other hand, have more cravings for sweetened fats such as chocolate, cakes, pies, puddings and brownies—especially during PMS. These calorie-packed foods can literally store up energy as fat and water in preparation for a potential pregnancy.

Food cravings are also fueled by our addiction to pleasure. "A euphoric or calming response is produced by certain foods that release morphine-like chemicals in the brain called endorphins. The mere touch of sugar on the tongue produces an immediate endorphin rush. Thus, we feel good immediately after eating a donut, because of the boost in the hormone, endorphins, which is followed by a lingering good mood induced by the slow-acting increase in the hormone serotonin, triggered by the carbohydrates," writes Elizabeth Somer, M.A., in her highly acclaimed book *Food and Mood* by Owl Books.

Due to this insatiable love of sweet things, the average North American consumes 156 pounds (about 71 kg) of sugar and other unhealthy sweeteners like high-fructose corn syrup annually, according to 1998 U.S. Department of Agriculture reports. That is an increase of 20 percent—31 pounds (14 kg) per person per year—over 1983 statistics. In 1993, we were eating about two-and-a-half pounds of sugar a week, per person. One-and-a-half pounds came from high-fructose corn syrup in overly processed foods. High-fructose corn syrup is six times sweeter than sugar and fast-food manufacturers do not use one-sixth as much—they use more. They know that sugar is addictive and it's an inexpensive preservative.

All processed foods, especially low-fat, fast foods, are full of high-fructose corn syrup in order to mask their unappealing flavor and taste. Between 1990 and 2000, the marketplace exploded with 3,000 to 4,000 new low-fat and fat-free, high-fructose corn syrup products per year. Be aware that "fat-free" does not mean problem-free.

Today, we North Americans get two-thirds of our sugar from processed foods. We also consume 30 million pounds of artificial sweeteners annually. This is approximately half of the world's annual production.

"OUT OF WHACK" HORMONES—IN A BIG SHOT OF INSULIN

Refined sugar, most artificial sweeteners, and processed carbohydrates cause the storage hormone insulin to spike sharply. Whatever isn't needed immediately is stored as fat. Fat cells can expand 1,000 times their size and eating sugars or artificial sweeteners (the only exception is the artificial sweetener called saccharine, marketed as Sweet 'n Low, but which is also unacceptable) causes the storage hormone insulin to sharply spike.

Carbohydrates is the scientific name for sugar. Carbohydrates represent energy that can be stored, and they are only stored by insulin. That is why you eat sugar and get fat. You now have endless access to the mighty caloric power of refined sugar and flour.

When we eat a refined carbohydrate like sugar, refined flour or a sweet treat, our insulin:

- uses 30 percent of the sugar as glucose (the body's primary fuel source) for immediate energy requirements;
- stores 30 percent of the sugar short-term in our liver or muscles as glycogen, an "on-demand" energy source, during the sleep cycle at night; and
- stores 40 percent of the sugar long-term as body fat.

Since we now consume, on average, about three pounds of sugar weekly, our stored sugar (glycogen) is never depleted. Now that our stores stay full almost continually, when we eat a processed carbohydrate or sugar, we cause a modern-day dilemma in a long-established feedback loop. As the sugar gushes into the portal vein between our liver and stomach, our pancreas responds with a big shot of the hormone insulin. This big shot of insulin balances our blood supply of glucose and simultaneously funnels the excess sugar to both the short-term and the long-term storage facilities. The problem is that the short-term facility is already full, so now it processes:

- 30 percent of the sugar, as glucose, for energy today, and
- 70 percent of the sugar, for long-term storage, as fat.

We repeat this scenario of storing unhealthy fat, stuck in "fast forward," day after day, week after week, month after month, and year after year. This results in hormone imbalances in the insulin-appetite control system, which, as we discuss below, accelerates aging and makes us more susceptible to degenerative diseases like cancer and heart disease.

Insulin decreases the blood sugar level, sometimes even pushing it below normal, while elevated insulin levels can linger in our blood for hours. Judith Rodin, Ph.D., of Yale University, feels the sugar-induced rapid rise in insulin might further arouse our hunger signals as the big hit of insulin gives our brain a euphoric feeling from rising endorphin levels, but our blood sugar is sub-elevated and homeostasis (our body's balance) now craves sugar to raise blood sugars.

Also, with our liver and muscle glycogen tanks full, there is really no place for our body to store the sugar from our next meal. Our body now works hard to burn the excess sugar, our cells' primary fuel mix, at the expense of previously stored fat. Eating high-carbohydrate foods when our glycogen tanks are full shuts down our fat-burning furnaces in the mitochondria of each and every one of our 100 trillion cells. Now we can't lose the fat we have.

Whole or real bioenergetic carbohydrates as colorful vegetables, ripe fruit or whole grains give you a lot of nutritional support with very few calories. They contain a powerhouse of many vitamins, minerals, water, protein, fiber and a little fat, including B vitamins that are necessary to make the very enzymes that will slowly digest low-density, natural complex carbohydrates and lower insulin secretion. You now experience appetite-control, sustained good moods and adequate zest. Congratulations!

In the example of white flour, the basis of all processed carbohydrates, the outside husk is stripped off during refinement leaving you with a pure starchy, sugar middle. Get the picture? Refined, sugary, salty, fried, processed foods would be an extinction-promoting accident in nature; treat them exactly the same way in your own life.

Your brain requires about 5 grams (1 teaspoon) of glucose (sugar) every hour to fuel its millions of biochemical interactions. Your body requires about 10 grams of glucose an hour to fuel its biological functions. The body must protect itself from excess glucose (sugar, fructose, sweeteners) consumption you take in from consuming refined foods. Consider how easy it is to overconsume sugar in processed foods, which severely upsets your homeostasis (biochemical balance), and your body's appetite-control hormones then spin out-of-control.

All of the following sugar-sweetened or synthetically sweetened foods swiftly "up-regulate" our body's appetite-control chemicals so that they malfunction. The result is an imbalance in blood-sugar levels and other nerve chemicals, which leaves us edgy; contributes to our emotional downhill spiral; makes us crave these foods even more; puts unwanted fat on our body; and wears out our glucose and insulin receptor sites so we cannot process this excess sugar in our blood.

THE SUGAR CONTENT OF CERTAIN PROCESSED FOODS

Fast-Food	Serving Size	Teaspoons of Added Sugar
Granola bar	1	1.8
Chewing gum	1 stick	0.75–1.5
Barbecue sauce	2 tablespoons	3.0
Wine	3.5 oz (110 mL)	3.0
Gatorade	1 cup	3.5
Spaghetti sauce	½ cup	4.0
Applesauce, sweetened	½ cup	4.0
Sherbet	½ cup	6.1
Muffin (commercial)	1	8.0
Low-fat blueberry yogurt	1 cup	8.5
Fat-free ice cream	1 cup	9.1
Coca-Cola	12 oz (375 mL)	9.3
Light cheesecake	1 medium slice, 7.0 oz (200 g)	11.5
Commercial cinnamon roll	1 medium	12.0
Fruit-flavored low-fat yogurt	1 cup	13.0
Chocolate shake	1 medium (12 oz/375 mL)	20

Most men (68 percent) and almost all women (97 percent) occasionally find it a battle to "say no" to a refined carbohydrate-rich snack such as a sweet treat. At least half the time, 85 percent of both women and men give in to those cravings. This causes insulin levels to rise to try to lower the rising blood-sugar levels. Judith Rodin, Ph.D., a professor of psychology and psychiatry at Yale University, produced research results revealing that people actually enjoy the sweet tastes more and are hungriest when their insulin levels are high. This is the vicious cycle—the more sweets we eat, the more sweets we crave. Sweets arouse our hunger signals and depress our satiety signals, and that in turn can lead to binge eating or eating disorders.

Not only are we destroying our health, but we're destroying the feedback loops that control appetite-mood centers. Feedback loops are delicate mechanisms that read a signal from one system in our body and send it back to another system.

Negative feedback loops read a signal and try to control the system with a "stop" message. Eating 150 pounds of sugar a year—all these tasty new convenience foods we have created—totally destroys our feedback loops.

The truth is, we do not require one single fast food for our well-being. There are no "essential" fast foods, but there are essential fats, proteins, fibers, vitamins, minerals and natural unprocessed carbohydrates. Your digestion, absorption, distribution and elimination processes have not changed in 100,000 years—only your food choices have changed. Stick to nature—that was Nature's plan for you before companies realized they could make enormous sums of money by dazzling you with their almost-irresistible processed fast foods. They entice you to binge, eat their synthetic "foods," and down you go!

Sustained high levels of any one hormone, in your hormone cascades, destroy the intricate balance in all hormone networks. This makes you maladaptive to your internal and external environments. You are now a threat to nature, as it puts you at odds with nature.

You can curb your cravings and avoid overeating simply by switching from a sugar-laden cinnamon roll to a fructose-filled apple. Strictly avoid processed fructose and high-fructose corn syrup in pop, sports drinks and processed foods. They are man-made and no substitute for natural fructose in fruits.

Eliminate refined "sweet treats" carbohydrates, which are counterproductive, by replacing them with "real food" carbohydrates, and you can cut out most obesity, most diabetes and most heart disease, and push escalating colon, prostate and breast cancer numbers into a declining tailspin.

What's more, filling up on sugary, fat-laden, salty fast foods significantly reduces our chance of consuming enough of the 50 vital nutrients we need for our hormones to work smoothly, for our sleep to be restorative, and for our energy and attitude to remain positive. When it comes to sugar, salt and fat—less is better for everyone.

THE SURVIVAL ADVANTAGE COMES IN AN APPLE—NOT A PACKAGE OF COOKIES

As a species, we evolved around food and the circadian rhythms of day and night or light and dark. The human body is an intimately integrated part of a larger biosphere, where everything is designed to be interactive. Maladaptive hormonal disharmony caused by willfully eating out of sync with your longstanding genetic predisposition to food is actually a self-extinction or accelerated-aging decision, a precursor to death.

When you start to eat out of rhythm with your design and you've lost the rhythm in your hormones (to direct all traffic by turning vital functions on or off instantaneously), bone marrow, spleen, lymphocytes and neurotransmitters, in your 100 trillion cellular, sub-cellular, molecular and even atomic levels, you have lost the survival advantage.

Once you lose your rhythm, you lose the split-second hormonal decision-making capabilities necessary to monitor and successfully sustain your survival.

Lose the supersymmetry and symphony of hormonal feedback loops and hormonal networks—and you promote an early extinction, even if it comes by your very own hands.

7

PHYTONUTRIENTS

For many years, researchers have recognized that individuals with diets high in fruits, vegetables, herbs, grains, seeds, nuts and legumes are less prone to a number of diseases, including heart disease, diabetes, cancer and high blood pressure, than those who follow diets laden with meat. Originally, many believed that it was the vitamin, mineral and enzyme contents of these plant-derived foods that were preventing malnutrition and disease.

In the 1990s, researchers discovered phytochemical compounds to which they attributed disease prevention. Finally modern science was discovering that nature, in its infinite wisdom, had designed plants to manufacture biodynamic disease-protective elements to successfully defend the plant, for its own survival, from strong sunlight, oxidation, viruses, bacteria, insects, disease and background radiation. Garlic and onions, for instance, contain potent sulfur compounds that act as bug repellents to keep the vegetable healthy. Likewise, carrots and apricots contain alpha-and beta-carotene, a vibrantly colorful plant pigment that protects them from potentially destructive, strong sunlight. All plants contain compounds that protect them from bacteria, viruses, pollutants, chemical invaders and insects.

When we eat plants, these very same biodynamic disease-protective elements, which researchers now call *phytonutrients*, predictably and measurably protect our bloodstream, cells, tissues, membranes, mitochondria, skin, organs and immune functions from the onslaught of man-made chemicals, toxins, automobile or factory emissions, chemical intruders, bacteria, pesticides, viruses, fungi, yeast, microbes, mutagens, food additives, free radical assaults and carcinogens. This has brought the plant-disease prevention connection to the forefront of serious worldwide nutritional research.

Researchers presently estimate that there are 30,000 to 50,000 of these phytochemicals, although only about 1,000 have been isolated so far. Of these, a mere 100 have been analyzed and tested. Scientists have given the elements a more "user-friendly" and more readily understandable name, phytonutrients. Phytonutrients, a word that comes from the Greek word *phyto*, meaning "from plants," are neither vitamin nor mineral. It is now believed that they are what defend and protect our 100 trillion cells from excessive wear and tear and the onslaught of degenerative diseases, such as cancer, heart disease, cataracts, arteriosclerosis and arthritis.

Our body has the innate ability to self-diagnose and self-heal. To do so, it requires the powerful biodynamic phytonutrients from colorful, plant-based foods. The latest discoveries in plant research that are sweeping the research community worldwide today, add up to an exciting revolution in science and medicine that now gives undeniable support as to why we should "return to the base of the food chain" to experience optimal emotional, mental and physical well-being. Returning to the base of the food chain means to cut out that middle step—the conversion of plant energy to animals—and eat plant energy directly.

Even more remarkable than the high estimated number of phytonutrients is the number of phytonutrients within a single unprocessed plant-derived food. Even the simple soybean, blueberry or Brussels sprout, for example, is a miracle of complexity far more intricate than the latest version of Windows, or any other sophisticated computer program.

A tomato is believed to contain an estimated 1,000 different phytonutrients. Every fruit, grain, legume, seed, nut, grass, sea vegetable and colorful vegetable tested has been found to be a veritable warehouse, jam-packed with these disease-preventive compounds. So the humble salad on our plate, or lentils in our bowl, or red peppers diced on our asparagus, or the pumpkin seeds in our oatmeal are offering us remarkable protection.

It appears that some of these recently discovered phytonutrients will fight not only deficiency-type diseases such as anemia, but also elusive, potentially fatal, age-related illnesses such as heart disease and cancer—which are responsible for 75 percent of all deaths in North America.

Unlike most vitamins, phytonutrients do not appear to be destroyed by preparation techniques such as chopping, grating, extracting, cooking or fermenting. Genistein, the powerful phytonutrient found in soybeans, is also found in soybean products that are cooked, such as miso, tempeh and tofu. Similarly, the phytonutrient sulforaphane, found in cabbage, remains intact even when the cabbage is made into coleslaw or sauerkraut. In fact, sometimes preparation is responsible for making phytonutrients more available to us. Lycopene in a tomato sauce may be made more bioavailable by the cooking process. The potent sulfur compounds from garlic or onions only become activated when they are chopped and exposed to air.

We must always make certain to eat a lot of our fruits and vegetables raw and to not overcook any of them. When we do cook vegetables, it should only be lightly, until "crunchy-tender," so we will be able to enjoy the benefits not just of the many bioenergetic phytonutrients, but of all the bountiful vitamins, minerals, enzymes, protein, fiber and other nutrients that fresh whole foods have to offer.

PHYTONUTRIENTS TAKE ON CANCER

Over 200 studies have examined the relationship between diet and cancer in various countries and cultures. When the data from these studies is combined, those that eat the lowest amount of fruit and vegetables develop various cancers 200 to 300 percent more than those of the higher consumption groups.

Progressive researcher Dr. Gladys Block and her colleagues at the University of California, Berkeley, analyzed all of the 170 controlled studies done to date on the effects of fruit and vegetables on cancer. Results from these studies revealed that the phytonutrients present provide protection against certain forms of this destructive disease.

TYPES OF CANCER
Number of Studies Showing Protection

Types of Cancer	Number of Studies Showing Protection
Lung cancer	24
Colorectal cancer	20
Stomach cancer	17
Esophageal cancer	15
Oral cancer	9
Cervical cancer	7

To understand how phytonutrients protect the body from cancer, it is important to understand that cancer formation is a multi-step process. Bioenergetic phytonutrients, formed during photosynthesis, block one or even more of the steps that lead to cancer. For instance, cancer can begin (initiate) when a carcinogenic molecule from the food we eat, or air we breathe, invades a cell. If sulforaphane, a phytonutrient found in broccoli, cauliflower, cabbage, broccoli sprouts and Brussels sprouts, also reaches the cell at the same time, it quickly activates a group of enzymes that whisk the carcinogen out of the cell before it can cause serious harm.

There are some phytonutrients known to prevent cancer in other ways. Flavonoids, found in citrus fruits and berries, keep cancer-causing hormones from latching on to cells in the first place. Genistein, daidzein and glycitein, found in soybeans, have been shown to inhibit angiogenesis, the process in which growing cancer cells create their own blood supply. Indoles, found in cruciferous vegetables like broccoli and cauliflower, cabbage, turnips and Brussels sprouts, boost immune activity and make it easier for the body to excrete toxins or chemical intruders. Saponins, as found in lentils and red kidney beans, prevent cancer cells from multiplying. P-coumaric acid, chlorogenic acid and lycopene, found in tomatoes, interfere with and prevent certain chemical unions that can create malignant tumors.

When you eat the fresh, colorful fruits, herbs, and vegetables teeming with bioenergetic phytonutrients, you are also protected by these powerful compounds. Nature wonderfully recycles her resources so these disease-preventing and health-promoting plant phytonutrients prevent and fight every disease known. Yes, it is absolutely true.

Phytonutrients have two cancer-preventing mechanisms. The first is their ability to block the initiation of the cancer process and the second is their capacity for suppressing the promotion of cells already initiated into the cancer growth process.

The following are three brief explanations of phytonutrient cancer initiator-blocking mechanisms. These explanations are the results of laboratory research in which disease-preventive phytonutrients are fed to laboratory animals and are able to prevent the development of experimentally induced malignant tumors. Also, phytonutrients are placed in cultures of living cancer cells, and are observed to inhibit or limit the growth of different human and animal lines of experimentally induced cancer. (I personally support only studies based on identified factors that impact distinct cultures or populations, not research done on laboratory animals.)

1. The sulfur compounds from garlic and onions; the dithiothiones and isothiocyanates from cruciferous vegetables; phenols in blueberries, raspberries and other fruits; green tea; several carotenoids, such as alpha- and beta-carotene or lycopene; and vitamin E and vitamin C, found in many fruits and vegetables, have strong antioxidant activity that scavenges and neutralizes free radicals and other electrophilic molecules before they can attack our cellular membranes, exposing our DNA or mitochondria to severe damage, which causes accelerated aging. This free radical attack, left unchecked, leads to a spiraling catabolic decline and degenerative disease.

   The mitochondria are the little energy furnaces in our cells that combine glucose or fuel with oxygen, the igniter, in a biochemical process called cellular respiration, which produces energy as ATP—adenosine triphosphate—our most basic form of energy. The natural byproducts or "smoke" from this biochemical process are corrosive little "free radicals," which literally smash into fine cell walls and eventually weaken and destroy them, leaving the cellular material open for further destruction. Cell walls can be "hit" by these free radicals up to 100,000 times a day. What happens if we get hit on the arm 100,000 times a day?

Exercise increases our mitochondrial oxidative stress and consequently produces an increase in free radical production. The harder we exercise or train, the more serious the problem is, and the more diligent we must be to ensure that we have a sufficient antioxidant arsenal in our bioenergetic whole food choices and antioxidant supplements.

Furthermore, free radicals are quickly formed through stress, excess sunlight, a hard workout or exercise regime, water or airborne pollution, veterinary residue from antibiotics or bovine growth hormones in animal products, pesticides, herbicides, late nights, lack of deep rejuvenating sleep, factory or car emissions and from the natural process of cellular respiration.

We cannot avoid the formation of free radicals, but we can minimize their destructive potential. Here is the clue! We already know it—just eat abundantly from nature's naturally low-calorie bioenergetic whole foods at each and every meal or snack, but practice portion control. The fewer calories we consume, the less energy is required to process the incoming food and the fewer free radicals we make. The fewer free radicals we make, the longer we live.

2. A large number of different phytonutrients interfere with the metabolism and activation of carcinogenic compounds. Indoles and dithiothiones from cruciferous vegetables; flavonoids in berries, squash, parsley and tomatoes; catechins in green tea; carotenoids in spinach, kale, Swiss chard, yams and sweet potatoes; sulfur compounds in garlic and scallions; protease inhibitors in soy sprouts; the Omega-3 polyunsaturated fatty acids in flax seeds, walnuts and fish oils; the plant sterols in wheat grass and barley grass; polyacetylenes and flavonoids in ginkgo biloba, bilberry, green tea, grape seed or skin, milk thistle and Siberian ginseng extracts—all stimulate enzymes that deactivate precarcinogenic compounds and prevent their transformation into a more dangerous form.

3. Soluble and insoluble fiber—from all fruit, vegetables, legumes, whole grains, herbs, seeds and nuts—in the intestines and stomach inhibit the uptake of pathogens and carcinogens from the gut into the circulatory system by absorbing them and excreting them harmlessly, preventing our cells from being exposed to dangerous carcinogenic substances.

What If the Carcinogenic Process Has Already Begun?

Should the initiation of cancer have already begun, phytonutrients have many channels through which they can suppress the process and inhibit the promotion of a precancerous cell to a malignant state. These bioenergetic phytonutrient compounds stimulate enzymes that convert the cell to a noncancerous form.

Examples of disease-preventing and cancer-promotion-inhibiting phytonutrients are as follows:

- Some carotenoids, such as alpha- or beta-carotene, quercetin, lycopene, lutein and liminoids in citrus fruits, help to lead a precancerous cell to differentiate into a nonmalignant form, or actually cause it to age quickly and become inactivated.
- Vitamin E in vegetable oils, nuts and seeds; protease inhibitors in soybeans or soybean products; isothiocyanates from cruciferous vegetables; phenolic acids from whole grains; and isoflavones from legumes, peas and beans reduce the growth and inhibit the proliferation of initiated, precancerous cells in experimental laboratory work.
- Vitamin C, vitamin E, zinc, selenium, alpha lipoic acid, CoQ10, the amino acid N-acetyl-cysteine and carotenoids neutralize or scavenge and absorb corrosive free radicals before they damage tissues or cells. This scavenging or neutralizing activity inhibits tumor promotion by reducing the turnover of precancerous cells and preventing them from rapid cell division.
- Glutathione-rich herbal extracts, particularly European bilberry, ginkgo biloba, milk thistle, full-spectrum grape seed and skin, green tea and Siberian ginseng, are generally found in a high-quality "green drink."

HOW MUCH DO WE NEED?

Both the Canadian Food Guide and the U.S. Food Pyramid now recommend six or more servings of vegetables a day and two servings of fresh fruit daily as a minimum. (One serving is equal to a one-half cup.)

Only 9 percent of the Canadian and American populations consume the minimum recommended number of servings of fruits and vegetables each day, almost 50 percent eat no fruit on any given day and 25 percent eat no vegetables at all on a daily basis. As many as 60 percent of children state that the only vegetable they consume, on most days, is French fries. Clearly, we are not giving ourselves the "survival advantage" generously offered to us in fruits and vegetables.

The first study that awakened the public to the importance of fruits and vegetables was published in the *American Journal of Clinical Nutrition* (1985, 41(1), 32–36). This study of 1,271 Massachusetts residents showed that the increased intake of green and yellow vegetables reduced cancer by 70 percent, compared to the low-vegetable-intake group. A high vegetable intake is associated with a decreased risk of various human cancers. Phytonutrients, as health-promoting nutrients, accelerate the anabolic state—but we need to eat them daily in bioenergetic whole foods. It's that simple!

CREATING "THE WORLD'S BEST DIET"

Both the Canadian and United States governments recommend that we consume six servings of vegetables. To have "The World's Best Diet," I suggest that we eat 13 servings from bioenergetic colorful salads and vegetables daily.

Both governments suggest two servings of fruit daily. For "The World's Best Diet," I believe that we should eat four servings of ripe fruit, berries or melons daily.

Both governments suggest six to 10 servings each day of processed, high-density carbohydrates like boxed cereals, bread, rice and pasta. This is too many calories from high-density carbohydrates. We know that their recommendation causes soaring insulin levels, mood swings and weight gain. I suggest that we eat three servings from organic whole grain bread or pasta, legumes, raw seeds and unsalted nuts, which are natural, low-density carbohydrates.

My recommendations allow us to voluntarily reduce our calorie consumption by 42 percent—but eat more anabolic vegetables, fruits, herbs, lean protein, seeds, nuts and sea vegetables, full of necessary vitamins, fiber, minerals, antioxidants and phytonutrients.

COMPARISON OF FOOD PYRAMIDS

World's Best Diet Food Pyramid

Labels (top to bottom): Essential Fats; Whole Grains; Low-Fat Protein; Fruits; Vegetables, Herbs, Sea Vegetables

U.S. Government Food Pyramid

Labels: Sugar and Fat; Dairy; Protein; Vegetables; Fruits; Grains and Starches

The main difference in the two pyramids is that I place much more emphasis on a variety of vegetables, herbs, sea vegetables, salads, fruit, essential fats and lean protein. It should be obvious which of the two pyramids will lead to a longer, healthier, hormonally balanced life. (As of 2001, the U.S. government is reviewing new dietary guidelines to replace the outdated 1941 "Recommended Daily Dietary Allowance" of nutrients, recognizing that recommendations should strive for optimal, not minimal, requirements.)

I am not promoting a short-term program, but advocating a lifelong food management system of unprocessed foods.

A COMPARISON OF "THE WORLD'S BEST DIET" AND GOVERNMENT DIETARY SUGGESTIONS IN TERMS OF TOTAL CARBOHYDRATE CONSUMPTION		
	Servings	Grams of Carbohydrates
World's Best Diet Recommendations:		
Vegetables, herbs, sea vegetables	13	75
Ripe fruit, berries, melons	4	40
Whole grains, legumes, nuts, seeds	3	30
Total	20	145
Government Recommendations:		
Vegetables	6	30
Fruit	2	20
Grains, pasta, rice	10	200
Total	18	250

HIDDEN PHYTONUTRIENTS IN PLANT-DERIVED FOODS

Here are my 25 favorite phytonutrients that we should go out of our way to eat on a daily basis—and they are all outrageously delicious!

Phytonutrient	Food Source	Protection Given
1. Allicin and allylic sulfides	Garlic, onions, leeks, chives, shallots	– sulfur content is antibacterial, antifungal, antiviral – reduces the risk of stomach and colon cancer
2. Anthocyanidins and cis-resveratrol	Dark grapes, berries, especially blueberries, bilberries, ginger, grape seed and skin extracts, plums, tart cherries, unsweetened grape juice, dry red wines	– highly effective antioxidants protect DNA in cells from damage, especially in the brain – keep capillary walls flexible and elastic, thereby regulating blood vessel action – anti-inflammatory – stop cancer cell formation
3. Carotenoids (alpha- and beta-carotene, lycopene, lutein and zeaxanthin)	Spirulina, chlorella, wheatgrass, green and black tea, all berries, acerola berries, carrots, sweet potatoes, spinach, lettuce, all peppers, tomatoes, apricots, Swiss chard, sea vegetables	– enhance immune function – balance blood sugars – kill pathogens we breathe, eat or drink in our food chain – protect GI tract from cancer – lutein has been documented to prevent macular degeneration in the eyes

4. Ellagic acid	Grape seeds and skins, apples, berries, cherries, nuts, seeds, acerola berries	– inhibits cancer cell growth – detoxifies cellular toxins and carcinogens – important "booster" of main network antioxidants
5. Bioflavonoids and flavonoids (anthocyanidins)	All herbs, fruit, vegetables, squashes, licorice root	– block cancer enzyme pathways – control nitric oxide levels – quench the hydroxyl radical
6. Fiber	Apple fiber, Nova Scotia dulse, whole grains, legumes, nuts, seeds, veggies, fruit, whole brown rice	– absorbs excess bile and other cancer-causing substances – prevents the reuptake of estrogen to improve estrogen balance – reduces serum cholesterol – improves healthy colon bacteria – releases sugar from foods slowly to keep blood sugar balanced
7. Indoles, diindolylmethane (DIM)	Broccoli sprouts, broccoli, Brussels sprouts, kale, Swiss chard, cabbage, cauliflower, arugula, watercress	– produce many enzymes in cancer-fighting mechanisms – diindolylmethane (DIM) is astonishingly protective – inhibit PKC "growth signals" that stop cancer cells from growing
8. Isoflavonoids (genistein, daidzein and glycitein), glucosinolates	Soy sprouts, soy beans, soy protein isolates, miso, tempeh, tofu, bee pollen, green tea, stinging nettle	– deactivate excess estrogen or testosterone, greatly lowering the risk of hormone-like cancers of the breast, cervix, uterus and prostate
9. Lignans	Organic flax seeds, whole grains, high-lignan flax seed oil	– block excess estrogen to reduce breast cancer
10. Lycopenes	Tomatoes, red grapefruit, watermelon, apricots, saw palmetto (herb), pumpkins, spirulina, chlorella, pygeum africum (herb)	– reduce or block the risk of prostate cancer and cancers of the digestive tract – reduce benign prostate enlargement

11. Monoterpenes	All citrus (including the white pulp and rings of organic citrus), milk thistle	—help increase liver enzymes that detoxify carcinogenic substances
12. P-coumaric acid and chlorogenic acid	Blueberries, berries, pineapple, strawberries, all peppers, tomatoes	—they detoxify and eliminate nitrosamines that cause cancer from second-hand cigarette smoke
13. Phenolic compounds	Turmeric (curcumin), celery, parsley, dill, fennel, coriander, ginkgo biloba, milk thistle	—protect cells from invading chemical intruders and toxins
14. Polyphenols	Green tea, bilberry, Siberian ginseng, bee pollen	—kill plaque-causing bacteria in the mouth —lower digestive tract pathogens
15. Protease inhibitors	Soy sprouts, beans, seeds, nuts, potatoes, rice, eggplant, fermented soy products	—kill cancer cells —powerful antioxidants
16. Quercetin	Bee pollen, yellow and red onions, yellow squash, shallots, red grapes, sweet potatoes	—inhibits tumor-stimulating enzymes and blocks tumor formation
17. GI flora ("friendly bacteria")	Active-culture yogurt, fermented veggies, FOS (fructo-oligo-saccharides), dairy-free probiotic cultures with FOS	—enhance immunity —protect intestines from toxins, chemicals, yeast and fungus
18. Omega-3 fatty acids	Flax seed, flax seed oil, hemp seed, hemp seed oil, organic borage oil, cold water fish, salmon, cod liver oil, DHA- and EPA-rich oil capsules (molecularly distilled) spirulina, chlorella, wheatgrass, alfalfa grass	—anti-cancer —anti-tumor —reduce cholesterol —anti-depressant effect —anti-inflammatory
19. Sulforophane	Cruciferous veggies like broccoli and cauliflower, especially broccoli sprouts	—neutralizes carcinogens —boosts the production of phase 2 enzymes
20. Glycosamino-glycans	Whole grains, seeds, nuts, legumes	—selenium-rich to make glutathione peroxidaze enzyme, which promptly

		eliminates harmful toxins and damaged molecules from our body
21. Polysaccharides and alginates	Sea vegetables such as Nova Scotia dulse, spirulina, chlorella, nori, kombu, wakame, etc.	−protect against radiation −absorb toxic metals and xenobiotics at the cellular level and discard them from the body
22. Soy protein isolates	Non-GMO water-extracted soy protein	−reset the anabolic drive −protect the breast and prostate from cancer
23. Whey protein isolates	Alphapure™, whey protein isolates, regular whey protein. (Alphapure is not denatured.)	−produce glutathione, serotonin and melatonin for the most powerful immune-boosting support and liver support known −re-establish our anabolic drive −90 percent bioavailable protein
24. Glutathione	Whey protein isolates, avocado, asparagus, okra, tomatoes, watermelon, grapefruit, oranges, cantaloupe, strawberries and meats, especially wild game	−maintains immuno-competence −reduces chronic inflammation of tissues −quickly binds to mutagens or cancer-causing chemicals from the environment and escorts them out of the body
25. Phosphatidyl choline (PC), phosphatidyl serine (PS), glyceryl-phosphoryl choline (GPC)	Organic, non-GMO soy lecithin granules are the only superior source	− necessary for the anabolic maintenance of the brain −necessary for memory, learning and an upbeat mood −a major fat subtype that keeps nerve and brain cell membrane integrity intact, yet fluid and anti-aging −potent methyl donors that effectively reduce the homo-cysteine content in our blood to protect our arteries, veins and heart

Hippocrates, the Greek physician who is known as the father of medicine, advised us to "let food be our medicine." I like to say that we should "eat as if our life depends upon it." It does.

8

ANTIOXIDANTS: THE FREE RADICAL POLICE

The human body uses oxygen to liberate energy from some proteins, carbohydrates and fats. A byproduct of this process, called oxidation, is a molecule missing one electron—a free radical. This free radical is corrosive, short-lived and unstable. It is a lethal force because it steals electrons from other molecules (making them unstable), damaging proteins and cell membranes and causing a build-up of cellular debris. In short, it causes cellular dysfunction, disease and premature aging. A free radical accelerates the catabolic state.

THE DAMAGING EFFECTS OF DAY-TO-DAY LIVING

In today's environment, we face an overwhelming number of free-radical-generating stresses, such as environmental pollutants, radiation, pesticides, herbicides, food preservatives, excess exposure to the sun, physical overexertion, illness, cigarette smoke, oxidized fats in foods, medications, alcohol, drugs, automobile exhaust, jet travel, late nights, barbecue smoke, paint fumes, carpet fumes, fluorescent lighting, fumes from toxic garbage dump sites and sulfur dioxide from far-off industrial fumes carried by the wind. On top of this, dust, dirt, parasites, bacteria, viruses, yeast, stale air in our homes or workplaces, fungicides and herbicides on foods, mercury in our dental fillings, PCBs, aluminum in cookware, antibiotic residues and various veterinary compounds (found in animal meats like poultry, turkey, red meat, farm-raised fish and dairy products) create a barrage of free radicals. Just think, more than 100,000 industrial chemicals (called xenobiotics) are used today and about 1,000 new chemicals are introduced worldwide each year.

Combine all this with the emotional stress we endure daily, and it is no wonder many researchers and health professionals feel we are facing "a free radical storm."

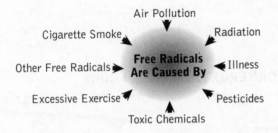

Air Pollution

Cigarette Smoke   Radiation

Other Free Radicals   **Free Radicals Are Caused By**   Illness

Excessive Exercise   Pesticides

Toxic Chemicals

Highly corrosive free radicals have an unpaired electron that initiates destructive chain reactions causing damage to cells.

The physical and mental deterioration typically associated with aging isn't necessarily a condition of human maturity, but of excess free radicals.

Stable molecules have electrons that are in pairs.

Dietary antioxidants help:

- maximize life span;
- prevent cell damage;
- slow the aging process;
- speed wound healing;
- prevent arthritis;
- protect against heart disease;
- prevent cancer;
- eliminate allergies;
- prevent mental deterioration;
- decrease endogenous free radical reactions.

Without antioxidants we would perish within hours, because of free radical destruction. Antioxidants are molecules that contain several easily removable electrons. Without destroying itself, the antioxidant is able to donate an electron to a free radical, thereby neutralizing its violent potential and rendering it harmless.

Antioxidant

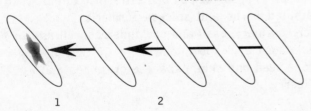

1   2   3

1. The highly corrosive free radical has one electron.
2. The antioxidant donates one electron to the free radical.
3. The free radical is now stable.

102 THE POWER OF FOOD

Without support against these free radicals or "oxidants"—"anti"-oxidant support—cells become severely damaged and can no longer function or reproduce properly. This can lead to every disease imaginable and accelerated aging.

FIGHTING BACK WITH BIOENERGETIC WHOLE FOODS

Antioxidants stabilize free radicals by giving them an electron to replace the one that was lost during oxidation.

In addition to those antioxidants our body produces on its own, nature has provided us with tens of thousands of antioxidants in the form of phytonutrients, which are found in bioenergetic whole foods.

When our daily menu is rich in bioenergetic whole foods, we have a constant source of protection. Happily, colorful vegetables and fruits supply antioxidants that not only protect our delicate cell walls from corrosion, but they tirelessly patrol our bloodstream, stepping in and out of the cells of all our organs, acting as toxic garbage cops. Your cells know what to do with every antioxidant. You only have to supply adequate amounts of them in your food choices.

My Favorite Anabolic Antioxidant Membrane Protectors

1. Colorful berries such as blueberries and strawberries. (Please note that strawberries are excessively sprayed with pesticides, so eat only organically grown strawberries.)
3. Non-GMO, organic soy lecithin granules full of phosphatidyl choline (PC) and phosphatidyl serine (PS).
4. Watercress and parsley.
5. Ninety-nine percent biologically active, undenatured whey protein isolates with sub-fractions.
6. Black cherries, sour cherries or unsweetened black cherry or sour cherry juice in moderation (4 oz or 125 mL serving size).
7. Organically grown and non-GMO soy sprouts and beans, and fermented soy as miso, tempeh and extra-firm tofu.
8. All non-irradiated herbs and spices—turmeric, black pepper, ginger, rosemary, basil and coriander, as well as herbal extracts such a ginkgo biloba, milk thistle, full-spectrum grape seed and skin, Japanese green tea and European bilberry.
9. Bee pollen.
10. Apricots, dark plums, prunes, red and purple grapes or any unsweetened fruit juices in moderation (4 oz or 125 mL serving size).
11. Carrots, tomatoes and red beets.

12. Yams, sweet potatoes and squashes.
13. All whole, organic, non-salted, raw seeds, nuts, legumes, whole grains and peas.

Membrane Protection

You can use the phytonutrients in bioenergetic whole foods to control the most fundamental aspects of your body's basic chemistry, the integrity of every one of your 100 trillion cell walls. Each cell contains fragile strands of deoxyribonucleic acid—that is, DNA—the genetic message system that directs all of our body's biochemical activities. One small nick in our DNA can destroy a cell. Or it can make a cell lose control and begin multiplying unusually, causing cancer.

Cell membranes are what give our body tissue its shape and hold everything together. A cell without a healthy membrane is like a ripe blueberry without its skin; it is fragile and decays quickly. If free radicals damage even a single molecule in a cell membrane, they can set off a chain reaction that, if not stopped, will destroy the cell and eventually all of your 100 trillion cells. Bioenergetic whole foods contain phytonutrients and antioxidants that get into the cell membrane and protect it from attack and degradation by corrosive free radicals.

Phytonutrient Bloodstream Protectors

Phytonutrients, a potent class of antioxidants, are powerful toxic garbage cops that roam our bloodstream tirelessly. They are powerful enough to eliminate thousands of different chemicals should they ever find their way into our bloodstream, and they even eliminate toxins before they can harm us.

Phytonutrients in our bloodstream are on constant patrol looking out for bacteria, viruses, parasites, fungi, toxins, cellular debris, pollutants and industrial chemicals—eliminating these toxic accumulated chemicals before you even know they are there. They remove the soot and grime from the innermost part of our body and bring them to the liver, colon and skin surface for elimination.

According to the book *Enzymes: The Fountain of Life*, written by Dr. Michael Williams, a professor of medicine at Northwestern University Medical School, we all have from 100 to 100,000 tumor cells floating around in our body at all times. If we consume a wide variety of colorful phytonutrients daily, they easily destroy each tumor cell by actively seeking them out, confronting them, dismantling and eliminating them before they can injure our 100 trillion cells and delicate tissues.

Phytonutrients Regulate Hormones

The third known way that phytonutrients ward off disease is by regulating hormones—most notably the female sex hormone, estrogen. They balance the amount of estrogens in the female body. When estrogen is produced at normal levels, it controls everything in a female body from menstruation to childbirth to aging normally.

When estrogen levels rise, they can stimulate hormone-related cancers like those of the breast and ovaries, says Dr. Leon Bradlow, Ph.D., director of biochemical and endocrinology at the Strang Cancer Research Laboratory in New York City.

One group of bioenergetic phytonutrients called isoflavones are very similar to natural estrogen and are called phytoestrogens. When women eat organic, non-GMO soy sprouts, soybeans, fermented soy products (such as miso, tempeh and extra-firm tofu) or water-extracted soy protein isolate powder, they are receiving the phytoestrogens genistein and daidzein. These phytoestrogens bind to the body's estrogen receptor sites. In PMS, where there is too much estrogen, these weak phytoestrogens block the escalation of the real estrogen hormones. In perimenopause or in menopause, where there is not enough estrogen being produced, these plant-derived phytoestrogens increase the beneficial estrogen 2-hydroxyestrone and decrease the levels of the dangerous 16-alpha-hydroxyestrone hormone, which is associated with breast cancer.

I strongly suggest that all women from the ages of 14 to 120 years of age get some of these critical phytoestrogens on a daily basis, without the indigestion of heated soy products. Non-GMO, certified organic soy sprouts are an excellent source.

THE ANTIOXIDANT NETWORK: A SUM GREATER THAN ITS PARTS

Phytonutrients found in whole foods act as powerful antioxidants in the body—not singly, but as a network. Though each phytonutrient has its specific protective action, its effectiveness is enhanced when it functions as part of a network. Phytonutrients synergize with each other, and even more importantly, recycle each other. As we discussed, when an antioxidant donates an electron to disarm a free radical, it becomes a free radical itself. Fortunately, if other antioxidants are present, the original electron donor can be "regenerated" or restored to its original antioxidant status.

"What makes network antioxidants so special is that they can greatly enhance the power of one another," states Lester Packer, Ph.D., director of Packer Lab at the University of California, Berkley, and co-author with Carol Colman of the book, *The Antioxidant Miracle.*

It is not single antioxidants in whole foods but the entire network that produces the manifold effects of preventing or reversing disease. It is the antioxidant network in whole foods that has the far-reaching consequences of reversing the catabolic drive and reinstating your regenerative anabolic drive. Forget the idea of a single antioxidant; it takes the whole network to effectively neutralize the lethal forces of free radicals and to efficiently "recycle" and keep each antioxidant in the network active.

An excellent example is lycopene, which is found abundantly in tomatoes and tomato-based products and credited with preventing prostate, lung and stomach cancer. But it isn't alone. According to a report by Dr. Edward Giovannucci of the Brigham and Women's Hospital and Harvard Medical School, in the *Journal of the National Cancer Institute* (Feb. 17, 1999), "Numerous other potentially beneficial compounds are present in tomatoes, and conceivably a complex interaction among multiple components may contribute to the anti-cancer properties of tomatoes." So in spite of the fact that antioxidants such as lycopene are available in supplement form, it is still best to eat the whole food version.

My Favorite Phytonutrient Bloodstream Protectors

1. Garlic, onions, scallions, shallots and chives.
2. The glutathione-flavonoid sub-network of the herbal extracts of European bilberry, ginkgo biloba, milk thistle, full-spectrum grape seed and skin, green tea and Siberian ginseng.
3. Organic green tea.
4. Flax, perilla or hemp seeds (or their fresh oils); organic borage oil; EPA- and DHA-rich fish oils or algae oils.
5. Sea algae such as spirulina and chlorella.
6. Alfalfa, barley and wheat grasses (freshly juiced or dry powders).
7. Broccoli sprouts, broccoli, cauliflower, Brussels sprouts and cabbage.
8. Kale, Swiss chard, spinach, dandelions and asparagus.
9. Extra-virgin, cold-pressed organic olive oil.
10. Green, red, yellow and orange peppers, and red beets.
11. Apples, grapes, prunes, watermelon and other fresh melons.
12. Sea vegetables (Nova Scotia dulse, wakame, kombu, nori, hijiki and arame).
13. Pink grapefruit, lemons, oranges, tangerines and limes (pulp and rind).
14. Organically grown and non-GMO soy sprouts and beans, and fermented soy such as miso, tempeh and extra-firm tofu.

Mixed Carotenoids as Network Antioxidants

Carotenoids constitute their own network, working synergistically with one another. They are the substance that gives fruits, vegetables, herbs and plants their orange, yellow and red colors. Green leafy vegetables are also high in carotenoids, but the color is masked by chlorophyll. Over 600 carotenoids have been identified to date.

Beta-carotene is one that has received a lot of attention. Beta-carotene converts to vitamin A in our body and is a powerful antioxidant that strengthens the immune system; maintains healthy epithelial tissues, such as skin, mucous membranes, urinary tract, and the lungs; aids in bone and tooth formation; and maintains normal vision. Alpha-carotene is another—but one that may be ten times more powerful than beta-carotene in protecting our body from skin, eye, liver and lung damage or cancer. Alpha-carotene protects us from skin cancer related to sun exposure because it quenches or neutralizes the very reactive free radical at the skin's cellular level before the sun can cause any damage. It acts as the skin's own internal "suntan lotion" and it appears to defend the skin from promotion or the initiation of melanomas on the skin.

Good sources of alpha-carotene are carrots, pumpkins, chlorella, squashes, spirulina, wheatgrass, and red, orange and yellow peppers.

Another carotenoid is lycopene, the red carotenoid found in tomatoes and berries that in addition to protecting the prostate, lungs and stomach as already mentioned, also protects the breast, pancreas, colon, rectum, esophagus and cervix from cancer.

Other types of carotenoids such as lutein and zeaxanthin, which are found in apricots, spirulina, yams, squashes, red beets, Swiss chard, chlorella, carrots, edible flowers, wheatgrass, spinach, kale and bee pollen, protect our eyes from cataracts and age-related retinal problems.

In addition to their antioxidant properties, carotenoids reduce cancer risk early on by their ability to enhance communication between premalignant cells and normal cells. The presence of carotenoids allows normal cells to send growth-regulating signals to premalignant cells. They also inhibit enzyme-generated "growth signals" that stop cancer cells from growing. It may be that carotenoids, once consumed in a colorful whole food, develop their potent metabolites such as apo-carotenoids and retinoids, which are the active carotenoid molecules that synergize as a network.

To optimize the networking of carotenoids, we should eat lots of fresh berries, such as blueberries, acerola berries, blackberries, strawberries and raspberries. Berries, and blueberries in particular, top the list of all fruits and vegetables for antioxidant power, and are the most potent dietary preventers of cancer, heart disease and neurodegenerative diseases.

Flavonoids as Network Antioxidants

Flavonoids are considered important boosters of the main network of antioxidants. They are extremely powerful antioxidants in their own right. Some are capable of quenching the hydroxyl radical, the most dangerous of the free radicals, capable of directly damaging DNA. Mixed carotenoids and flavonoids are nature's main network antioxidants.

Flavonoids' "boosting" role certainly deserves attention. Proanthocyanidins and anthocyanidins from full-spectrum grape seed and skin extract, as well as European bilberry extract, significantly boost or regenerate levels of vitamin C, vitamin E and glutathione.

One of the most important functions of flavonoids is their ability to control the levels of nitric oxide, which is extremely harmful when in excess. It accelerates aging and promotes a quick catabolic dive.

There are very good reasons to think that a high daily dose of flavonoids—from organic alfalfa, barley and wheatgrass (luteolin and apigenin), berries (carotenoids), apples (apigenin), onions (quercetin), tomatoes (lycopene), green tea (polyphenols), grape seed and skin extract or dry red wine (proanthocyanidins), miso (genistein), garlic (sulfides), organic 70 percent cocoa (chocolate in moderation), one cup daily of organic black coffee; and from water-extracted herbal extracts of bilberry, ginkgo biloba, milk thistle, full-spectrum grape seed and skin extracts and Siberian ginseng—might give us lifelong freedom from heart disease, cancer, cataracts and the nightmarish neurodegenerative diseases such as Alzheimer's and Parkinson's diseases.

Since the supplement industry has given us a C-complex and a B-complex, we should soon also have E-complex, and even a flavonoid complex. Once supplement manufacturers understand the networking concept, it will only be a matter of time. The world's first "network" antioxidant, protect+, and the world's first "network" anti-glycated end product, A•G•E. inhibitors™ are now available.

Apigenin: A Potent Flavonoid: Apigenin is a flavonoid found in parsley, onions, apples, basil, tea, peas, alfalfa grass, barley grass, wheatgrass, feverfew, grapefruits and oranges.

Based on a study of 21 different flavonoids to determine their effect on the growth of human breast cancer cells, apigenin was shown to be the most effective anti-proliferative. A related study, reported in *Endocrinology* (October 1998), demonstrated that flavonoids such as apigenin bind to estrogen receptor sites on cell membranes in order to prevent over-proliferation of these cells in response to excess estrogen, a potential initiator of breast cancer.

Furthermore, a study conducted by Dr. M. Richter, Ph.D., on colorectal cancer cell lines, reported in *Nutrition and Cancer* (Vol. 34, 1999), demonstrated that apigenin and quercitin (a flavonoid found in onions and full-spectrum grape seed and skin extract) were shown to interfere with epidermal growth factor cell stimulation. The researchers speculate that these flavonoids are the primary components in fruits and vegetables that reduce the risk of colorectal cancer by interfering with the cancer cell growth factor signaling pathway. The epidermal growth factor signal transduction pathway is an essential component of both cancer cell growth and differentiation.

In a study on human promyelocytic leukemia cells, apigenin, as well as the flavonoids genistein and daidzein (from soy products), was the most potent inhibitor of toxic free radical byproducts generated by these leukemia cells. The scientists, led by Dr. D. Giles, Ph.D., stated that the antioxidant effects of these flavonoids protect against human cancers.

Luteolin: Another Disease-Preventing Flavonoid: Luteolin is found in many of the same foods that contain apigenin, especially alfalfa, barley, wheatgrass and citrus fruits. It produces effects similar to apigenin, but has its own unique beneficial properties as well.

Several studies show that luteolin reduces excess estrogen formation by suppressing the aromatase enzyme and blocking estrogens from breast cell receptor sites. This suggests that luteolin may help prevent breast cancer.

Do Flavonoids Protect Us from Cancer?

How important are flavonoids in protecting us against cancer? Cancer researchers in Spain, Drs. Garcia and Closas, Ph.D.s, who conducted a human epidemiological study showed a 56 percent reduction in stomach cancer among those individuals who consumed the highest levels of flavonoids. The results of this study seem to indicate that the well-established protective effects of fruit and vegetables could, in part, be due to the presence of flavonoids.

Optimizing the Network

When we eat a wide variety of organic, colorful bioenergetic whole foods such as vegetables, fruits, herbs, grains, sea vegetables, nuts, seeds, grasses, bee pollen, legumes and salads, we provide our bodies with a whole range of antioxidants. This ensures that the complex interaction between them can take place and that those damaged in the line of duty can be quickly and efficiently regenerated and restored.

Boosting Network Antioxidants

If you use supplemental antioxidants such as alpha lipoic acid, non-acidic vitamin C as an ascorbate mixed with bioflavonoids, N-acetyl cysteine, vitamin D-3, mixed tocopherol vitamin E, mixed carotenoids (alpha- and beta-carotene, lutein, etc.), CoQ10 with tocotrienols (which are similar to tocopherols in vitamin E except they are more mobile than vitamin E and distribute themselves more evenly throughout membranes, as tocopherols tend to cluster), and 99 percent biologically active whey protein isolate, they should all be consumed together with 1/2 tablespoon of "high-lignan" organic flax seed oil and 1/2 teaspoon of organic borage oil. You are now "boosting" the levels of all the other network antioxidants and together they are much more effective (synergistic) than taken separately. Take your antioxidant supplements, fish oil capsules and borage oil with a protein shake each morning.

Furthermore, there exists an extremely potent glutathione-flavonoid sub-network found in quality water-extracted herbal extracts that increase glutathione levels in your cells, tissues and liver. They include full-spectrum grape skin and seed extract, Siberian ginseng extract, European bilberry extract, milk thistle extract, green tea extract and ginkgo biloba extract. Use these six concentrated, water-extracted, standardized herbal extracts daily to broaden your antioxidant network from whole foods and organic medicinal herbs.

High-quality "green drinks" are your most convenient way to consume this extremely protective glutathione-flavonoid sub-network of water-extracted, herbal extracts.

Dr. Lester Packer, with a group of researchers at Berkeley and another group at Yale, used alpha lipoic acid and vitamin E succinate in combination with vitamin D-3 (cholecalciferol) to make leukemia cells differentiate (become normal cells as opposed to cancer cells). For the first time, they showed that lipoic acid activates an enzyme called capase, which kills leukemia cells. They also showed that lipoic acid suppresses the "cancer gene" c-fos. Vitamin E and alpha lipoic acid both require the natural form of vitamin D, which is vitamin D-3, not the synthetic version, which is vitamin D-2 (ergocalciferol), to initiate and support these positive effects. Researchers at the University of Toronto published research results in the February 2001 edition of the *American Journal of Clinical Nutrition* (vol. 73) that 62 percent of North Americans are deficient in vitamin D. They suggest supplementing with 4000 IU per day of vitamin D-3. However, during sunny months unprotected sun exposure in the early morning or late afternoon is by far the best way of getting your vitamin D.

Vegetables and fruits provide the ideal mixtures of phytonutrients and antioxidants that work together in a network fashion, synergistically enhancing one another.

To maintain high blood plasma levels of phytonutrients, regular intake of phytonutrients should be part of each of your three meals and two snacks every day. Blood levels of phytonutrients reflect dietary intake over the last 48 hours. It does not appear that the body has any long-term phytonutrient storage mechanisms.

When you eat a wide variety of organic, colorful whole foods such as vegetables, fruits, herbs, grains, sea vegetables, nuts, seeds, grasses, bee pollen, legumes and salads, you ensure optimal recycling of key antioxidants by continually consuming a whole range (network) of crucial antioxidants in your delicious food choices.

GLUTATHIONE: A POWERHOUSE OF PROTECTION

There are a myriad of chemical reactions within our body that require catalysts to bring them about. One such catalyst is the enzyme. There are thousands of kinds of enzymes and each one makes a particular chemical reaction possible. Certain enzymes, for example, make digestion possible. Others cause the biochemical interactions that allow us to see, hear or fight invading toxins. Some enzymes initiate the release of the special Omega-3 fatty acids in our system, while others help to synthesize hormones such as melatonin, serotonin, dopamine and cortisol.

Likewise, enzymes tackle toxins in the form of bacteria, viruses, parasites, fungi and carcinogens that have been escorted to our liver to be eliminated from our system before they cause serious injury to our cells. A Phase I enzyme is secreted, which binds an oxygen molecule to the toxin. This is good, but remember that oxygen is unstable and can cause free radical production. The toxin and oxygen combination can become even more active than the actual toxin was when it entered the body. It is critically important that our body quickly adds a Phase II enzyme to the toxin-oxygen combination as this stabilizes the oxygen and prevents it from becoming a corrosive free radical.

According to Dr. Paul Talalay of Johns Hopkins University, "The vast majority of cancer-causing chemicals are not carcinogenic in and of themselves. But when they enter cells and are acted on by Phase 1 enzymes, these relatively innocuous substances are converted to highly-reactive compounds that can damage our DNA, setting in motion the process that leads to cancer."

However, if the liver is healthy, as soon as a Phase I enzyme attaches an oxygen molecule onto the toxin, a Phase II enzyme is immediately attached to the toxin also, thus neutralizing the oxygen and hooking the toxin onto a carrier molecule, which carries it out of the cell and eliminates it from our system. If the level of Phase II enzymes is high, reactive toxic chemicals are intercepted and a carrier molecule transports them out of the cell before they do any damage. The most important carrier molecule that destroys and eliminates toxins is glutathione.

Enzymes benefit from inducers found in phytonutrients that cause the body to make an abundance of Phase II enzymes. For instance, broccoli and broccoli sprouts contain the phytonutrient sulforaphane, which is "an exceedingly potent booster of Phase II enzymes," says Dr. Talalay. Phytonutrients such as sulforaphane cause the release of a key protein known as Nrf2, which then switches "on" the production of a dozen or more toxin-busting enzymes, according to Dr. Thomas Kensler, an environmental toxicologist, writing in the March 2001 edition of the Proceedings of the National Academy of Sciences.

Another phytonutrient called thiols (organic sulfur derivatives also known as mercaptans) was studied by two of the world's foremost antioxidant researchers, Dr. Lester Packer and Dr. Chandan K. Sen of the Ohio State Medical Center, the results of which were released in early 2000. Thiol homeostasis has numerous roles in biological systems, including a role in coordinating antioxidant defenses. Two thiols, N-Acetyl-Cysteine (NAC) and alpha lipoic acid, have both been found highly effective in enhancing the regeneration and activity of glutathione, especially during oxidative stress such as exhaustion, fighting an illness or a flu or during oxidative stress induced by intense exercise.

(**a**) Toxin enters your bloodstream and is taken to the liver.

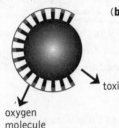

(**b**) The toxin is acted on by Phase I enzymes and has an oxygen molecule attached to it.

toxin

oxygen
molecule

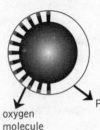

(**c**) If the diet is high in phytonutrients, then Phase II enzymes are activated by Nrf2 proteins that neutralize the oxygen, attaching the toxin to a large carrier molecule like glutathione, which carries it out of the cell and eliminates it from the body.

Phase II enzyme

oxygen
molecule

Glutathione is the most important antioxidant inside the cell. Among its many functions, it primes DNA synthesis for cell division and switches on the enzymes that repair DNA. These enzymes literally travel up and down the DNA strands fixing damage done to DNA by free radicals or invading toxins. Glutathione also regulates the genes involved in producing chronic inflammation that can lead to arthritis, autoimmune diseases and cancer. Glutathione helps to control the levels of steroid hormones and prostaglandins by sulfating them in the liver, thus making them water-soluble for easier excretion. It also stimulates the production of interleukin 1 and interleukin 2 and increases the proliferation of lymphocytes, important components of our immune system.

Glutathione may also be one of the most important keys to healthy longevity. People with the lowest glutathione levels have the highest premature mortality levels. Those individuals who have lived to 100 years of age have been repeatedly found to have higher levels of glutathione than would be expected for their age.

Increasing Our Glutathione Intake

We can easily boost our intake of glutathione. Of course, consuming it as part of naturally occurring antioxidant networks in bioenergetic whole foods is important to maximizing its potential.

All berries, oranges, grapefruits, cantaloupe, watermelon, bananas, apples, peaches, pears, avocados and tangerines are loaded with glutathione. Vegetables such as carrots, yams, lettuce and other leafy greens, cucumbers, tomatoes, asparagus, okra, cabbage and green peppers, and nuts such as walnuts, peanuts, almonds and sesame seeds, are also good sources. Special undenatured whey protein isolate powder will also significantly raise glutathione levels in our cells, tissues and liver.

A combination of herbal extracts from ginkgo biloba, European bilberry, milk thistle, full-spectrum grape seed and grape skin extract, Japanese green tea and Siberian ginseng consumed together can also elevate glutathione levels.

Supplementing to Raise Glutathione Levels

Athletes who need to maintain their immune functions at optimum in spite of the high oxidative stress of rigorous training will benefit from maintaining high levels of glutathione and of a vitamin E-complex especially high in gamma tocopherols.

Likewise, sufferers of oxidative stress such as cancer, atherosclerosis and AIDS will require glutathione. Any serious infection or illness depletes the level of glutathione in plasma, as well as in cells and tissues. The faster glutathione levels are restored, the better.

Be careful if you are orally taking more than 500 mg of a single glutathione precursor like N-acetyl-cysteine (NAC). The volatile sulfur in NAC can oxidize quickly and become toxic.

Cysteine's potential toxicity can be easily avoided by simultaneously using other network antioxidants with it, such as 100 mg of alpha lipoic acid, 50 mg of selenium, 1,000 mg of non-acid vitamin C-complex as ascorbates combined with bioflavonoids, and 400 IU of a vitamin E-complex high in gamma tocopherol. If you take more than 100 mg of alpha lipoic acid a day, take 100 mcg of biotin for each 100 mg of alpha lipoic acid. Your biotin is best taken in a vitamin B-complex.

If you are in chemotherapy or radiation therapy, it is imperative that you check with your oncologist before taking glutathione precursors or reduced L-glutathione itself. Since glutathione is so protective against toxic substances, such as those used in chemotherapy, as well as against the effects of radiation therapy, it may, according to the thinking of most oncologists, cancel out the effect of the chemotherapy or radiation therapy.

Clinical experience seems to indicate that network antioxidant supplementation, including glutathione, in concert with a daily protein power shake of undenatured whey protein isolates, will make it possible for patients to tolerate higher doses of chemotherapy by reducing their nasty side effects. Look for an oncologist who is open-minded and flexible to review this information.

In the case of radiation therapy, it is a clinically well-known fact that cancer cells have higher glutathione levels than normal cells and are much more protected from radiation than normal tissues. Glutathione precursors or L-glutathione supplementation will therefore protect healthy, normal cells from radiation therapy.

For a list of North American physicians who are open and flexible, consult the *Directory of Innovative Doctors*, which is available by calling the Life Extension Foundation at 1-800-841-5433.

While you read this book, sulfur dioxide from far-off industries, ozone, auto exhaust, gases from synthetic paint or carpets in your home and fumes from ordinary household detergents and cleaners are right now combining with dust, dirt, microbes, background radiation and oxidative stress, and are literally attacking you. You may not notice them, but they have isolated you. Lester Packer, Ph.D., says that most people do not inherit "cancer genes"; rather, they have a genetic weakness in their detoxification system. Glutathione is an extremely important part of the detoxification system, and thus of your defenses against cancer and degenerative diseases in general. He calls it the "ultimate antioxidant."

Supplementing With Smart "Network"Antioxidants

Phytonutrients found in bioenergetic whole foods act as powerful antioxidants—not singularly, but as a network. Each vitamin or phytonutrient has a specific protective action, but its effectiveness is enhanced when it functions as part of a network. Phytonutrients and vitamins synergize with each other, and, more importantly, recycle each other. They greatly enhance, boost and regenerate the active power of each other.

Researcher Brad J. King, M.S. MFS, has formulated the most comprehensive "network of protection" in a remarkable network antioxidant formula called protect+. I personally use it and highly recommend that you use four capsules a day—one at each meal and one before sleep. The protect+ capsules contain:

1. Beta-carotene (pro-vitamin A)
2. Vitamin C (calcium ascorbate)
3. Vitamin E (d-alpha-tocopheryl succinate plus beta, delta and gamma tocopherols)
4. Selenium (HVP chelate)
5. N-acetyl cysteine (NAC)
6. Full spectrum grape extract
7. Alpha lipoic acid
8. CoQ10
9. Citrus bioflavonoids
10. Lycopene
11. European bilberry

Part IV

MAKING THE CONNECTION: A RETURN TO WELL-BEING

9

FACING THE FACTS: ASSESSING YOUR HEALTH

OUR AGE FACTOR

Our chronological age is the age based on our birth certificate or driver's licence. But this doesn't really represent how old we are—that is, to what extent our body has actually aged. At 40 years of age, one person runs a marathon race while another is on the couch, overweight, exhausted, eating processed "foods" and watching the race.

Biological age is a concept developed by researchers to quantify how an individual compares biologically with the "average" of his or her chronological age. It is important because, essentially, it is the only measurement that counts.

There is a correlation between chronological age and biological age—but they are pretty much irrelevant to researchers. Every person has a unique biological rate of aging. How many times have you guessed a person's age only to be surprised that they are much younger or older than your guess? Our biological age is determined 15 to 20 percent by the genes we inherited and 80 to 85 percent by our lifestyle—what we eat, how we exercise, our total stress factor and our disposition to life. Our biological age can be altered quickly—decreased with anabolic good habits and increased with catabolic poor habits.

To keep our biological age low we need to:
- eat bioenergetic whole foods;
- balance the pH in our body so we are more alkaline and less acidic;
- remove excess and corrosive free radicals and keep them from damaging our sensitive cells and the energy factory within them, our mitochondria;
- reduce insulin levels;
- reduce blood glucose levels;
- reduce stress and cortisol levels; and
- get 8.25 to 8.5 hours of sleep in a dark environment each night.

I have designed a questionnaire for you to answer to help you determine your biological age, regardless of your chronological age. This will tell you if you are accelerating the aging process or slowing it down. Answer each question as honestly and accurately as possible.

DIETARY LEVEL

1. Do you eat three meals and two snacks every day?

never	once a week	twice a week	every day
3	2	1	0

2. How many servings of vegetables or salad do you consume daily? (1 serving = ¼ cup)

none	one per day	two per day	three to four per day	five or more
5	4	1	0	−1

3. How often do you consume fish oil supplements, algae oil supplements, flax seeds or oil, hemp seeds or oil, or eat salmon, tuna, sardines or mackerel?

never	once a month	once a week	daily	twice a day
3	2	1	0	−1

4. How many servings of fruit do you eat daily? (1 serving = ½ cup)

none	1 per day	2 per day	2+ per day, and 1 is a serving of berries
3	1	0	−1

5. How many glasses of water do you drink a day?

none	1 per day	3 per day	8 per day	10+ per day
4	2	1	0	−1

6. How often do you consume sea vegetables, culinary herbs or herbal teas?

never	once a week	twice a week	daily
3	2	1	−1

7. How often do you eat barbecued or fried foods?

daily	a few times a week	a few times a month	never
3	2	1	−1

8. How often do you consume processed foods with white flour, sugar, artificial sweetener; soft drinks; fast foods?

2+ times a day	once a day	once a week	never
3	2	1	−1

9. How often do you add table salt to your food?

on all foods	once a day	a few times a week	never
3	2	1	−1

10. How many alcoholic beverages do you drink?

daily	4 per week	2 per week	occasionally	avoid
4	3	2	1	−1

ACTIVITY LEVEL

11. How often do you exercise for 30 minutes or more?

never	once a week	3 times a week	5+ times a week
3	2	1	−1

12. How often do you do 30 minutes of aerobics plus 15 to 30 minutes of weight-bearing exercises?

never	sometimes	2–3 days a week	4 days a week
3	2	0	−1

13. Do you get 8.5 hours of sleep a night?

never	sometimes	once a week	nightly
3	2	1	−1

14. Do you sleep deeply all night and awake rested?

never	sometimes	once a week	nightly
3	2	1	−1

15. Do you have large, easily eliminated bowel movements?

never	once a week	3 times a week	daily	2+ times daily
4	3	2	0	−1

16. Do you experience constipation?

daily	once a week	once a month	never
3	2	1	−1

SUPPLEMENTATION

17. Do you take a multivitamin-multimineral supplement?

never	once a week	several times a week	daily
2	1	0	−1

18. Do you take any extra antioxidants such as selenium, vitamin C, CoQ10 or grape extract?

never	once a week	several times a week	daily
2	1	0	−1

19. Do you use any herbal supplements?

never	once a week	several times a week	daily
2	1	0	−1

20. Do you use a "green drink"?

never	once a week	several times a week	daily
2	1	0	−1 .

21. Do you use whey or soy protein isolate powders?

never	once a week	several times a week	daily
2	1	0	−1

STRESS LEVEL

22. At home, driving in traffic or at work do you experience anxiety or stress?

all day	a few times a day	a few times a week	almost none
3	2	1	−1

23. Do you smoke or are you exposed to second-hand smoke?

all day	a few times a day	a few times a week	almost never
3	2	1	−1

24. Do you use recreational drugs for a "high"?

daily	once a week	once a month	never
3	2	1	0

25. Do you get angry, moody or confrontational?

daily	once a week	once a month	almost never
3	2	1	0

26. Do you get fearful or depressed?

daily	once a week	once a month	almost never
3	2	1	0

MEDICAL LEVEL

27. How many individuals in your immediate family have or have had cancer, diabetes, depression, obesity, heart condition, high cholesterol or high blood pressure?

3 or more	2 or more	1	none
2	1	0	−1

28. How many of the ailments described in question #27 have you had?

3 or more	2 or more	1	none
3	2	1	−1

29. Do you experience headaches, upset stomach, blurry vision, hearing difficulty, gall bladder attacks, colds, flus, yeast infections, bladder infections, viral infections or bacterial infections?

2+ times a month	once a month	2+ times a year	almost never
3	2	1	−1

30. Have you ever been exposed to heavy metals in mercury dental fillings or from pesticides, herbicides, sprays, commercial household cleaners or lawn sprays?

daily	weekly	monthly	almost never
3	2	1	0

Calculating Your Biological Age Factor

Add your scores up from each section to calculate your biological age factor:

Dietary Level: _____

Activity Level: _____

Supplement Level: _____

Stress Level: _____

Medical Level: _____

Biological Age Factor: _____

Interpreting Your Score

This is an overall index or screen of where you are on the aging scale. If you want to know your biological age, add this factor to your chronological age. More sophisticated and specific tests can be done by your medical specialist.

1. Biological Age Factor of 25 or More

If your Biological Age Factor is 25 or more, you are at very high risk of developing serious degenerative diseases. You are on a rapidly declining catabolic free-fall caused by an accelerated-aging lifestyle. Your level of emotional and psychological stress is sapping your energy levels, and this is exacerbated by a combination of poor diet and sedentary lifestyle. You are on the verge of a life-threatening disease.

Act immediately with the effective anti-aging regimen recommended in this book.

2. Biological Age Factor of 15 to 25

If your Biological Age Factor is between 15 to 25, you have silently deteriorating biological and hormonal systems that are triggering brain cell degeneration. Change your lifestyle before you undergo a more profound catabolic declining spiral. Diet and exercise need to have structure and discipline. Carefully review your strategies for diet, exercise, sleep and stress management. Avoid processed "foods."

You still have time for intervention into your advanced aging and dysfunctional hormonal harmony before these habits become more entrenched, making it difficult to modify later. Avoid alcohol, smoking and recreational or street drugs. Please be wise, this is your "last chance." Follow the recommendations outlined in this book diligently—you will never regret it.

3. Biological Age Factor of 5 to 15

If your Biological Age Factor is between 5 and 15, your lifestyle choices need some modification as they heighten the risk of serious health problems. Chances are you will get worse without immediate intervention. You are forcing yourself into an early, dreadful midlife crisis, and you are prone to gaining weight. As growth hormone (GH) levels drop: skin begins to sag, muscle mass is harder to maintain, eyesight worsens, hair thins and vitality diminishes. There is a decreased sense of well-being, and the low-energy syndrome settles in, affecting cognitive abilities, memory, initiative and alertness.

4. Biological Age Factor of 0 to 5

If your Biological Age Factor is between 0 and 5, your general overall health is good, but you can still make improvements in your health and fitness. You need to begin minimizing, then avoiding, those lifestyle and dietary factors that promote aging—begin to live and "eat smart."

You can reduce your biological age by five to eight years in 30 days simply by following the recommendations in this book. In their book *Shed Ten Years in Ten Weeks*, Dr. Julian Whitaker and co-author Carol Coleman write that you can reduce your biological age by 10 or more years in just 10 weeks. Intensify your commitment to your optimum well-being. Follow the recommendations in this book carefully and decrease your bad habits with proactive intervention. The time to begin is now.

5. Biological Age Factor of –10 to 0

If your Biological Age Factor is between –10 and 0, you are in hormonal harmony with healthy lifestyle factors in the key areas of diet, exercise, stress management and supplementation. Increase your vigilance and maintain your optimum health. Take off that extra 5 or 10 pounds by stretching and doing hatha yoga or Tai Chi, which will make you more agile, flexible and less sluggish. Exercise four days a week, sleep 8.5 hours a night, and reduce stress to balance cortisol-to-DHEA levels.

Detoxify your liver twice a year. Continue to avoid environmental or agrichemical toxins and substitute with natural-based products whenever possible.

6.Biological Age Factor of Less than –10

If your Biological Age Factor is lower than –10, your general health is superior. Congratulations! Do not become obsessive with your health but do maintain a hormonally supportive lifestyle. You are defying the classic view of aging. With your hormonal supersymmetry and superior well-being, earnestly investigate your spiritual growth. This is a rare and unique opportunity. This is a human being's greatest frontier—to be proactive in prayer, pondering, meditation, reading, hiking in nature, star gazing, writing poetry, going on retreats, deepening and enriching oneself.

Help your family, friends or community by reaching out to those who really need an emotional, psychological, physical or spiritual boost.

FIVE TESTS YOU WANT TO PASS

Testing your blood for four vital values and finding your percentage of body fat can tell you a lot about your current state of health and your risk of developing a serious health problem. I strongly recommend that you get a simple blood chemistry profile completed through your physician. Be sure to take the blood test after an overnight fast in order to obtain accurate values.

Your blood is the focal point to determine how successful you are with your dietary strategy. Your blood is an honest critic; it hides nothing and tells no lies. Your blood test results will inform you if you are in an anabolic drive and aging slower than your chronological age—or you're in a catabolic drive with your age accelerating faster than your chronological age.

You change the oil in your car every three months to keep your motor clean and in a high-performance status. You should check your overall health with these blood tests once a year to check on your aging progress. You can tweak your dietary strategy to optimum anabolic status if your results are not satisfactory, and then you'll see the results in the next round of blood tests.

Test One: Glycosylated Hemoglobin Levels

Both excess glucose and excess cortisol in the bloodstream can accelerate your aging. This test will tell you if you are controlling blood glucose levels and minimizing cortisol production. The higher the level of glycosylated hemoglobin found in red blood cells, the more excessive glucose tends to react with proteins to form compounds called AGEs (advanced glycated end products). AGEs are cross-linked compounds of protein and glucose, forming into sticky deteriorated proteins (this is bad). Their formation is accelerated by excess free radicals in your system. The more AGEs you make in your body, the faster you age because glucose-modified proteins are much "stickier" and adhere to the surfaces of arteries and capillaries, hastening an increase in arteriosclerosis, impotence, blindness and kidney disease. The brown age spots on your skin contain lipofuscin (also called amyloid plaques), a cross-link of protein and fat. The amyloid protein is a natural part of the brain, but it appears that the increasing glycosylation of this protein accelerates its amyloid accumulation, leading to Alzheimer's disease.

Eating too many calories, especially high-density, processed carbohydrates that are sweetened, will cause an increase first in blood glucose levels and then in insulin. As increased insulin lowers the glucose levels, it forces the hormone glucagon (which tries to restore blood glucose levels) down, which then forces your body to secrete more cortisol (stress hormone) as a backup system to ensure adequate blood glucose levels to your brain. Increased cortisol levels and increased insulin levels destroy the ventromedial neurons (VMN) in the hypothalamus (hormonal control center in the brain), which promotes hormone dysfunction and miscommunication. Excess cortisol also kills cortisol-sensitive cells in the thymus gland resulting in decreased immune function. Meanwhile, those increased blood glucose levels increase the production of AGEs.

These three events (increased glucose and insulin, the formation of AGEs and the elevation of cortisol levels) are among the primary biological markers of the aging process.

Your glycosylated hemoglobin levels should be less than 5 percent. People with Type 2 diabetes who form AGEs more quickly than the average person and die sooner than the average person, have glycosylated hemoglobin counts of between 7 and 11 percent. Their goal is to reduce this level to below 7 percent, and thus reduce the chance of long-term complications.

The level of insulin in your bloodstream should be less than 10 µU/mL. This is a measurement of fasting insulin.

Test Two: Total Cholesterol

Healthy individuals with sustained cholesterol levels of 150 mg and below enjoy clean arteries. Your ideal is to keep your total blood cholesterol level at 150 mg or below. A healthy range for total cholesterol is between 110 and 150 mg.

Your HDL "good" cholesterol levels should be at least 70 mg for optimal lifespan. If you keep your cholesterol at 150 or below, your HDL value will be between 30 and 70.

Your LDL "bad" cholesterol levels—which rise from eating saturated fat in animal products, eggs and full-fat dairy—should be 130 at the maximum, but ideally between 80 and 120.

Test Three: Triglycerides

After you eat a meal, your liver processes fat into triglyceride molecules that travel through the circulatory system to be stored as body fat or used in building cell membranes. Elevated triglycerides are a risk factor for heart disease and other health problems. Sugar, alcohol, dietary fat, and a lack of exercise can all raise your triglyceride levels.

The ideal range for triglycerides is between 60 to 90.

Test Four: Fasting Triglyceride to HDL Cholesterol Ratio

The higher the fasting-triglyceride-to-HDL-cholesterol ratio, the greater your chance of a heart attack. HDL is known as the "good" cholesterol because it is associated with a decreased risk of heart disease. Triglycerides is another name for fat. High fasting-triglyceride-to-HDL-cholesterol ratio is another indicator of elevated insulin levels and also means you have lots of the "bad" or dangerous, small, dense alterherogenic LDL particles that are closely associated with heart disease.

The ratio should be below 2, and ideally below 1. If your ratio is 3 or 4, you are accelerating aging.

Test Five: Percentage of Body Fat and Body Mass Index

Your weight is not really important. Weight measures muscle, bone, organs, skin—and fat. The important measure is your percentage of body fat. Close to 40 percent of North American adults are overweight, and nearly 30 percent of North American children are overweight. Excess body fat is directly related to increased insulin levels. Adult males should average about 15 percent body fat and females about 22 percent. If your current body fat is above these percentages, you are accelerating your aging process and encouraging a catabolic hormonal nosedive. The sophisticated calculation of body fat is the BMI, or body mass index. You can compute your BMI by dividing your weight in kilograms by the square of your height in meters.

A BMI from 19 to 26 is in the healthy range, while 27 and above puts you at risk for hypertension, diabetes and cardiovascular disease.

How to Determine Your Body Mass Index (BMI)

1. Multiply your weight in pounds by 0.45 to get your weight into kilograms (e.g., 150 pounds x 0.45 = 67.5 kilograms).
2. Multiply your height in inches by 0.025 to get your height in meters (e.g., if you are 5'10" tall, that is 70" x 0.025 = 1.75 meters).
3. Square the number you calculated in Step 2 (e.g., 1.75 x 1.75 = 3.063).
4. Divide your weight in kilograms (the number you calculated in Step 1), by the square of your height in meters (the number you calculated in Step 3). (For example, 67.5 divided by 3.063 = 22.04.) This is your BMI.

WHAT THE TEST RESULTS MEAN:

Test	Anabolic Revitalization, Slow Biological Aging	Catabolic Decline, Accelerated Aging
Glycosylated Hemoglobin	– Less than 5%	– More than 7%
Total Cholesterol	– Total cholesterol 150 mg and below	– Above 200 mg/dL
	– HDL above 70 mg/dL	– Below 50 mg/dL
	– LDL between 80 and 120 mg/dL	– Above 120 mg/dL

Triglyceride to HDL Cholesterol	– Less than 2	– 4 or more
Fasting Insulin	– Less than 10 µU/mL	– More than 15 µU/mL
BMI (Body Mass Index)	– Between 19 to 26	– More than 26

Additional Blood Tests You May Take	Anabolic Revitalization	Catabolic Decline
Glucose	– Between 75 and 100 mg/dL	– Above 150 mg/dL
Iron	– Under 100 mcg/dL	– Above 120 mcg/dL
DHEA	– Above 225 mcg/dL	– Below 150 mcg/dL
Homocysteine	– Under 7 micro mol/L	– 8 to 10 micro mol/L
C-Reactive Protein	– Below 1 mg/L	– Above 1.5 mg/L

DO YOU NEED TO LOSE WEIGHT?

To keep from gaining excess weight or to lose those extra pounds we may have already gained, we need to relearn some important things our ancestors understood, such as sleeping when it is dark and rising when it is light, and eating foods by season that are as close to their natural state as possible. We must learn to "eat in harmony with our longstanding genetic predisposition to food."

Instead, we stay up late at night, or we indulge in late-night carousing and eat excessive sugar in the form of processed, high-density carbohydrates. We raise insulin levels. The longer our blood insulin levels stay high, the more likely we are to accumulate excess body fat and battle a weight problem. After our late-night binging, we want to sleep in late the next morning to sleep off excess sugar or get ready to procreate because excess sugar means it is autumn and feasting time in preparation for winter's famine.

> Why does alcohol have the effect that it does? Because it's a high-density carbohydrate. Like all excess or processed carbohydrates, it causes changes in our appetite and affects our mood, eating patterns, sleeping patterns, thought processes, memory and personality.

Balance and Moderation

If you want to lose fat permanently, repeat this mantra: balance and moderation. The only three basic food groups that were, and still are, necessary, are protein, fats and carbohydrates. If we live on only one food group to the exclusion of the other two, our natural synchronicity for the quick and accurate balance of our internal-survival switches with hormones is destroyed, "out of whack," so we accelerate aging, pain, disease and an early extinction—death.

Reduce Fat Intake:

All calories are not treated equally by the body. Let's say you eat a large order of French fries. If you have not exercised that day, your glycogen storage tanks are already full. Your body now will burn the excess carbohydrates for energy and immediately stop burning fat. Now your body keeps all of its stored fat, along with all the fat that soaked into the potato during frying.

The bottom line for eating the French fries is you'll keep all the body fat you presently have plus an additional 150 calories worth of fat from the fat in the fries.

The body resists using its stored fat for energy unless it absolutely has to. Dr. Susanne Holt, Ph.D., at the University of Sydney observed: "Fatty foods are not satisfying, even though people expected them to be." We think the reason is that the body sees fat as a fuel which should only be used in emergencies—it stores it in the cells instead of breaking it down for immediate use. Because it doesn't recognize the fat (in food) as energy for immediate use, the body does not tell the brain to cut hunger signals so we go on wanting more.

How do we know how much fat we're eating? The new Nutrition Facts label is shown here. It has to appear on all packaged foods. Look carefully at the line, Calories 90, Calories from Fat 30. Divide the total calories (in this case 90) by the calories from fat (in this case 30). If the result is less than 5 (it is 3 in this case), don't buy the food as it is more than 20 percent fat. An answer of 5 or more is what we want; it means that the food gets 20 percent or less of its calories from fat. Many failed dieters believe they are following low-fat nutrition, when in fact they are being fooled by false food labeling. Even "low-fat" milk is really high in fat.

How does low-fat milk get away with its name? The dairy industry got an exemption from the new labels. Nevertheless, an 8 oz glass of low-fat milk (2 percent) serves you a hefty 33 percent of its calories from fat. Especially beware of the slew of "reduced fat" products. Under the label laws "reduced fat" means 25 percent less fat than the original product. Oreo cookies for example are 44 percent fat calories. The new Reduced Fat Oreos are legally labelled as such, but still loaded—with 33 percent of their calories from fat. Reduced fat cold cuts can still be 60 percent fat. Also "light" and

Nutrition Facts

Serving Size ½ cup (114 g)
Servings Per Container 4

Amount Per Serving	
Calories 90	Calories from Fat 30

	% Daily Value
Total Fat 3 g	5%
Saturated Fat 0 g	0%
Cholesterol 0 mg	0%
Sodium 300 mg	13%
Total Carbohydrate 13 g	4%
DietaryFiber 3 g	12%
Sugars 3 g	
Protein 3 g	

"lite" foods, that have to be one-third less fat than the original, can still be 40–50 percent fat calories. Only trust the Nutrition Facts panel on food labels— it is scientifically and legally correct.

Reduce High-Density Carbohydrate Intake

Chronic high-density carbohydrate consumption—in the form of processed foods—causes accelerated aging, and you not only store much of it as fat, but you hit menopause or andropause sooner. Concentrate on low-density carbohydrates (vegetables, fruit and whole grains) in your diet. See Chapters 10 and 11 for more on carbohydrate consumption.

Reduce Sugar Intake

Our species, Homo Sapiens, had to evolve constantly to meet the challenges of hungry predators and a hostile environment in order to survive. When our ancestors came across wild fruit or wild berries such as strawberries, they ate all they could. Their bodies had developed an internal chemical monitor system of hormones that could turn chemical reactions "on" or "off" quickly, so their bodies were in balance or what we now call homeostasis. Their body had to learn how to handle the large influx of glucose that got into their bloodstream. They ran their bodies on glucose as a fuel and, as their descendants, we do also.

When our bloodstream has excess glucose circulating, the beta cells in our pancreas secrete the hormone insulin. Insulin has the triple job of "turning on" the chemical switch that delivers glucose to our cells for energy and "turning off" that chemical switch when cells are saturated with glucose, and then "switching on" a storage enzyme (lipoprotein lipase), to store the rest of the glucose, long term, as body fat in adipose tissue.

Blood-sugar controls both our appetite and mood. Insulin lowers blood-sugar levels when they rise too high. Insulin also ushers blood-sugar into our cells for energy and maintains blood-sugar levels in a process called homeostasis.

Sustained high levels of any one hormone, in our hormone cascades, destroys the intricate balance in all hormone networks. This makes us maladaptive to our internal and external environment. We are now at odds with nature.

Chronic high levels of insulin (a vital anabolic hormone, which in excess becomes dangerous), as an example, lead to stubborn obesity, diabetes, heart disease and cancer.

Choose the Right Sugar: Our ancestors ate fructose, a sugar found naturally in fruit. Unlike refined sugar, fructose as found in fruit does not trigger the insulin response and subsequent food cravings. One clear example comes from a study in which participants drank a beverage sweetened with either fructose, glucose or aspartame (tradenamed Nutra Sweet). People who drank the fructose-sweetened drink ate fewer overall calories and less fat than did the other people.

Fructose is absorbed more slowly than glucose or sucrose (which is 50 percent glucose and 50 percent fructose). Fructose must travel to the liver to be converted to glucose, and then it enters the bloodstream. Fructose does stimulate insulin, but not nearly as dramatically as table sugar.

We can curb our cravings and avoid overeating simply by switching from a sugar-laden cinnamon roll to a fructose-filled apple. We must strictly avoid processed fructose and high-fructose corn syrup in pop, sports drinks and processed foods. They are man-made and no substitute for natural fructose in fruits.

If we eliminate refined "sweet treats" carbohydrates, which are counter-productive, and replace them with "real food" carbohydrates, we not only reduce our chances of obesity, but of diabetes, heart disease and colon, prostate and breast cancer as well.

Dieting: It Gets Worse

Dieting has never worked and never will work. It is estimated that 95 percent of all dieters put the weight back on—if not more—within one year of ending "the miracle diet guaranteed to lose four pounds a night while you sleep."

When we diet, our body only recognizes a "famine mode" and does what it has always done—slows down our metabolism to conserve its portable energy stores from fat. We mainly lose critical water, muscle and bone.

Once we begin eating again, we "feast" as our body will store fat at a greater capacity than before the diet, because it now recognizes that there still are "famines."

Revving the Fat-Burning Engine

Daily exercise or exercise at least five times a week actually helps to regulate blood-sugar levels, and provides a nifty endorphin rush without all those sugars, fats, salt and excess calories. Aerobic activity such as walking, jogging, swimming, spinning, rowing or bicycling should be done for half an hour or more at 60 percent of your maximum heart rate. (An intensity greater than this will build your heart, but you will not burn fat.) Exercise is an important consideration for controlling our cravings as we also offset unhealthy cravings with natural, unprocessed, bioenergetic whole foods. This is the basic equation to both cutting caloric intake and increasing caloric expenditure.

Getting Enough Exercise: Data gathered by B.E. Ainsworth Ph.D, et al., published in *Medical Science Sports Exercise 25* in 1993, studying Harvard graduates, demonstrates that we need approximately 2,100 calories of exercise-related expenditure per week. This is 300 exercise-related calorie expenditures per day. What does it take to burn 300 calories per day?

For most people, a brisk walk for little more than half an hour per day will meet their calorie-expenditure requirements. This form of exercise also generates nearly a 70 percent reduction in the incidence of breast cancer in women. Adding weight training will make you more fit, enhance your independence and give you greater functionality later in life. If you maintain your lean muscle mass and muscle strength, you will be able to walk, move about freely, get up and down, as well as continue to exercise well into your senior years.

MINUTES REQUIRED FOR VARIOUS ACTIVITIES TO BURN 300 CALORIES PER DAY

Activity	Average female	Average Male
Bicycling	35	25
Jogging slowly	40	30
Using rowing machine	30	24
Spinning	30	24
Using stationary bike	35	30
Swimming	35	30
Walking briskly	45	35
Walking slowly	90	75

If you drink a "green drink" in water before you exercise, you will force your body to burn 22 percent more of its calories from fat, preserving your blood glucose and muscle glycogen levels for an extended exercise period. You'll also have the added bonus of burning more body fat while exercising. For many hours after, your resting metabolism rate (RMR) will increase and continue to remain elevated and will burn calories for a full 12 hours.

We must eat the way nature intended us to, long before companies realized they could make enormous sums of money with their processed foods. They entice us, and down we go!

Our digestion, absorption, distribution and elimination processes have not changed in 100,000 years—only our food choices have changed.

Weight Loss Is Only a Minor Adjustment Away

The most important piece of advice I can give you is to persuade you to eat fewer highly salted and sweetened processed foods, especially the low- or no-fat synthetic "foods," which are also full of unhealthful chemical additives and devoid of protective nutritional factors. Begin eating bioenergetic whole foods that are in harmony with your longstanding genetic predisposition to food. These real foods are both a source of high-quality fuel, and a positive feedback loop of hormonal modulators of mood, abundant energy and mental acuity.

The good news is it takes only minor adjustments in your current eating pattern to produce improvements in your energy, thinking and mood—quite often dramatic ones! More good news is that the taste for sugar and salt is a learned one, which means it can be unlearned or totally replaced by a new habit.

The neurotransmitters galanin and endorphins, made in the hypothalamus of the brain, encourage us to eat fat. When we diet or several hours have passed between meals, the breakdown of body fat releases fat fragments called free fatty acids that travel to the brain and to the hypothalamus and trigger the release of galanin. Elevated galanin levels, in turn, trigger cravings for fat-containing foods from ice cream to French fries. Reproductive hormones like estrogen, the stress hormone cortisol and elevated insulin levels "turn on" galanin. This should explain the food cravings that often accompany premenstrual syndrome in women, which occur when estrogen levels swell in the menstrual cycle. In addition to increasing our cravings for fat, galanin affects how much of that dietary fat is stored as body fat.

Galanin levels are low in the morning, start to rise by early afternoon, and peak in the evening when our galanin-induced desire for fattier foods is highest. This is the body's attempt to store fat as long-term energy to survive the overnight "famine."

Remember that our food preferences, desires, cravings and loves are literally hardwired into our basic instincts for survival and safety. What we eat directly and indirectly affects all our hormones and neurotransmitters, which in turn influence our energy levels, moods, food cravings, stress levels, sleep habits and inherited genetic traits. Choose wisely!

Follow These Ten Tips to Lose Weight

1. Drink eight to 12, 8 oz (250 mL) glasses of water daily between meals. Constantly prehydrate. Drink two or three cups of unsweetened herbal tea daily.
2. Never eat after 7:30 p.m. or your pituitary gland will not secrete growth hormone (GH) to burn fat and build lean muscle mass, while you are in deep sleep.
3. Never go more than three hours without eating a meal or snack and have some protein at three meals (the average man should consume 35 grams of protein per meal and the average woman about 27 grams).
4. Eat all the salads and steamed, "crunchy-tender" vegetables you want. Try eliminating potatoes, rice, bread, bagels, buns and "sweet treats." Avoid processed high-density carbohydrates completely. Use only 1 tablespoon of extra virgin olive oil daily and 1 tablespoon of organic flax seed oil on your salads or veggies. Use fish oil supplements containing the essential fatty acids

rich in DHA and EPA, or, for vegetarians, algae supplements rich in DHA and EPA, which are heart and brain-healthy. Use 1/2 teaspoon of borage oil, which gives you 500 mg of GLA.

5. Always eat before you feel too hungry, so that you won't be so likely to binge or overeat. A "green drink" between meals satiates hunger and food cravings.

6. The fewer excess calories you eat, the slower you age and the greater your longevity. Eat moderate portions at each meal. By consuming bioenergetic whole foods women should get about 1,400 to 1,800 calories a day, and men 2,000 to 2,400 calories.

7. Sleep 8.5 to 9.0 hours every single night in a totally dark room with no light contamination. Try to go to sleep as soon after sundown as possible.

8. Don't forget the excess fat in your foods is stored directly as body fat. The composition of stored fat in your body is similar to the fat in your diet. Mediterranean cultures, who derive most of their fats from olive oil and fish, and Asian cultures, who eat a lot of soy foods and fish, have the healthiest fats stored in their bodies.

9. Exercise three to four times a week at a gym. Have an exercise fitness consultant design a special program for your needs and capabilities. Be sure to do 30 minutes of aerobics and 15 to 30 minutes of a wide variety of weight resistance, anaerobic exercise at each session. The timing of exercise is everything. Exercise in the morning, and the earlier the better. Morning exercise raises your resting metabolism rate (RMR) and you continue to burn fat for a full 12 hours. If you exercise in the evenings and then go to bed, you lose most of the fat-loss effect, because sleep causes your metabolic rate and body temperature to decline.

10. There is a powerful herbal combination called lean+ that appears to effectively open fat cells and encourages the fat-releasing hormone (hormone-sensitive lipase) to shuttle stored fat in adipose cells to the mitochondria to be burned as fuel. This formula also reduces the production of acetyl coenzyme A, a compound necessary for excessive fat to be stored in the body. lean+ increases the ability of the liver and muscles to synthesize and store glycogen, thereby suppressing appetite. The formula is outlined in the following Protein Recipe for Weight Loss.

A second supplement called conjugated Linoleic Acid (CLA) was shown in the June 2000 issue of *The Journal of Nutrition* to reduce the overall fat pad weight by up to 32 percent in female rats. In a second study, rats fed CLA showed reductions in fat pad weight within seven days. The reduced fat pad size was due to smaller adipose (fat cell) size rather than a reduced fat cell number. The researchers concluded that not only does CLA shrink fat cells, but that it promotes weight loss even in relatively lean individuals. Superior formulas contain 74–82 percent CLA.

Protein Recipe for Weight Loss

- Put 8 oz (250 mL) of pure water in a shaker cup.
- Add 2 level scoops of undenatured Alphapure™ whey protein isolate powder or soy protein isolate powder.
- Shake for five seconds. Drink and enjoy.

This formula contains only 108 calories and no sugars so you will take in 30 grams of bioavailable protein and burn body fat for energy. You will trade body fat for lean muscle mass with this recipe. The cost is about $2.20 per serving.

To maximize fat burning and reduce your fat stores quickly, 20 minutes before your protein shake, take four capsules of a weight-management herbal formula containing hydroxycitric acid (500 mg), citrus aurantium (325 mg), grapefruit juice powder (200 mg), coleus forskohlii (100 mg), cayenne (100 mg), gugulipid (75 mg), alpha lipoic acid (50 mg) and green tea (350 mg). This herbal combination turns "off" the fat-storage hormone lipoprotein lipase and turns "on" fat-shuttling hormone-sensitive lipase efficiently, quickly and safely. Hormone-sensitive lipase shuttles fat from adipose cells via L-carnitine to the mitochondria in the muscle tissue to be burned as a fuel source.

Protein Recipe for Lean Muscle Growth
- 8 oz (250 mL) of plain, organic hemp milk, rice milk, goat's milk, fat-free cow's milk, almond milk or oat milk
- 2 scoops of undenatured Alphapure™ whey protein isolate powder
- 2 heaping tablespoons of plain organic yogurt or BioK+
- 2 tablespoons of ground flax seeds
- 1 cup (250 mL) of fresh or frozen blueberries or another berry or combination of berries
- 2 tablespoons of bee pollen ground in a coffee grinder
- 2 tablespoons of soy lecithin granules
- three capsules of A•G•E inhibitors™
- two capsules of a "friendly bacteria" acidophilus mix emptied into the shake, or take two enteric-coated capsules with your power protein shake

  This formula gives you a full 35 grams of undenatured protein and approximately 450 calories. The cost is about $3.50 per serving.

Notes on blending:
- Blend all ingredients in a blender, except the protein powder.
- Put blended liquids in a hand-held shaker cup with a lid, add the protein powder and shake for ten seconds—this leaves the whey sub-fractions intact and undenatured.

One half hour before you exercise, drink a high-quality "green drink" that contains no fructose, sweetener or sugars (use water as the liquid). This will make your tissues alkaline so you can work your muscles longer until they become restricted by lactic acid and pyruvic acid buildup, which is the rate-limiting factor of exercising. Herbal anabolic activators naturally build muscle quickly.

To allow your protein power shake to be extremely effective at burning body fat and building lean muscle mass, use an herbal anabolic activator to reach your goal but not your limits. Take three capsules, 20 minutes before your protein power shake, containing Ekdisten (500 mg), Samambaia (400 mg) and stinging nettle (1,000 mg).

How to Control Your Appetite

The body has checks and balances on brain activity when it has had enough to eat. Cholecystokinin (CCK) is a hormone found in both the brain and the small intestine that aids in digestion and relays the message of satisfaction—"stop eating." The more CCK you release, the slower you digest your food, the sooner you feel full, the less food you eat.

AIDS and cancer patients with high CCK levels and low endorphin levels can lose their appetites, which contributes to the wasting syndrome associated with both diseases. Those with eating disorders such as bulimia have low levels of CCK, which can help to explain why they don't feel full even when they've eaten large amounts of food.

Glucagon tells us we have eaten enough protein.

The brain has feedback systems to tell the body when it has had enough to eat called the appetite-control loop:

- NPY (neuropeptide Y) is the neurotransmitter that encourages us to eat carbohydrates. NPY levels drop and serotonin levels rise after eating a meal containing carbohydrates, stopping our carbohydrate cravings.
- Galanin levels are balanced by eating a little fat.
- CCK is released from the intestines, after a meal containing protein, sending messages of satiation to the brain.
- Elevated insulin levels, in the blood after a meal, "switch off" NPY levels and turn on corticotropin-releasing hormone (CRH) to curb hunger, especially during stress and long-term dieting.
- Exercise helps to normalize endorphin levels ("feel good" hormones).
- Stress elevates cortisol levels, which increase our preference for fatty foods.

If your eating habits are fueled by modern-day processed foods, you can quickly, through a few simple dietary and life-style changes, influence what foods appeal to you. Adjusting both your appetite-control and mood-control hormones, as well as your neurotransmitters, can have dramatic effects on your skin texture, weight, sustained energy, sleep patterns, food cravings, clarity of thinking and personality.

10

THE PRINCIPLES OF EATING SMART: THE WORLD'S BEST DIET

When most of us think of the word "diet," we think of a short-term plan involving extreme and sometimes bizarre food restrictions or prescriptions in order to lose excess weight in as little time as possible. But at one time, before the Weight Watchers, and Scarsdales of the modern world, "diet" referred to the food and drink we routinely consumed. And so it should. Short-term and extreme weight-loss plans don't generally have long-term health benefits.

As I mentioned earlier, I am not advocating an overnight solution to whatever ails us, but rather a *lifelong food management system* that will ensure our optimal well-being.

There is no need to flip-flop from diet to diet to diet. We must simply eat in harmony with our longstanding genetic predisposition to food—food that is natural, whole and bioenergetic. We must follow the natural circadian rhythm both daily and seasonally. And we must build a physical and emotional routine that will benefit and not harm our health.

If we do, we will be delivering all of the nutrients to our 100 trillion cells necessary for self-diagnosis and self-healing. We will achieve hormonal balance. We will boost our mood, remain vigilant, calm and alert. We will live a longer, healthier life.

The lifelong food management system that can achieve all of this, I like to call "The World's Best Diet." It is based on four important, but easily understood, principles: adaptability, moderation, variety and balance. Let's explore these further.

Adaptability

We must adapt, the way our Paleolithic ancestors did, to the world around us. Adaptability is our most powerful tool for optimum health. Today, we have more work and greater stress, and we are surrounded by a much harsher environment characterized by polluted air, water and soil and subsequently contaminated food. So we need to eat much more conscientiously than prehistoric man did in order to survive.

We need to return to those foods that are grown organically, and eat them in sync with our daily and seasonal circadian rhythms. We also need to adapt our lifestyle to the cycle of the day and cycles of seasons. That means getting a good night's sleep in complete darkness. It also means reasonably eating as much bioenergetic, whole, colorful, fresh food that is in season as we can.

Make sure the food you eat adheres to the nutritional guidelines in this book, looks appealing, satisfies your hunger and gives you pleasure. Have gratitude for food.

Be an alchemist in your own kitchen. Food preparation and cooking are a creative art. Imagine aromas and flavors in your mind—then translate them into practical meals both you and your dearest ones will enjoy. You need to imagine, picture in your mind, and anticipate the smell, look and taste of what you want to prepare. Pay strict attention to every detail of food cleaning, chopping, cooking and artfully displaying fresh, bioenergetic colorful, whole food. Bring these vast numbers of variables together and create your own spontaneous preparations, rather than referring to recipes.

I advise you to change some of your eating habits to improve your health and avoid the midday doldrums. I am concerned about the eating habits of children. If they get great satisfaction and become accustomed to the tantalizing taste of unhealthful, processed, fast foods—those habits may persist throughout their life. This phenomenon is called "programming," intelligently predetermined by seductive, compelling, slick billion-dollar advertising. How can our children stand up to them? Set a healthful example for your children's sake. You must adapt wisely and so your children must adapt wisely to survive well. It is that basic. It always has been about adaptability, it is about adaptability, and it will always be about adaptability. Early extinction is simply not being able to adapt well to the environmental cues at hand.

I personally never eat at fast-food restaurants or take-outs. I am very happy eating healthily and I want you to be also. I stand by that statement.

Today, genetics and lifestyle are colliding. Can we be creatively adaptable?

Moderation

We should eat as much as our body needs, and not more. This voluntary calorie restriction that will ensure our body does not take in extra calories, gain unnecessary weight, or produce an abundance of free radicals.

We should eat appropriately sized meals so that we feel full for three hours after each meal and not hungry in between. This means our appetite-control hormones will be balanced and we won't crave foods we don't need and we won't feel compelled to binge—but more about this later.

Moderation also means that we will limit or omit attractively packaged processed fast foods, and foods that are high in salt, sweeteners and destructive trans-fatty acids.

Salt: There is nothing wrong in satisfying a craving for salt, except the foods we typically turn to are often loaded with fat and sugar or sugar substitutes.
The taste of salt is appealing to people of all cultures. However, most people consume much more salt than they need, which means at least a portion of our craving is due to habit. Salt has a habituating effect that comes close to addiction. We only notice how dependent we are on it once we seriously start cutting down.

The fact is, salt intake above a certain level is harmful. Research proves that excess salt consumption:

• shortens lifespan;
• contributes to osteoporosis; and
• causes the body to retain excess fluid.

Furthermore, there has been considerable controversy over salt's contribution to high blood pressure. A *New York Times* article (October 3, 1995) printed research results that demonstrated that salt raises blood pressure levels.

Women, during the two weeks prior to their periods, might experience increased cravings for salty foods. The female hormone estrogen increases the anti-diuretic hormones, vaso-pressin and aldosterone, which cause fluid retention. Some women can gain up to 10 pounds of added water weight during this time of month, which triggers their salt cravings to help maintain the additional water concentration in the body.

There is a delicate sodium/potassium balance in our body. When we eat too much salt (sodium chloride), we raise our sodium levels and simultaneously deplete the potassium level in our 100 trillion cells. Potassium neutralizes some of the toxic effects of excess sodium intake—but as it is depleted, excess sodium causes chaos in our cells' biochemistry.

All natural, bioenergetic foods contain a perfect balance of sodium and potassium. Processed foods have tipped the scales heavily in the favor of sodium. North Americans consume 80 percent of their daily dietary sodium from processed foods such as cheese, crackers, luncheon meats, soups, soy sauces, desserts and other sauces.

Our body naturally contains more potassium than sodium, at a ratio of about two to one. Those of us weaning ourselves off of table salt may require additional potassium, in supplements of 99 mg a day, to reset the sodium-potassium balance. Bioenergetic whole foods high in potassium that naturally reset this balance are beet greens, acorn squash, avocados, apricots, blackstrap molasses, yams, whole grains, soybeans, Swiss chard, sunflower seeds, salmon, lean meats, tomatoes and spinach.

We can use sea salt with added potassium to reduce sodium levels, but I have other suggestions. We can reprogram our taste buds by either cutting back or by trying one or more of the following suggestions to soothe salt cravings:

- substitute lemon juice for salt in cooking or in salads;
- season with low-sodium, wheat-free soy sauce or low-sodium miso;
- season with Bragg's Liquid Aminos;
- boost flavor with bioenergetic herbs and spices like rosemary, thyme, oregano, fenugreek, curry, turmeric, sage or lemon peel;
- substitute high-fat and high-salt grated Parmesan cheese with Sapsago cheese, a hard, low-salt cheese from Switzerland made from skim milk, spices and herbs; and
- use salt-free seasonings such as Spike, salt-free all-purpose herbal seasonings or Nova Scotia dulse.

If you choose to use some salt, use Celtic sea salt, not iodized table salt. It is the cleanest, most mineral-rich sea salt. A great alternative is to mix 20 percent Celtic sea salt with 80 percent of an herbal salt-free mixture like Spike or salt-free Mrs. Dash.

So how much salt do we need? Dr. Derek Denton of the University of Melbourne, Australia, reported in *Nature Medicine* (October 1996) that humans evolved to handle 2 or 3 grams of salt a day. Most people, children and adults, in North America average between 10 to 15 grams a day. I suggest 1 to 2 grams daily.

I myself have no salt in my kitchen. I use each of the above suggestions every day instead. I receive 1 to 2 grams of organic sodium daily by following the dietary strategies outlined in this book.

Sugar: As with salt, we have to be very careful with our intake of sugar. Children become sugar addicted and turn into sugar-addicted grown-ups. Excess sugar leads to diabetes, and to abnormally high cholesterol levels by encouraging the production of very low-density lipoprotein. It also encourages existing cancers.

When we eat grains, legumes, vegetables or fruits, the normal digestive enzymes in our mouth, stomach, intestines and pancreas slowly break down the complex sugar in these foods to more easily absorbed sugars like sucrose, fructose and glucose.

As soon as these sugars enter our bloodstream as blood glucose, a negative feedback loop kicks in. Insulin is secreted from the pancreas into the bloodstream and excess glucose is converted to glycogen and stored in the liver or muscles "short term." If there is any excess glucose in the bloodstream once the "short-term" fuel tanks are full, the remainder is converted to fat and stored as adipose tissue, "long-term" storage.

Cancer cells love sugar and use more of it than normal cells do. Cancer cells force the liver to produce more and more glucose for them from stored glycogen; this process also triggers the breakdown of fat and muscle cells. The result is abnormal glucose tolerance and increased glucose production in people with cancer, which results in the breakdown of fat and muscle resulting in a terrible wasting syndrome.

I strongly suggest you avoid refined white table sugar as much as possible—because the refining process involves the use of potentially mutagenic chemicals. There is also some evidence that sugar may inhibit immune function.

Instead of refined sugar, we can use a small amount of unpasteurized raw honey, which also has some medicinal properties. Honey is 30 percent sucrose, 40 percent fructose and 30 percent glucose. We may also use small amounts of organic, unsulphured blackstrap molasses, fructo-oligo-saccharides (FOS), barley malt or brown rice syrup, which are acceptable on the glycemic index. Agave nectar, a liquid sweetener, is a good substitute for corn syrup.

My absolute preference for a sweetener is the herb stevia—not the white crystalline extract, but the chopped green leaves. Stevia has no calories and does not cause any insulin response. It is a dream-come-true for diabetics, athletes, those trying to lose weight, and conscientious eaters like you. There are several books available that explain stevia in detail, as well as several excellent cookbooks full of stevia recipes. I highly recommend *Stevia Sweet Recipes* by Jeffrey Goettemoeller and *Nature's Sweetener Stevia* by Rita Elkins.

Eggs: Eggs have received a bad rap over recent years, but when eaten in moderation they do provide some unique health benefits.

Free-range, organic eggs produced by chickens that were fed flax seeds are a complete protein because they contain all nine essential amino acids in the right proportion. One egg provides only 75 calories with 7 to 8 grams of balanced protein and 250 mg of cholesterol per yolk—and also 700 mg of lecithin that emulsifies or neutralizes the cholesterol. The yolk supplies Omega-3 fats, which are essential for brain development, and DHA—but the amount is highly dependent upon what the chicken was fed. Regular supermarket eggs contain on average only 1 mg of DHA. Organic, free-range chickens that are fed flax seeds may contain as much as 20 mg of DHA per egg and are referred to as high-DHA eggs.

Eggs also contain huge supplies of the antioxidants superoxide dismutase (SOD) and catalase, which "quench" or neutralize superoxide, a free radical that is extremely destructive to our cells. SOD and catalase are complicated long-string amino acids, with SOD comprised of 150 units and catalase over 500. Because SOD and catalase are so complicated, oral supplementation is an inefficient way to boost cellular levels, but eggs are the "eating smart" way.

There are numerous studies that indicate eggs actually improve your blood cholesterol profile. Eggs raise your "good" high-density lipoprotein (HDL) levels of cholesterol. Egg yolks are also a source of two powerful phytonutrients, lutein and zeaxanthin, which filter out blue light to prevent age-related macular degeneration that destroys sharp, detailed vision. Protect the delicate DHA fatty acids and preformed cholesterol in egg yolks from oxidizing due to the heat of frying and only eat them poached, soft- or hard-boiled, but do not overcook eggs to the point where the blue-green sulfur has separated from the yolk.

Finally, egg yolks are a powerhouse of the sulfur-bearing amino acids that we need for superior immune responsiveness. The yolks contain vitamin B12, which is generally lacking in plant foods, and choline, the building block of the brain neurotransmitter acetylcholine, which improves short-term memory and boosts abstract thinking.

I recommend three to nine quality eggs a week, unless you are experiencing any type of inflammation. If that is the case, I then recommend that you avoid the arachidonic acid (AA) content of the yolks, but do eat the white of the eggs. Arachidonic acid encourages the development of the pro-inflammatory prostaglandin-2 (PGE2).

Avoid salmonella by buying free-range, organic chicken's eggs rather than eggs produced in massive factory-like conditions, where chickens are raised in over-crowded and possibly unsanitary settings and may be fed animal protein parts, fish scraps, antibiotics and hormones. They are kept in tiny cages under lights that never go out to force them to lay eggs at a much higher rate than is natural.

There is no nutritional difference between brown- and white-shelled eggs.

Variety

Variety is also key to maintaining "The World's Best Diet." We should eat a large variety of bioenergetic whole foods daily to ensure that we have covered all of the nutritional bases. Their treasure chest of organic vitamins, minerals, phytonutrients, carbohydrates, proteins, fats, fiber, water and antioxidants will strengthen our muscles, bones, blood vessels, connective tissues, bloodstream, organs and glands. These special foods give your body ultimate protection from viruses, bacteria, fungi, invasive yeast, intruding environmental or agrichemical toxins, petrochemicals and a host of ever-present carcinogens.

Variety also means eating something raw at each meal and snack—raw nuts and seeds, vegetables, sprouts or herbs. Utilizing raw bioenergetic foods ensures that our body will receive all the live enzymes, organic water and soluble and insoluble fibers that it needs. Fresh vegetable juices in moderation are a great source of active phytonutrients and antioxidants, but limit the carrots and beets.

Plant and animal food products have plenty of enzymes in their natural state. Unfortunately, food enzymes are destroyed at 122° Fahrenheit (50° Celsius). That is the reason I suggest you eat some raw food at each meal. Have seeds and nuts on your oatmeal at breakfast; tomatoes, onions, red peppers, herbs, sunflower-seed sprouts and grated carrots on your sandwich at lunch; or a colorful salad or shredded beets and herbs to garnish your dinner protein entrée. All these "live foods" provide those essential enzymes.

Living foods have live enzymes—proteins that initiate biochemical reactions such as digestion in the same way a spark plug initiates combustion. Pull the spark plugs from your car's engine, and your car won't start. Without the enzymes in raw foods, the body lacks the digestive "spark plugs" to easily break down foods.

Fruits, however, should be eaten separately, not mixed with most proteins, or with any salads, vegetables, grains or fats. The only exception is berries, especially phytonutrient-rich blueberries, either fresh or frozen, which can be added to a protein power shake at breakfast. Every single nutrient found in fruits is also found in vegetables. Therefore I recommend only two servings of organic fruit daily, with one being fresh or frozen berries in your breakfast power protein shake.

My preference is that you purchase certified organically grown fruit, vegetables and grains whenever possible to avoid the unhealthful residues of pesticides, herbicides and fungicides.

If you use conventionally grown fruits and vegetables, it is especially important to wash them carefully, removing outside leaves and peeling them when appropriate.

The ten most contaminated kinds of produce, with unacceptable levels of agrichemical residues are:

1. strawberries
2. peaches
3. apricots
4. cherries
5. green beans
6. celery
7. spinach
8. grapes from Chile
9. cantaloupes from Mexico
10. apples

Try to purchase these fruits and vegetables as organically grown or, if not available, wash them very carefully and minimize consumption.

Balance

To achieve balance within ourselves, we must balance our diet as well. This means eating the right foods in the right proportions at the right times of day. If you do this, you will be able to synthesize, transmit and receive high-fidelity messages in the hormonal Internet between your brain and body—throughout your entire life. This is a state of hormonal balance that can only be achieved by the food you eat, the water you drink, the stress you reduce and the restorative deep sleep you get in the dark cycle of each night.

You can protect your finely crafted cellular mechanisms from dysfunction and chronic disease. Consequently, you can quickly drive down your risk for heart disease, mental decline, osteoporosis, the roller coaster ride of emotional "ups and downs," diabetes and cancer into a declining tailspin.

The end result is that you'll live a longer, healthier life. Hopefully, with this energetic gift of health you can, physically or mentally, be able to contribute something good in your own unselfish way, for all humanity—whether anyone ever knows you have or not!

THE WORLD'S BEST DIET IN ACTION

We need to eat a balance of carbohydrate, protein and fat in all three of our meals with a suggested 55:25:20 ratio, which means that 55 percent of our total daily calories comes from carbohydrates, 25 percent from protein, 20 percent from fat. Each of our three meals will vary to supply the proper nutrients for homeostasis and hormonal supersymmetry. But, by the end of the day, our proportions should total 55:25:20.

Today, the average North American adult is eating 35 percent of his or her calories from processed carbohydrates, 25 percent from protein and a whopping 40 percent from mostly unhealthy fats. It's no wonder life spans in North America fail to improve in spite of the advances of modern medicine. Unlike our ancestors, who had limited access to fatty foods according to Dr. Boyd Eaton, co-author of *The Paleolithic Prescription*, we have unlimited access to fat and typically overeat it because of an evolved appetite-control mechanism that drives us to eat it whenever available.

THE TYPICAL NORTH AMERICAN LOW-NUTRIENT DIET IN 2001

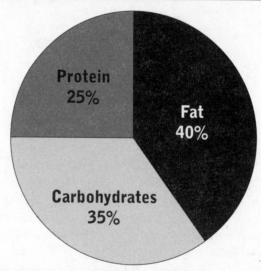

Protein 25%

Fat 40%

Carbohydrates 35%

With every medical specialty claiming great advances in North America, there should be more healthy longevity and less premature death. In comparing different countries' life expectancies at birth, surely you would think we should be top of the list. But we are not.

LIFE EXPECTANCY AT BIRTH FOR DEVELOPED COUNTRIES IN 1990, LISTED BEST TO WORST		
Country	Male	Female
Japan	76.4	82.1
Switzerland	75.2	82.6
Spain	74.8	81.6
Italy	74.5	81.4
Sweden	74.7	80.7
Netherlands	74.2	81.1
France	73.4	81.9
*Canada	74.0	80.7
Norway	73.3	80.8
Germany	73.4	80.6
Austria	73.5	80.4
Belgium	73.4	80.4
Australia	73.5	79.8
England	73.3	79.2
*United States	72.1	79.0
Portugal	70.9	78.0

Source: K.G. Kinsella, 1992.

The problem is, "Our bodies weren't designed for today's never-ending abundance of easily digested carbohydrates and fat, along with no activity," says George Armelagos, Ph.D., professor of anthropology at Emory University.

To ensure your meals follow the 55:25:20 ratio, begin by dividing your plate into three equal portions with a fourth equal but separate portion in a bowl.

Portion 1: About one-third of your plate should be protein. You do not need to count calories or make complex calculations. You only need to use your palm and your eye. One serving size of plant-based protein is equivalent to 2 cups (500 mL) and for animal-based protein, about the size and thickness of your palm.

THE WORLD'S BEST HIGH-NUTRIENT DIET COMPOSITION

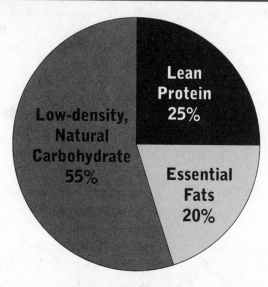

You should work with a knowledgeable physician or qualified nutritional consultant to determine the best ratio for yourself based on extensive blood tests. Each of us has biochemical individuality specific to our biological and physiological needs, and this ratio may change throughout your life.

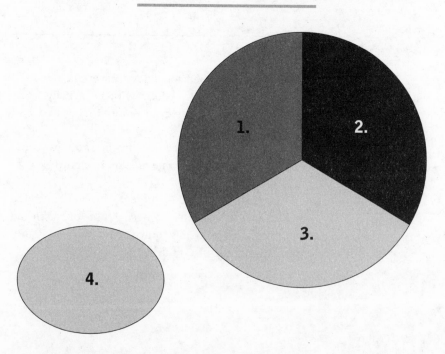

Acceptable protein sources are shown in the table below.

Animal-Based Protein	Lacto-Ovo Vegetarian	Vegetarians
• Whey protein (isolate powder)	• Whey protein (isolate powder)	• Soy protein (isolate powder)
• Soy protein (isolate powder)	• Soy protein (isolate powder)	• Raw seeds and nuts
• Chicken	• Fat-free yogurt	• Nutritional yeast
• Fish	• Low-fat cheese	• Legumes
• Turkey	• Free-range, organic eggs	• Peas
• Lamb	• bee pollen	• Whole grains
• Wild game	• Raw goat's milk	• Bee pollen
• Eggs	• Raw seeds and nuts	• Soy beans
• Low-fat cheese	• Nutritional yeast	• Grasses
• Fat-free yogurt	• Legumes (lentils)	– alfalfa
• Raw seeds and nuts	• Peas (split peas)	– barley
• Soy beans	• Whole grains	– wheatgrass
• Legumes	• Soy beans	• Sea vegetables
• Peas	• Grasses	– spirulina
• Grain	– alfalfa	– chlorella
• Grasses	– barley	– Nova Scotia dulse
– alfalfa	– wheatgrass	• Extra-firm tofu
– barley	• Sea vegetables	– tempeh
– wheatgrass	– spirulina	– miso
• Bee pollen	– chlorella	– soy burgers
• Sea vegetables	– Nova Scotia dulse	– edamame (green soy beans)
– spirulina	• Extra-firm tofu	
– chlorella	– tempeh	
– Nova Scotia dulse	– miso	
• Extra-firm tofu	– soy burgers	
– tempeh	– edamame (green soy beans)	
– miso		
– soy burgers		
– edamame (green soy beans)		

Portion 2: About one-third of your plate should be low-density carbohydrates such as colorful vegetables, lightly steamed to "crunchy-tender." Acceptable vegetables are:
- artichokes, asparagus, acorn squash, avocado;
- beets, beet tops, bamboo shoots, bean sprouts, bok choy, broccoli, Brussels sprouts;

- green beans, yellow beans, peppers (green, yellow, orange, red);
- cabbage (red or green), cauliflower, celery, collard greens, cucumber, carrots, fresh corn;
- dandelions;
- eggplant, endive, escarole;
- greens, beet tops;
- jalapeño peppers;
- kale;
- lettuce (romaine, leaf, butternut, bibb, mesclun and mizuna);
- leeks;
- onions (all types), okra;
- parsnips, potatoes (red, yellow, white and purple);
- radishes, radicchio, red beets;
- sauerkraut, scallions, shallots, snow peas, spinach, Swiss chard, squash (butternut, spaghetti), sunflower sprouts;
- tomatoes, tomato sauces, chili sauce, salsa, turnips, turnip greens;
- water chestnuts, watercress; and
- zucchini.

Use a stainless steel food grater to add colorful vegetable shreds of raw red cabbage, squash, yams, sweet potatoes, turnips, beets, carrots, garlic and onions. And add fresh herbs and spices (such as parsley, watercress, ginger, rosemary, tarragon, thyme, mint, oregano, cumin, curry, mustard seed, turmeric, basil, marjoram, sage, salsa, cilantro and chili powder) to your protein and vegetables.

I strongly suggest you avoid raw or cooked common button mushrooms (Agaricus bisporus), popular in North America, because of the possible carcinogenic toxin they may contain. Do eat fresh or dried Asian mushrooms such as shiitake (Lentinula edodes), oyster mushrooms (Pleurotus spp), enoki-dake (Flammulina velutipies) and maitake (Grifola frondosa).

Shiitake and maitake are available dried, in a capsule and as a supplement, to give your immune system a boost with their phytonutrient immunologically active polysaccharides, if needed.

Portion 3: The final third of your plate should be comprised of low-density carbohydrates as colorful, zesty, creative salads. Use a variety of fresh herbs in your salads. Make your salads both flavorful and visually appealing by adding grated carrots or beets, sliced onion or pepper rings, soy beans or lentils, or sunflower, sesame or pumpkin seeds that have been dry roasted in a heavy skillet for several minutes.

Your salad can be an entire meal by adding steamed "crunchy-tender" vegetables to the salad and topping it with your protein. This type of salad is outrageously delicious and should be eaten in a large bowl so its aroma and visual presentation can be maximized.

Acceptable salad ingredients are the same as the vegetable selection.

Use 1 tablespoon of extra-virgin olive oil on your salad with 1 teaspoon of fresh lemon, salt-free herbal seasonings, Nova Scotia dulse and a salt-free, non-irradiated all-purpose blend of dry herbs.

Portion 4: The bowl should contain low-density carbohydrates such as whole grains that are used as condiments. Whole grains are rich in soluble fiber, but should be used in moderation.

Acceptable grains and grain products are:
- Essene sprouted breads (usually in coolers of health food stores);
- whole-grain boiled bagel (small);
- sourdough whole-grain breads (two slices); avoid wheat and try breads from rye, spelt, amaranth, rice, millet or buckwheat;
- hot cooked grains such as millet, rice (basmati or brown), barley or quinoa, buckwheat or Kasha, bulgur wheat or couscous (1 cup/250 mL);
- whole-grain pasta (1 cup/250 mL);
- sprouted wheat wrap-ups (two);
- whole-grain pita bread (one piece);
- popcorn (4 cups/1 L);
- corn or sprouted wheat tortilla (two); and
- cereals such as oatmeal, multi-grain cereals or cream of rice (1 cup/250 mL).

Timing

When we eat is just as important as what we eat. Erratic eating habits—or skipping a meal—will undermine our energy level.

There is wisdom in the adage "Breakfast is the most important meal of the day." A good night's sleep raises dopamine and cortisol levels, which rouse us in the morning. Our body will use the "short-term" fat storage fuel mix, glycogen, available in our muscles and liver to get us physically going. But by mid-morning the storage has been depleted, energy levels fade, and we begin to feel drowsy and most likely irritable. The morning's demands cannot be met with vigor, and the stress on an underfueled body raises the corrosive stress hormone cortisol, as well as other stress hormones.

Refueling in the morning when we rise is critical. Dr. Wayne Callaway, M.D., associate clinical professor of medicine at George Washington University, observes that breakfast increases the metabolic rate by 25 percent and makes us feel good.

Edmund R. Burke, Ph.D., author of *Optimal Muscle Recovery* writes, "In addition to providing energy for muscle contraction, glucose is a vital source of energy for the brain and nervous system." No wonder you feel so drained and mentally exhausted by late morning. When you do not eat breakfast, your brain and nervous system take a rapid nosedive. "In fact, 50 percent of the glucose supplied by the liver is used strictly for brain and nervous system function."

Dr. Sarah Leibowitz, Ph.D., professor of psychology at Rockefeller University, found that neuropeptide Y (NPY) levels are highest in the early morning. NPY is the neurotransmitter that measures the glycogen stores, somewhat like a chemical "dip-stick." NPY sparks the appetite for carbohydrates to replenish the depleted "short-term" fuel storage levels drained while we slept.

A body that has exhausted the last of its glycogen fuel supplies and is struggling to meet the demands of the day, experiences stress that will trigger the release of the stress hormones cortisol and norepinephrine (a derivative of adrenaline) from the adrenal glands. Stress also triggers NPY and galanin production and activity—both powerful brain chemicals that spark our appetite. This increases our cravings for carbohydrates and fats, and often leads to overeating and unwanted weight gain.

In desperation, you may reach for a donut and coffee—which temporarily reduces your drowsiness, but in an hour you'll lose the energy gain and mental power. This can start the vicious cycle of craving processed carbohydrates to alleviate your weariness and mental fatigue, and you become addicted and reach for another coffee and muffin as a mood and energy-altering fix. That is how easily we get hooked and these cravings are only met with high-calorie foods and weight gain.

If you have been skipping breakfast, start eating it from now on, even when you are not hungry. It will take you only three weeks to reset your appetite clock, once you begin.

The very best energy-boosting breakfasts mix one part protein to two parts low-density complex carbohydrates, with a little fat high in long-chain Omega-3 essential fatty acids, high in DHA and EPA . After exercising, your very best energy-boosting breakfast is one part protein to four parts low-density complex carbohydrates, with the same long-chain Omega-3 fats.

The higher the NPY levels, the greater the urge and the more you will enjoy the carbohydrates. Your carbohydrate cravings diminish as NPY levels decrease and your appetite control center becomes balanced.

RECOMMENDED DAILY BREAKFAST

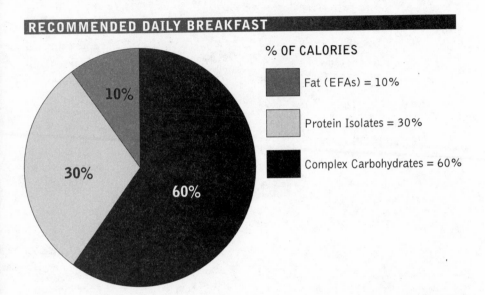

% OF CALORIES

Fat (EFAs) = 10%

Protein Isolates = 30%

Complex Carbohydrates = 60%

RECOMMENDED BREAKFAST AFTER EXERCISING

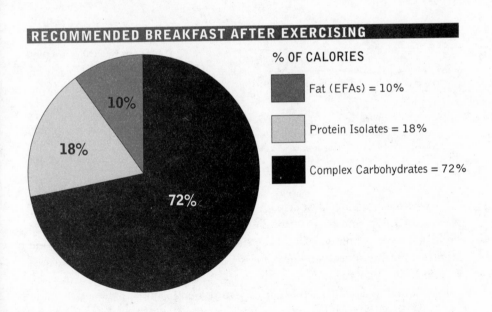

% OF CALORIES

Fat (EFAs) = 10%

Protein Isolates = 18%

Complex Carbohydrates = 72%

THE IDEAL BREAKFAST PROMOTES HORMONE HARMONY

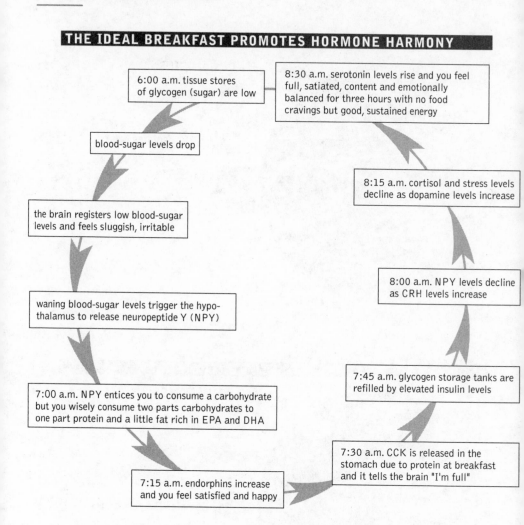

6:00 a.m. tissue stores of glycogen (sugar) are low

8:30 a.m. serotonin levels rise and you feel full, satiated, content and emotionally balanced for three hours with no food cravings but good, sustained energy

blood-sugar levels drop

8:15 a.m. cortisol and stress levels decline as dopamine levels increase

the brain registers low blood-sugar levels and feels sluggish, irritable

8:00 a.m. NPY levels decline as CRH levels increase

waning blood-sugar levels trigger the hypothalamus to release neuropeptide Y (NPY)

7:45 a.m. glycogen storage tanks are refilled by elevated insulin levels

7:00 a.m. NPY entices you to consume a carbohydrate but you wisely consume two parts carbohydrates to one part protein and a little fat rich in EPA and DHA

7:30 a.m. CCK is released in the stomach due to protein at breakfast and it tells the brain "I'm full"

7:15 a.m. endorphins increase and you feel satisfied and happy

A well-balanced breakfast actually helps us to control our appetite. We have a built-in checks-and-balances brain meter that registers when we have had enough to eat. Cholecystokinin (CCK) is released from the protein in the stomach and intestines, sending a message of satiation to our brain. Elevated insulin levels after the meal also "turn off" NPY and "turn on" corticotropin-releasing hormone (CRH), which further curbs our appetite.

Studies have shown that protein, when combined with carbohydrate, almost doubles the insulin response and increases the rate of glycogen synthesis by 30 percent. However, protein stimulates the chemical release of CCK in the stomach and intestines, which slows the rate of gastric emptying. This is the rate at which our stomach contents are emptied into the intestines. Therefore, too much protein at breakfast slows fluid and electrolyte replacement, because fluids must first leave the stomach and enter the intestines to be absorbed into the bloodstream.

By carefully balancing carbohydrate and protein to a critical ratio, which Dr. Burke calls "the optimum recovery ratio or OR^2," we successfully balance the two opposing hormones insulin and glucagon. This ratio is four parts complex carbohydrate to one part protein after exercising in the morning, or two parts carbohydrate to one part protein for breakfast if we have not exercised before breakfast. Fat intake is minimized at breakfast because fat, like protein, stimulates CCK, which has a negative effect on gastric emptying. A four-to-one ratio after exercise enhances the insulin response to refill glycogen storage tanks without affecting the rate of gastric emptying.

Combining a little highly absorbable protein with fiber-rich complex carbohydrates at breakfast helps to keep us full, satisfied, energized and happy for three full hours, until having a snack at about 10:00 a.m. Researchers at the Massachusetts Institute of Technology (MIT) found that too much protein at breakfast leads to fatigue and sleepiness. Likewise, researchers at the Wageningen Agricultural University in the Netherlands compared the results of high-protein, high-fat breakfasts of bacon and eggs—to breakfasts of small amounts of protein, with a smidgen of fat and complex carbohydrates. The high-protein meal led to hunger, lethargy, increased food cravings and overeating at lunch time. The complex carbohydrate (four parts after exercising or two parts for a breakfast not following exercise) to bioavailable protein (one part), along with a little fat, made participants feel energized, full, happy and satiated.

When too much protein is consumed, between 40 and 50 grams at breakfast, the body converts the excess to fat and increases the blood levels of ammonia and uric acid. Ammonia and uric acid are toxic metabolic waste products that make us feel sluggish and sabotage our morning's performance.

There is one exception I must draw your attention to. If you are a serious athlete, you want to gain maximum lean muscle mass and shed fat, to accelerate peak performance. To accomplish this you must eat every three hours to keep your amino acid pool full and available to your muscles. Have two to three power protein shakes daily with 35 (women) to 40 (men) grams of protein in each.

If you are a serious body builder, I would follow Michael Colgan, Ph.D.'s excellent calculation. To both maintain present muscle and grow new muscle at optimum potential, Dr. Colgan suggests serious, elite athletes' protein consumption should be 1.9 grams per kg of body weight.

The Best Breakfast Plan

The best dietary strategy for breakfast is:

1. Rehydrate with 8 to 32 oz (250 mL to 1 L) of room-temperature water, with a dash of fresh lemon or lime juice, and drink it through a straw, as soon as you wake up. Place the water by your bedside just before you go to sleep.
2. Fifteen minutes later have a "green drink," supplying you with 1,000 mg, if not more, of phosphatidyl choline (PC) and 60 mg of phosphatidyl serine

(PS), the building blocks of the brain-stimulating neurotransmitter acetyl-choline. This kick-starts your positive mental acuity. Have this "green drink" in water, supplying about 35 calories and zero sugars, or with just 4 oz of unsweetened juice.

A "green drink" should contain the glutathione-flavonoid subnetwork of these six herbal extracts:

- milk thistle;
- Siberian ginseng;
- ginkgo biloba;
- Japanese green tea;
- European bilberry; and
- full-spectrum grape seed and skin extract.

Glutathione is the most important cellular antioxidant and must be replenished in the morning to protect your energy factories, the mitochondria in each cell, from excessive "wear and tear," called oxidation.

3. Have a healthful, light breakfast of a power protein shake that takes five minutes to prepare. This will fuel you right through the morning hours with energy and a perfectly balanced hormonal symphony—homeostasis—until your 10:00 a.m. snack of zesty raw vegetable sticks to keep your blood sugar balanced.

You must not drink a protein shake too quickly, but slightly chew each mouthful before swallowing, to begin the process of digestion. You may choose to also consume a thin slice of whole-grain bread with just 1 teaspoon of almond butter if you feel hungry after consuming the power protein shake.

A healthful addition is 1 tablespoon of high DHA/EPA cod liver oil or krill oil, or two fish oil softgels of salmon, sardines, anchovies or mackerel oils, or six to nine algae-extracted oil capsules—all rich in brain- and heart-healthy DHA and EPA. This gives you 5 grams of fat, and about 45 calories from fat. This small amount of fat keeps levels of the neurotransmitter galanin steady as the hormone leptin "turns off" galanin secretion when fat is eaten so you do not crave fats. Sarah Leibowitz, Ph.D.'s research demonstrates that to survive, our hunter-gatherer ancestors developed a built-in appetite system for fat, the long-term storage fuel. This appetite is regulated by galanin, which rises as the day progresses and triggers a desire for fatty foods at dinner. It is lowest in the morning and highest at dinner. Leptin is the hormone monitoring your fat deposits and it turns galanin "on" or "off."

Galanin, along with other hormones, converts dietary fat into body fat. As galanin levels go up, body fat goes up. Galanin and endorphins (the euphoric or pleasurable feeling hormone) coexist in the same nerve cells. Both sugar and fat release endorphins in the brain for a natural euphoric feeling. Galanin drives you to eat ice cream or chocolate, and your endorphins make it a pleasurable experience. That is why it is hard to eat just one cookie or one spoonful of ice cream.

A MORNING "GREEN DRINK" INCREASES MENTAL ACUITY

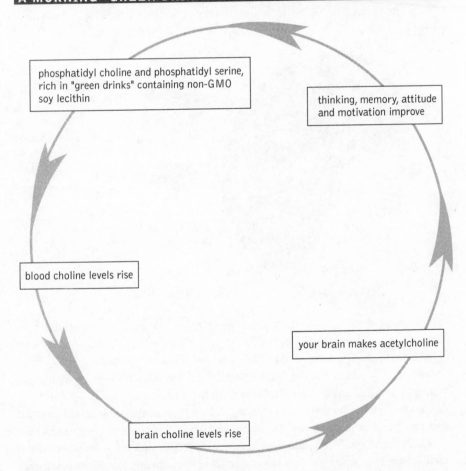

phosphatidyl choline and phosphatidyl serine, rich in "green drinks" containing non-GMO soy lecithin

thinking, memory, attitude and motivation improve

blood choline levels rise

your brain makes acetylcholine

brain choline levels rise

Final Thoughts on Breakfast: This is our most important meal for jump-starting our body in the morning and to initiate hormonal harmony. Nancy Clark, M.S., R.D., author of *Nancy Clark's Sports Nutrition Guidebook: Eating to Fuel Your Active Lifestyle*, writes, "The biggest mistake people make is they eat too little early in the day, start craving sweets by mid-afternoon, and end up eating anything in sight."

The right foods, at the right time for breakfast, could be one answer to fighting depression, stress, a lack of energy, an inability to concentrate, or the inability to fall asleep quickly.

Make a lifelong commitment to be your healthiest—physically, mentally and emotionally. If you slip, don't get down on yourself; just make your next meal well balanced. It is the rate of recovery that is so important.

Lunch

Our lunch should be eaten at about noon, about two hours after our mid-morning snack.

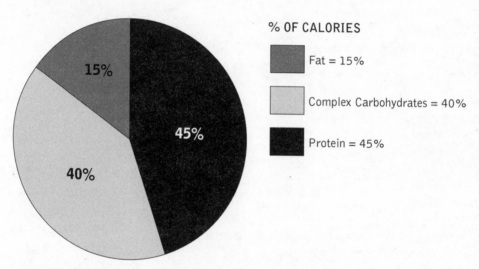

% OF CALORIES

Fat = 15%

Complex Carbohydrates = 40%

Protein = 45%

Whether we are at school, in an office, working outdoors, at home, traveling or eating in a restaurant, this is the meal at which we should emphasize lean protein and low-density carbohydrates that are minimally processed.

The ideal lunch would be a crisp salad, two servings of vegetables steamed "crunchy-tender" and a lean source of protein.

The vegetables should be contrasting colors such as the red-orange of yams and the green of broccoli; the yellow of squash and the red of beets; the green of Swiss chard with the yellow of beans; the deep purple of cabbage with the vivid orange of carrots; or the pungent red, yellow or white of onions contrasted to the green, orange and red of sweet peppers.

The vegetables and salad can be mixed together with a dressing. The dressing I make daily consists of 1 tablespoon of extra-virgin olive oil, 1 teaspoon of fresh lemon or lime juice, salt-free herbal mixes and some fresh culinary herbs (such as basil, lovage, parsley, cilantro, thyme, rosemary, mint, sage and Nova Scotia dulse). You can also add fresh minced ginger or exotic spices such as curry, chili peppers, turmeric, black pepper, horseradish or mustard.

To this dressing, I add 1 tablespoon of seaweed gomasio from Eden Foods. This is a combination of organic, dry-roasted sesame seeds combined with three sea vegetables (kombu, nori and Nova Scotia dulse). This is an ingredient combination suggested by George Ohsawa, the Japanese patriarch of macrobiotics.

If you are out at a restaurant, ask the server to request that the kitchen uses no salt or sauces on your vegetables.

You can add your protein source now to balance your carbohydrates. You can add a chicken breast broiled without the skin, an extra-firm tofu steak, double tempeh patties, three hard-boiled eggs (eating only two of the three yolks), fat-free cottage cheese, soy beans, baked salmon, baked beans or lentils, fat-free yogurt, almonds, dry-roasted peanuts or sunflower seeds.

If the salad or vegetable selections are marginal, you can quickly mix a "green drink" in water or unsweetened juice to get all your vegetable nutrients with no sugar and only 35 calories. A single serving of the most superior "green drinks" is equivalent to six servings of fresh, organic salads or vegetables. When you are traveling, studying, trying to meet family obligations, working to meet a deadline or racing through a busy schedule, you can mix your "green drink" and your whey or soy (or both) protein isolate powders for a world-class, easily digested, five-minutes-to-prepare lunch.

Women should consume 30 grams of protein and men 35 to 40 grams at lunchtime to meet the protein demands of the afternoon.

Protein sources at lunch should emphasize abundant food sources of the neurotransmitter phosphatidyl choline (PC) for a neurological boost, for clear, focused, elevated mental acuity.

Lunch should also contain high amounts of the amino acid tyrosine—which, along with magnesium and vitamin B6, makes the "stay-sharp" hormone dopamine. High dopamine levels in early afternoon keep us alert, vigilant, motivated and able to energetically compete successfully. Large amounts of the amino acid tryptophan will help make the serotonin hormone that is necessary for mental balance, good moods, behavior modification and clarity.

Eating "smart" at lunch can increase dopamine and serotonin levels to increase anabolic capacity and anabolic drive so your afternoon commitments are met with enthusiasm, zest and mental clarity.

You can also have one or two cups of plain, caffeinated or decaffeinated green tea before your lunch.

HORMONE-BALANCING LUNCH SUGGESTIONS

Selected Food	PC* Umol/kg	Calories	TYR* (mg)	TRYP* (mg)	Fat (g)	Carbs (g)	Protein (g)
"Green drink" with 97% oil-free lecithin and phosphatidyl choline (PC)	75,000	35	1,070	400	2.0	12.0	3.0
Fat-free cottage cheese (1 cup/250 mL)	500	30	1,490	300	0.5	5.0	26.0
Soy beans (1 cup/250 mL)	40,000	300	1,092	420	15.0	17.3	29.0
Chicken breast without skin	18	185	970	310	7.2	0.0	29.3
Fat-free yogurt (1 cup/250 mL)	38	30	601	65	0.5	14	13.1
Beans baked (1 cup/250 mL)	420	380	385	169	13.0	53.9	16
Peanuts, dry roasted (1 oz/28 g)	4,960	160	363	62	13.9	164	6.6
Hard-boiled egg white (one)	0	16	135	42	0.0	0.3	8.5
Hard-boiled whole egg (one)	52,000	77	261	76	5.2	0.3	8.7
Raw almonds (1 oz/28 g)	5,000	174	169	45	14	6.0	7.1
Cauliflower, steamed (1/2 cup/125 mL)	2,750	15	24	19	0.1	2.5	1.5
Whole-grain bread (one slice)	352	71	60	60	1.0	11.0	3.1
Spinach, steamed (1/2 cup/125 mL)	05	21	18	36	0.2	3.4	2.8
Broccoli, steamed (1/2 cup/125 mL)	07	22	19	24	0.3	4.0	2.5

*PC = phosphatidyl choline, TYR = tyrosine, TRYP = tryptophan.

Dinner

The dinner meal should contain ample bioenergetic, low-density, natural carbohydrates; a moderate amount of protein; a small amount of fat; ample natural fibers from several sources—and should total about 500 calories.

Carbohydrates: Dinner should be built around complex carbohydrates with an idea of what lean protein might accompany it. A crisp salad, a medley of colorful vegetables lightly steamed in bamboo containers, or assorted fresh vegetables sautéed or roasted are all excellent choices.

Whole-grain pasta cooked al dente; brown or basmati herbal rice; whole-grain bread, buns or sprouted wheat wraps; cooked whole grains such as millet, amaranth, quinoa, kamut, buckwheat or wild rice; oven-baked red potato, orange yams and yellow sweet potato "fries"; a baked potato with salsa or baked yam; curried sweet potato with fresh green tender peas; savory Swedish poppy seed dandelion coleslaw; cool gazpacho with chickpeas; garlic linguine with broccoli and roasted yellow peppers; gingery carrot-rosemary soup; snappy green beans with fresh dill and whole pan-roasted almonds topped with broccoli sprouts—all would make delicious additions.

As would a stir-fry with wild rice, soba noodles or rice noodles; a lovely marinara sauce on kamut pasta; Indian cumin spiced cucumber raita; feta Greek salad; Russian beet spinach salad; steamed winter squash with walnuts and pine nuts; or a savory guacamole with sunflower sprouts.

Fats: For the fat source, I highly recommend 1 to 2 tablespoons of extra-virgin olive oil on the salad or vegetables. Always stir fry in water and add the olive oil at the very end to add flavor and aroma, without heating the oil. One-half tablespoon of hemp or flax seed oil may be used in place of the olive oil.

Protein: Protein sources are endless. It can be hummus from chickpeas; lentils with kale or Swiss chard; Mexican pinto beans with tangy salsa and cilantro garnish; eggplant-walnut-baked extra-firm tofu; miso soup with green onions and green peas; or tempeh topped with grated carrots, beets and turnips.

Or it can be baked tarragon-lemon ginger salmon; a lime garlic paprika chicken breast cooked without the skin and with subcutaneous fat removed; roasted turkey with assorted herb rub; or water-packed, low-sodium, solid white albacore tuna.

You may try thick soups or stews such as fragrant asparagus soup with poached eggs or roasted vegetable stew with watercress and soybeans. I like thick winter root stews with yams, turnips, parsnips, roasted garlic, red onion, parsley, herbal extra-firm tofu, and topped with watercress, chopped red peppers, chopped green onions and pan-roasted sunflower seeds.

Wraps are a quick and easy dinner to make along with a salad. Thai wraps with peanut sauce and chicken slices or a spicy black bean burrito wrapped in a 12-inch (30 cm) sprouted wheat tortilla are crowd pleasers.

One dish that not only is a breakfast staple—but is also a perfect dinner ratio meal is a hot seven-grain cereal, millet, oatmeal or cream of rice, mixed with 15 grams of protein of either whey protein isolate powder or soy protein isolate powder, to enhance the protein-to-carbohydrate ratio. Top any of these grains with 1 tablespoon each of almonds, flax seeds, sunflower seeds and pumpkin seeds. One tablespoon of bee pollen and 4 tablespoons of organic, plain, fat-free yogurt are optional. You can do what I do. I grind the flax seeds in a coffee grinder for five seconds, then add them on top of the cooked grain. Try doing this with all the seeds and nuts to ensure you will digest them.

Fiber: All of these suggestions contain about 15 grams of both soluble and insoluble fiber from natural sources. Fiber is the indigestible part of whole foods that makes up much of the bulk of stool. We can all benefit by eating more of it.

Insoluble fiber includes cellulose and lignin, which occur in whole grains, and hemicellulose, which is slightly soluble in water and occurs in vegetables, fruits, seeds, nuts and whole grains. Collectively, these fibers protect the health of our intestinal tract, gently scrubbing it clean, increasing stool bulk and decreasing its transit time.

We require 40 grams of fiber a day to keep our intestinal tract clean and healthy.

I do not recommend taking fiber supplements as powders, pills or as brans. They may interfere with the absorption of minerals, and can impede bowel movements unless a large quantity of water is drunk with them. Just simply eat more vegetables, fruits, whole grains, seeds, nuts and herbs, and you will have all the fiber you need from whole foods.

Fiber is critical at dinner because it remains in our small and large intestine while we sleep. During deep sleep, when growth hormone is being released in spurts, our body is actually cleaning out all the biochemical cellular debris from the hard work they just did all day. Eventually, by early morning, our body escorts all the waste material to our intestinal tract as "garbage disposal." It is the fiber that literally soaks up the waste, binds it and eliminates it safely from the bowel. For superior inner hygiene—we can keep our intestinal tract clean with many sources of fiber. If we do not eat enough fiber, much of the waste material in our "garbage disposal" does not get excreted but accumulates in the intestinal tract as a putrefying, hardening crust. The buildup of this material prevents the body from being able to absorb nutrients from food, as the putrefying material blocks the "portals of entry" on intestinal walls.

This may be the primary reason we put weight on so easily in North America. If the "portals of entry" are blocked, we eat and eat but the brain is not able to detect nutrients being absorbed and thus it encourages us to keep eating in desperate hope of finding the vitamins, minerals, fats, carbohydrates and protein necessary for survival. This is sheer stress—desperate stress to our body—and promotes an early extinction. Putrefying material gives off toxins that the intestines absorb in a process called autointoxication.

Transit time is how long it takes after food is eaten until its residues are excreted through the anus. The shorter the transit time, the less the food residues will putrefy before being expelled from your body, and the less will be resultant autointoxication.

Transit time should be about 12 hours. It takes eight hours for food to travel through the stomach and small intestine, and the remainder of the transit time is spent in the colon. The average transit time for North Americans is 24 to 30 hours.

Dietary fiber from bioenergetic whole foods lowers the levels of two fatty substances in the blood known as cholesterol and triglycerides. Reducing the blood levels of both is highly beneficial to good health.

You should have three, well-formed, easily eliminated, bowel movements each day. If you are eating enough fiber and drinking enough water, your stool should ideally float on top of the water. Dysfunctional bowel movements and autointoxication are surprisingly prevalent.

No Late-Night Meals

Late-night cravings for sweet-and-creamy foods like ice cream or salty-and-greasy foods like potato chips are most common when we skip dinner, avoid lunch, or eat too many sugary foods throughout the day. These cravings are mostly conditioned responses: the more often we snack at night, the stronger our body's craving to snack night after night.

We should try not to eat dinner after 7:30 p.m. This will allow insulin levels to decline by 10:00 p.m., when we are ready for deep sleep. Once our glycogen storage tanks are full, to supply the brain and millions of night-time metabolic processes with the fuel-mix blood glucose, we can have an uninterrupted night, without the urge to refuel mid-sleep.If we eat later than 7:30 p.m., insulin levels will still be high when we go to sleep and high insulin levels drive down melatonin and growth hormone levels, which means we are accelerating aging and promoting a catabolic decline. Melatonin is our strongest anti-cancer hormone and a powerful antioxidant.

If we do eat dinner by 7:30 p.m., our glycogen storage tanks are full by 10:00 p.m., which allows high-fidelity hormonal synthesis and an anabolic, life-regenerative hormone cascade to follow.

Your Elegant Hormonal Cascades

5:00 p.m.	1. The neurotransmitter galanin begins to rise, signaling the enzyme lipoprotein lipase to store fat as a "backup" energy source for the long night's deep sleep—"a famine period."
8:00 p.m.	2. Serotonin levels rise from the complex carbohydrates eaten at dinner, leaving us feeling satisfied, satiated and calm; neuropeptide Y (NPY) levels decline.
	3. Dopamine levels decrease as our brain prepares for sleep.

4. Cortisol levels and norepinephrine levels decline sharply as our mental functions, stress, alertness and energy levels decline as the competition of the day is removed.

5. The brain's feedback loop tells the body it has had enough to eat, as cholecystokinin (CCK) is released from the intestines after dinner and sends a message of satiation to the brain. This feedback loop turns "on" corticotropin-releasing hormone (CRH) in the brain, which curbs appetite and suppresses NPY.

   The hormone galanin, notified by leptin hormonal levels, which acts as a fat-monitoring "dipstick," is kept in check by eating some, but not too much, fat.

   The appetite-control symphony of hormones and neurotransmitters have elegantly cascaded following our built-in checks-and-balances chemicals, to promote sleep and rejuvenation at a cellular level, once it gets dark.

9:00 p.m.   6. Melatonin is synthesized in the pineal gland from serotonin once sundown begins and the rose-yellow-orange light spectrum, as photons, is brought into our bloodstream by the cryptochrome cells on our skin that measure light and dark. Melatonin puts us into a deep sleep if our bedroom is dark. Light dramatically reduces the amplitude of the circadian melatonin rhythm. Insulin levels decline. The body's core temperature declines in circadian temperature rhythm during this revitalizing, cool "shut down" phase.

1:00 a.m.   7. Growth hormone (GH) is secreted in spurts for the next five to six hours to reinvigorate all of our 100 trillion cells.

8. Glucagon rises as insulin has declined to feed the brain and diverse metabolic processes with the fuel-mix blood glucose, stored in the "short-term" fuel storage tanks of the liver and muscles. This allows us to sleep without refueling with food during the night.

3:00 a.m.	9.	Prolactin is secreted for a calm mind and central nervous system so we may sort out and deeply integrate life—between the subconscious and conscious mind. This is an excellent time to meditate or pray.
6:00 a.m.	10.	Cortisol levels and dopamine levels begin to rise with the green spectrum light of the early morning, as photons brought into our bloodstream by the cryptochrome cells on our skin that monitor light and dark to rev up our biochemical systems make us alert and motivated to function at optimum.
6:30 a.m.	11.	Neuropeptide Y (NPY), as a neurotransmitter, rises to urge us to eat low-density carbohydrate to replenish glycogen fuel tanks depleted during the night, supplying our brain and body with a glucose fuel mix while we slept, sparing us from interrupting our deep sleep to "hunt" or "gather" food.
	12.	The neurotransmitter phosphytidyl choline (PC) rises to activate the successful transmission, across synaptic intersections or gaps, for brain messages, instructing how our 100 trillion cells should function optimally.

All hormones and neurotransmitters function in a harmonious balance biologists call homeostasis and quantum physicists calls supersymmetry. Our bioenergetic food choices and living in sync with the circadian rhythms of night (dark) and day (light) allow us to function in optimal physical, mental, emotional and spiritual harmony.

Erratic eating and sleeping habits can cause our hormones to be topsy-turvy and be way "out of whack"—an imbalance that contributes to chronic disease, a self-propelled early extinction event.

HOW MUCH DO YOU NEED EVERY DAY?
Choose your level of activity from the table below and plug the number into the equations shown to get your exact daily calorie and macronutrient requirements.

CALORIE REQUIREMENTS BASED ON DAILY PHYSICAL ACTIVITY	
Level of Activity	**Multiplier**
(a) Sedentary	1.0
(b) Light activity (walking)	1.1
(c) Active (exercise four hours a week)	1.2
(d) Very active (exercise five or more hours per week)	1.3
(e) Strength athlete (exercising for maximum muscle growth)	1.5
(f) Elite athlete	1.5

Three-Step Exact Daily Calorie and Macronutrient Requirement

Step 1: Calculate Your Daily Calorie Needs: Multiply your present weight by a factor of 15 if you wish to maintain your current weight and 10 if you wish to lose weight. Multiply the result by the Physical Activity multiplier. For example:

(a) 120-pound active woman who wants to maintain her weight:

120 x 15 = 1,800 x 1.2 = 2,160 calories required daily

(b) 160-pound man who does light activity and wants to lose weight:

160 x 10 = 1,600 x 1.1 = 1,760 calories required daily

Step 2: Calculate the Number of Calories from Carbohydrates, Protein and Fat: I am recommending that we take 55 percent of our calories from carbohydrates; 25 percent of our calories from protein; and 20 percent of our calories from fat. Therefore, our examples would show:

(a) 2,160 total calories x .55 = 1,188 calories from carbohydrates

2,160 total calories x .25 = 540 calories from protein

2,160 total calories x .20 = 432 calories from fat

(b) 1,760 total calories x .55 = 968 calories from carbohydrates

1,760 total calories x .25 = 440 calories from protein

1,760 total calories x .20 = 352 calories from fat

Step 3: Calculate Daily Minimum Needs in Grams: If you would prefer to work with grams, there are 4 calories in every gram of carbohydrates; 4 calories in every gram of protein and 8 calories in every gram of fat. Therefore, our active woman would require 297 grams of carbohydrates; 135 grams of protein; and 54 grams of fat. Our man with some weight to lose would need 242 grams of carbohydrates; 110 grams of protein and 44 grams of fat.

Athletes Need More Protein: It takes a lot more protein for our body to grow new drug-free muscle than to just keep the muscle it has. Gains will depend on genetic type, our age, and how long we have been seriously training with weights. Athletes don't exercise—they train. Avoid anabolic steroids that build weak and unnatural muscle constructs that do not form part of the normal contractile apparatus of muscle. They form temporary constructions that are never as strong as they look and disappear rapidly when the drugs stop. Build drug-free muscle from high-BV diverse protein sources daily, spaced among three meals and a 10:00 a.m., as well as a 3:00 p.m. protein snack.

To build muscle, we must be in a positive nitrogen balance. Nitrogen leaves the body primarily in the urine. Nitrogen lost by excretion must be replaced by nitrogen taken in from food. Protein contains a fairly large concentration of nitrogen. Generally, healthy adults are in a nitrogen equilibrium, or zero balance—that is, their protein intake meets their protein requirement. A positive nitrogen balance means the body is retaining dietary protein and using it to synthesize new protein tissues. If more nitrogen is excreted than was consumed, the nitrogen balance is negative. The body has lost nitrogen—and therefore protein. A negative nitrogen balance over time is a dangerous catabolic drive, leading to muscle wasting and disease.

Strength training enhances nitrogen retention. In other words, protein is retained and used to synthesize new tissue.

Have your health professional run a routine blood chemistry panel, which contains a number for your blood urea nitrogen (BUN) level. Protein is the only food that contains nitrogen. The BUN number can be a marker of protein breakdown by oxidation or the elimination of urea by your kidneys. Either one can indicate an early protein problem. If the number is very low, it may mean you are not eating enough protein. A high-normal value can mean a pronounced breakdown of protein (if kidney function is normal), or be a marker of excessive protein intake. Track it over time and correlate it with your protein intake.

ONE FINAL THOUGHT

It is important that we enjoy dinner and let go of the anxiety and stress of the day. It is also critical to say, or sing, a grace before dinner to experience and demonstrate gratitude for the life-sustaining food that maintains our well-being. And pray for those without food!

I personally say a grace over every food, snack or meal I eat, no matter where I am, or what the conditions are.

11

CARBOHYDRATES: OUR HIGH-OCTANE FUEL SUPPLY

Carbohydrates are the leading nutrient fuel for our body. They are broken down during digestion into glucose, which circulates in our bloodstream and is used by our brain and nervous system for energy. If our brain cells are deprived of glucose, our mental acuity immediately suffers. If our muscles are deprived of glucose, our physical stamina and energy likewise suffer.

I highly recommend that we stock up on colorful vegetables, salads, herbs, sea vegetables and a moderate amount of fruit rather than bread, rice, potatoes and pasta. Always remember that any food that is not a protein or a fat is a carbohydrate.

CARBOHYDRATES: NOT ALL CREATED EQUAL

Very low-density carbohydrates like vegetables, herbs and sea vegetables are powerhouses of vitamins, minerals and fiber and contain little sugar. They take up a lot of room on our plate and add color with few calories. Even on a voluntary calorie-restricted diet, we can eat large amounts of vegetables and salads, so we never feel deprived. And the fewer the calories we eat, the fewer the free radicals we produce, the slower we age—and the greater our healthy longevity.

Their fiber content slows down the entry rate of any carbohydrate, as sugar, into the bloodstream, thereby lowering insulin secretion.

Fruits are also low-density carbohydrates, but contain more sugar than vegetables, and are in a slowly metabolized form called fructose.

Vegetables and salads should be our primary source of low-density carbohydrates, supplemented with lesser amounts of fruits.

High-density carbohydrates like refined sugar and starch have much less fiber and more readily available sugar than very low-density or low-density carbohydrates in vegetables or fruit. The amount of carbohydrate in a commercial cinnamon roll, for example, is equivalent to 6 cups of steamed vegetables or 3 cups of phytonutrient-rich berries. And it contains 12 teaspoons of added sugar, virtually no nutrients, and 670 calories. Six cups of powerful steamed vegetables, on the other hand, contain virtually no sugar, but a storehouse of fiber, vitamins, minerals and only 250 calories.

> One trick I've learned is that fat carries the aroma, and sugar the sweet taste in high-calorie, processed foods. A craving for something sweet or creamy could be fueled by a desire for something tasty. What I do is add non-caloric spices such as vanilla, cinnamon or nutmeg to fat-free plain organic yogurt, which appeases the aroma, and the desire for fat and sweet, without adding unwanted calories.

I strongly recommend that you obtain 55 percent of your total daily calories from complex, low-density carbohydrates. On a diet of 2,000 calories, at least 1,100 of those calories should come from natural, or slightly processed, complex carbohydrates. If you are an elite athlete, I recommend that 60 percent of your calories be from complex, low-density carbohydrates.

Restrict Processed Carbohydrates

Boyd Eaton, Ph.D., M.D., an expert in the diet of early humans and co-author of *The Paleolithic Prescription*, states that 99 percent of our genetic structure was formed about 40,000 years ago. Furthermore, 99 percent of Homo sapiens' genes were formed before the advent of agriculture, 10,000 years ago. Our genes, which control all facets of our life, are the same as those of our early ancestors. It takes almost 100,000 years for any major genetic alteration to become a permanent part of our genes and cells. Processed carbohydrates from grains and sugars have only been in our food supply for 10,000 years. Therefore, it will take another 90,000 years before we can fully adjust to a high-density carbohydrate diet.

Presently, we are not genetically programmed to consume a diet high in simple, high-density carbohydrates from processed or refined foods.

CARBOHYDRATE SOURCES

Food	Amount	Carbohydrates (g)	Calories
Fruit			
Orange	1 medium	15	62
Berries (blueberries)	1 cup	20	70
Apple	1 medium	21	81
Melon (watermelon)	1 medium piece	25	100
Apricots (dried, unsulphured)	¼ cup	25	107
Banana	1 medium	28	109
Vegetables			
Lettuce	1 cup	05	15
Tomatoes	½ cup	10	25
Sunflower sprouts	1 cup	11	25
Peas	½ cup	13	47
Winter squash	½ cup	10	47
Carrots	1 medium	10	48
Yams, sweet potatoes	1 medium	12	49
Beets	1 medium	13	50
Legumes			
Soy beans	1 cup	34	200
Lentils	1 cup	40	230
Pinto beans	1 cup	52	236
Black beans	1 cup	4	240
Navy beans	1 cup	54	296
Pasta and Starches			
Soba noodles (buckwheat)	1 cup	29	156
Spaghetti (al dente)	1 cup	40	197
Baked potato, with skin	1 large	46	201
Baked yam, with skin	1 large	49	206
Brown rice	1 cup	46	218
Grains and Cereals			
Cream of wheat	1 cup	27	129
Cream of rice	1 cup	27	129
Oatmeal, plain	1 cup	34	150
Oatmeal with 1 tbsp each of sunflower seeds, almonds, flax seeds	1 cup	75	362
Granola, low-fat	1 cup	76	364

Food	Amount	Carbohydrates (g)	Calories
Breads			
Essene bread (sprouted)	⅙ loaf	20	110
Matzo	1 sheet	24	112
greens+ bar	1 bar	16	115
Whole wheat	2 slices	26	138
Pita pocket, whole wheat	1	35	170
Tortillas, sprouted wheat	1	35	170
Spelt-rye, sourdough	2 slices	35	175

Carbohydrate Pitfalls

We can help lower cortisol levels, boost our natural defenses, calm ourselves and curb the negative effects of stress on our body and mind by fueling our body with the nutrients it needs to stay healthy, rather than succumb to cravings for starches and sweets.

When we choose protein, fat or carbohydrates to eat, we should eat only bioenergetic whole foods. We thereby avoid excessive calorie consumption and reduce both our fat and sugar intake. This will keep our anabolic drive going— especially during stressful times.

It takes willpower to give our body what it needs rather than what it might be craving.

In times of stress, the hormone cortisol rises and scrambles our appetite-control chemicals. Cortisol lowers serotonin levels (our "stay calm" hormone), reduces dopamine levels (our "stay alert" hormone), but turns "on" the production of neuropeptide Y (NPY). At a time when we need mental, physical and emotional reserves, we may make a poor choice and grab a convenient, attractive, tasty processed food—spurred on by rising NPY levels that urge us to eat a sweet or salty snack or processed grains. The serious dilemma is that these processed snacks—like muffins, potato chips, candy, chocolate bars, French fries, cinnamon rolls, milk-shakes, ice cream, donuts, alcohol, pretzels, bagels and soda pop—compromise our health as they replace nutritious foods, or add unwanted calories and hydro-genated fats full of dangerous trans-fatty acids (TFAs).

Larry Christensen, Ph.D., of the University of South Alabama, reports that people suffering from emotional stress feel better if they are trained to eliminate sugar, fat and coffee from their diets. In fact, during stress, if we cut back on sugar or fat and use a "green drink" to raise the levels of the neurotransmitter acetylcholine (or consume an apple, a piece of watermelon, an herbal relaxing tea such as chamomile, or have a power protein shake with whey isolates), cortisol levels drop dramatically and the stress is mitigated.

MOOD AND FOOD AND BACK TO MOOD: THE WRONG CHOICE

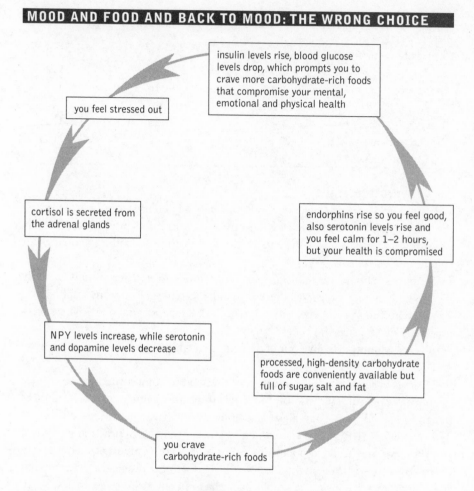

insulin levels rise, blood glucose levels drop, which prompts you to crave more carbohydrate-rich foods that compromise your mental, emotional and physical health

you feel stressed out

cortisol is secreted from the adrenal glands

endorphins rise so you feel good, also serotonin levels rise and you feel calm for 1–2 hours, but your health is compromised

NPY levels increase, while serotonin and dopamine levels decrease

processed, high-density carbohydrate foods are conveniently available but full of sugar, salt and fat

you crave carbohydrate-rich foods

THE GLYCEMIC INDEX OF CARBOHYDRATES

The rate at which carbohydrates are broken down to simple sugars and enter the bloodstream is called the glycemic index. Eating foods with a glycemic index below 60 tends to conserve insulin, energy and moods, balances hormones and adds to our anabolic capacity and anabolic drive. Food binges and overeating are actually encouraged by foods with a glycemic index of 75 or over. It is the blast of insulin from foods with a high index number of 75 or over that drives hunger cravings and causes a sudden release of the hormone insulin, which then causes all other hormones to decline, so we experience mood swings, irritability and weight gain.

Insulin (a storage hormone) stores at least 40 percent of the sugar digested from processed carbohydrate foods—as fat. Foods with a glycemic index of 75 or more are enhancers of the rapidly declining catabolic drive.

We should select our daily foods from bioenergetic whole foods with a glycemic index of 60 and below. Occasionally eat, if necessary, a food choice up

MOOD AND FOOD AND BACK TO MOOD: THE RIGHT CHOICE

the craving stops, insulin levels stay balanced in "homeostasis" and you have enhanced your mood as well as added to your mental, emotional and physical well-being and boosted your anabolic drive

you feel stressed out

cortisol is secreted from the adrenal glands

endorphins rise so you feel good, serotonin levels rise so you feel calm for three hours, the brain chemical acetylcholine rises so you feel mentally alert

NPY levels increase, while serotonin and dopamine levels decrease

you mix a "green drink" in pure water or an unsweetened juice or you mix a protein shake with berries as the carbohydrate

you crave carbohydrate-rich foods but you're trained to eat foods high in the amino acid tyrosine, which raises dopamine levels, as well as raising your serotonin levels with low-density, natural carbohydrates

to 80 but never those over 80, except in the case of carotenoid-rich, colorful carrots, which I encourage you to eat.

Note: Bioenergetic anabolic whole foods have the inherent ability to keep our blood sugar levels even (homeostasis), or normal, so we have no ups or downs but only a constant energy supply at our command, and an even, balanced mental disposition. They are whole foods with a glycemic index of 60 or lower. They are anabolic because they do not cause the pancreas to secrete a lot of the hormone insulin and they favor building lean muscle mass over storing energy as fat. High glycemic index foods with a rating of 60 or above are catabolic and cause our energy to fluctuate, induce definite mood swings and promote food addictions. High glycemic index foods are a definite contributor to the acceleration of aging, an early degenerative-disease model.

THE EFFECT OF FOOD'S SUGAR METABOLISM ON BLOOD SUGAR LEVELS

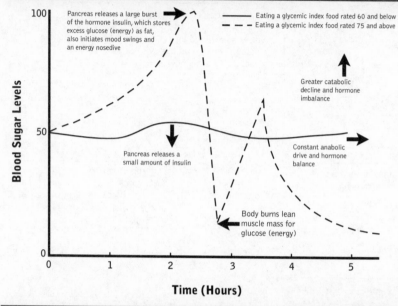

Pancreas releases a large burst of the hormone insulin, which stores excess glucose (energy) as fat, also initiates mood swings and an energy nosedive

——— Eating a glycemic index food rated 60 and below
– – – Eating a glycemic index food rated 75 and above

Greater catabolic decline and hormone imbalance

Pancreas releases a small amount of insulin

Constant anabolic drive and hormone balance

Body burns lean muscle mass for glucose (energy)

Blood Sugar Levels

Time (Hours)

THE GLYCEMIC INDEX OF CARBOHYDRATE FOODS

Fruits		Legumes and Proteins	
Raisins	70–95	Green beans	45
Watermelon	60	Pinto beans	40
Pineapple	60	Lentils	40
Banana	60	Split peas	40
Mango	50	Lima beans	40
Kiwi	50	Soy lecithin, miso, tempeh	35
Grapes	50	Extra-firm tofu	35
Peach	45	Black beans	35
Pear	45	Azuki beans	35
Apples (or sauce)	40	Garbanzo beans	30
Plum, prunes	40	Kidney beans	30
Orange	40	Soy beans (or milk)	30
Apricot	30	Non-GMO soy protein isolate	15
Cherries	25	Whey protein isolate powder	15
Pink grapefruit	25		
Acerola berries	20		
Blueberries	20		
Strawberries	20		
Blackberries	20		
Raspberries	20		
Cranberries	20		

Dairy

Ice cream	80
Yogurt with fruit	35
Organic milk	30
Dry curd, no-fat cottage cheese	15
Organic plain yogurt	10

Fresh or Dried Herbs

Basil	20
Fennel seeds	20
French lavender	20
Lemon balm	15
Marjoram	15
Milk thistle	15
Mint	15
Parsley	15
Rosemary	15
Sage	15
Tarragon	15
Thyme	15
Watercress	15
Commercial dandelions	10

Healthy Herbal Extracts

Full-spectrum grape extract	15
Ginkgo biloba	10
Milk thistle	10
Siberian ginseng	10
Green tea	10
European bilberry	10
Garlic	10
Licorice root	10
Stinging nettle	10
Quercitin	10

Seeds and Nuts

Almonds	25
Sunflower seeds	20
Sesame seeds	20
Pumpkin seeds	20
Dry-roasted peanuts	20
Walnuts	20
Pine nuts	15

Vegetables

Baked potato	95–100
Cooked parsnip	95
Cooked carrots*	80–95
French fries	80
Corn	80
Beets	60
Raw carrots	60
Onions	50
Yam, sweet potato (baked)	50
Green peas	45
Artichokes	25
Asparagus	20
Wheatgrass	15
Alfalfa grass	15
Barley grass	15
Fresh tomatoes or sauce	15
Kale, Swiss chard	15
Squashes	15
Celery, peppers	15
Various lettuces	15
Sea vegetables:	15
wakame	15
kombu	15
nori	15
chlorella	15
Nova Scotia dulse	15
spirulina	15

Beverages

Carrot juice*	80
Orange juice	60
Black cherry and apple juice	50
Fresh vegetable juice	45
Tomato juice	40
Pink grapefruit juice	40
Green tea	10
"Green drinks" (greens+)	10
Pure water	0

Sweeteners

Maltose	100–150
Glucose	100
High-fructose corn syrup (avoid)	80
Honey (processed)	75
Sugar (refined)	75
Unrefined raw honey	60
Organic unrefined brown sugar	60
Unprocessed blackstrap molasses	60
Barley malt	55
Organic brown rice syrup	55
Organic, grade C maple syrup	55
Fructose (avoid)	20
Stevia (herb)	0
FOS (fructo-oligo-saccharides)	0

Grains, Breads, Cereals and Sweets

Cornflakes	100+
Rice cakes	100+
French bread	100+
Milk chocolate	95
White bread	95
White rice	85
Whole-wheat bread	85
Pretzels	80
Bagels	80
Candy bars	80
White flour	75
Crackers	75
Boxed breakfast cereals	75
Organic chocolate 70% cocoa	70
Corn tortilla	70
White-flour spaghetti, pasta	60
Pita bread	55
Brown rice	55
Wild rice	55
Oatmeal	55
Popcorn	55
Whole-grain breads	45
Whole-grain pastas	40

Exotic Spices

Cardamom	20
Cinnamon	20
Cloves	20
Mustard seed	15
Cayenne	15
Paprika	15
Peppercorns	15
Saffron	15
Nutmeg	15
Cloves	10
Coriander	10
Chili powder	10
Allspice	10
Turmeric (curcumin)	10
Curry	10
Garlic, ginger	10

*Yes, cooked carrots are high on the glycemic index, but this is really misleading. Do not avoid eating raw or steamed "crunchy tender" carrots. When you make a vegetable juice, never use more than one medium-sized carrot. This is a maximum amount. Make the remainder of your juice from watercress, parsley, kale, wheatgrass, ginger, celery, peppers, beets, spirulina or chlorella (sea vegetables), or better still, a powdered "green drink" can be added to the final juice. Purchase it in a health food store as low-temperature-dried green powders.

Do We Crave High-Glycemic Foods?

As I mentioned, eating foods with a glycemic index of 75 or more causes irritability, mood swings and excess weight gain. These are signs of an insulin imbalance and that other heart disease risk factors can be expected to follow. It may also indicate a carbohydrate addiction.

In many cases, overweight individuals eat less than normal-weight individuals—our weight does not necessarily reflect how much we eat. If we are overweight and have a family history of weight or eating problems, high glycemic index foods eaten frequently throughout the day, as well as inadequate fruit, vegetable, water and lean protein intake, stress and a sedentary lifestyle combined, can have devastating effects on our cardiovascular health, mental and physical well-being and longevity.

High glycemic index foods cause far too much insulin to be secreted from the pancreas to try to "bring down" the large and imbalanced amount of glucose that enters the bloodstream after these foods are eaten. We may then experience blood sugar swings. We may feel hungry and irritable eating these foods and reach for more food or drink high on the glycemic index, keeping the insulin-releasing cycle going while we then develop blood sugar swings, cravings, weight gain, mood shifts and eventually insulin resistance.

Say "No" to Sugar Substitutes: Avoid foods that contain artificial, non-sugar sweeteners and sugar substitutes. They actually act as powerful triggers for insulin release. The downside to all artificial sweeteners is that none of them help curb carbohydrate cravings, boost moods or help to manage weight. I personally avoid all of these sugar substitutes, such as Nutra Sweet®, Equal, Saccharin, acesulfame potassium (Sunett®), maltodextrin, dextrose, maltrose, high-fructose corn syrup, sucrose, etc. The addition of manufactured fructose or high-fructose corn syrup to foods, especially sports drinks, may accelerate diarrhea, gas and abdominal pain. Avoid it! On the other hand, naturally occurring fructose in colorful fruit is perfectly safe and advisable to eat!

Check labels carefully, especially whey and soy protein isolate powders. Some of them contain one or more of these sugars and sugar substitutes. They cause too much insulin to be secreted from the pancreas, so the protein is not fully absorbed into the lean muscle tissue. Part of insulin's job is to trigger the promotion of protein synthesis in muscle tissue. If the insulin is being overtaxed to deal with sugar or another sweetener, then its muscle synthesis is compromised. Furthermore, it is my theory that sugar (glucose) or sugar substitutes (like fructose and acesulfame potassium) ferment in the acidic stomach, forming more sugars and alcohol. These sugars and alcohols promote the overgrowth of the unfriendly yeast called candida albicans in our small intestine.

Sugar substitutes did not exist when our body evolved over the last 100,000 years. Our body was made to handle the "real" sugar it finds in whole foods and to this day it will treat anything that tastes sweet as if it contained real sugar. Trouble is, insulin gets secreted but finds no incoming "real sugar" for the insulin to work on. So insulin looks for the only sugar it can find, the sugar in our blood that we desperately need for sustaining energy. With all sugar substitutes, we experience a steady energy decline and mood swing as insulin clears out this critical and necessary amount of glucose from our blood and stores 40 percent of it as fat in our cells. So, in addition to the loss of our critical anabolic drive, we also put on weight.

The only sweetener that I feel is suitable is the herb stevia rebaudiana (glycemic rating of 0). The following natural sweeteners can also be used in moderation: brown rice syrup (55), barley malt (55), unpasteurized, unprocessed raw honey (60), unprocessed blackstrap molasses (60).

Check at health food stores for the herb stevia, not white crystalline stevia extract, and for books that explain how to use it as a sugar substitute.

The Benefit of Combining Protein with Carbohydrates

One important consideration is to always eat some protein at each of our three meals. Protein with a carbohydrate food will slow down the rate of digestion of that food and literally lower its glycemic index, as the protein slows down the breakdown of that food to glucose (blood sugar).

The body wants homeostasis (metabolic balance), which means our blood sugar or energy supply stays constant, as do our vital control-program hormones such as glucagon, insulin, thyroid hormones, estrogen and testosterone, so we do not experience mood swings and depressive letdowns. Low glycemic index foods like vegetables, salads and fruit provide energy in a slow and sustained-release form, reducing hunger and facilitating the smooth use and storage of calories. It is very difficult to over-consume low-density carbohydrates such as salads, vegetables and fruit because their very high fiber, water, vitamin and mineral levels slow their rate of entry into the bloodstream, thereby maintaining the best possible insulin control. High glycemic index foods like bagels, white rice or French bread provoke strong insulin responses, increasing the exposure of our body to the harmful effects of excess insulin. These high glycemic index foods do provide bursts of energy, but are generally followed by hunger, fatigue, restlessness, severe mood swings and depleted energy.

This does not mean high glycemic index foods are all bad and low glycemic index foods are all good. We must consider that the proportion of high glycemic index foods in the diet is an important variable when evaluating health risks. As an example, 1 cup of cooked pasta has the same amount of carbohydrates as 12 cups of broccoli. At any given meal, keep the total glycemic load low.

Factors Affecting the Glycemic Index

What we must consider is the chemical nature of the carbohydrate in a particular food. Notice that white bread and commercial whole-wheat bread are very high on the scale. Why? Well, it is not because of the bioenergetic whole food wheat—it is all because of the processing. Once the outer husk of the wheat is removed and the starch in white bread or rice cakes is puffed up by heat or the leavening action of yeast, the surface area of the starch has been increased, allowing digestive enzymes a greater surface to work on more quickly; and so the starch is broken down to sugar quickly.

It is interesting to note that individuals sharing my Italian heritage enjoy pasta cooked al dente, which may appear to be slightly undercooked to some. White pasta cooked al dente is a moderate glycemic index food since digestive enzymes cannot break it down quickly, whereas well-cooked pasta that is slightly "mushy" is digested more quickly and is rated a high glycemic index food.

Another factor influencing the glycemic index is the presence of fiber, because the hard-to-digest fibrous walls around seeds, nuts, beans, legumes, vegetables, fruits and whole grains—as well as the cellulose in the whole, unprocessed plant cell wall—slows down digestive enzymes keeping them from reaching the starch too quickly. Fiber acts as a physical barrier to digestion, but when bioenergetic whole foods are processed or finely milled, this natural effect is lost.

Another factor influencing the glycemic index is the amount of fat in a food. Fat slows the rate of emptying from the stomach and also slows the rate of digestion of a starch. As an example, French fries have a rating of 80, while a white baked potato is 100. Adding fat to potatoes to make French fries slows down the rate of digestion, lowers the glycemic index, protects us a little more from the harmful effects of high blood sugar and excessive insulin secretions—but adds excess fat that makes us fat and adds destructive trans-fatty acids.

Andrew Weil, M.D., in his book *Eating Well for Optimum Health*, promotes the use of apple cider vinegar or lemon juice because they increase gastric acidity, which automatically slows stomach emptying and digestion whenever we do consume a simple carbohydrate dessert that is high on the glycemic index. However, I have another suggestion for you. Simply mix 1 scoop of Alphapure™ whey protein isolate powder (about 15 grams of protein) in 8 oz (250 mL) of water and consume this protein shake before consuming the "rare" dessert. The protein will slow down the rate of sugar metabolism and significantly lower the glycemic index of the dessert to keep insulin balanced.

We generally eat complex meals that contain carbohydrates, protein, fats, fiber and micronutrients. We can easily balance the high glycemic index effect of meals in which we have bread or tortillas by including a low glycemic index food like beans (e.g., pinto), peas (e.g., split peas) or legumes (e.g., lentils), thereby keeping the total glycemic load low.

So do not be misled by those writers who issue blanket condemnations of high glycemic index foods. These writers may want us to avoid cooked carrots, which have an index of 80 to 95. To measure the glycemic index of a food, volunteers are fed 50-gram portions of each food. Carrots are only about 7 percent carbohydrate, so to get 50 grams we would have to eat 1.5 pounds (about 750 grams) of cooked carrots at one meal. Not a likely situation. Carrots may be high on the glycemic index, but you could never eat enough of them to cause a sharp insulin spike. Carrots are jam-packed with protective phytonutrients, especially the carotenoid pigments such as alpha- and beta-carotene, which are potent cancer fighters. Suggesting that we avoid cooked carrots would be just unsound nutritional advice—not good for health and longevity.

The rule of thumb is to avoid the disastrous effects of consuming refined and processed carbohydrates such as rice cakes, cookies, cakes, squares, croissants, crackers, bagels, boxed cereals and white bread that are the unwise choice offerings of the fast-food and processed-food industries. This has made 70 percent to 75 percent of the North American population very sensitive to processed carbohydrates, a condition we now call, in this modern day, "carbohydrate sensitivity."

Remember, it is the kind of carbohydrate we eat that is most critical, not whether we eat carbohydrates. Simply stay with the foods, as staples, that have a glycemic index of 60 or less, except in the case of carrots, which I do want you to eat.

THE SATIETY INDEX

The glycemic index only measures the blood glucose-raising effects of a single food. There is another more important index we must consider called the satiety index. This index measures the ability of a single food to satisfy our appetite and hunger. It may surprise you, but potatoes rank highest, followed by oatmeal and pasta.

Baked potatoes, yams, sweet potatoes, oatmeal and al dente pasta do not contain any cholesterol and are very low in fat. We will not gain weight eating them in moderation because they are so filling that most people simply won't be able to eat enough of them to make themselves fat. A medium serving of each is only 105 calories. Just do not add fatty sauces. These foods are the most filling for the least calories and force our body to release stored fat to burn as fuel.

Dr. Susanne Holt, of the University of Sydney, demonstrated the superiority of complex carbohydrate foods over high-protein and high-fat foods in satisfying hunger. It's not calories that matter. Foods scoring highest on the satiety index contain fewer calories per gram than cheese, steak or pizza. Holt also noted that complex bioenergetic carbohydrates improve alertness and satisfy our hunger, as well as balance our blood sugars. Processed carbohydrates leave people feeling grumpy, aggressive and slightly dissatisfied or disappointed.

In the table below, all foods are compared to white bread that is assigned the number 100. The higher number denotes foods that provide the greatest satiety.

THE SATIETY INDEX OF FOODS

Baked potatoes, yams, sweet potatoes	323	
Oatmeal	209	
High alpha whey protein isolate powder	205	
Non-GMO soy protein isolate powder	205	
Unsweetened "green drinks"	203	
Oranges	202	
Apples	197	
Berries (all types)	195	
Whole grain pasta	188	E
Fish	185	A
Chicken, turkey	175	T
Beans, peas, legumes	165	
Whole grain bread	160	
All vegetables	155	
Free-range organic eggs	155	
Brown rice	150	
Low fat cheese	150	
Air-popped popcorn	150	
White rice	132	
White pasta	119	A
Crackers	127	V
Cookies	120	O
French fries	116	I
White bread	100	D
Candy bars	70	
Donuts	68	
Cake	65	
Croissants	47	

Most of the phytonutrient-rich carbohydrate foods that are bioenergetic whole foods are low in calories. They appear on the satiety index with numbers 150 or above. Eat only those foods with an index number of 150 or greater. Only fat-laden, sweetened, processed carbohydrate foods that contain concentrated calories—such as croissants, donuts, pastries, French fries and cookies—will make us gain weight rapidly.

SHAPING OUR DESTINY

Keeping these two indexes in mind, I prefer that we bake yams or sweet potatoes in place of white baked potatoes, use brown or basmati rice over regular white rice, and organic whole-grain breads over white breads. Now we are getting the best of both indexes without the fat—and with more nutrients, fiber and phytonutrients.

It is the kind of carbohydrate we eat that is critical, not whether we eat a carbohydrate. Our diet can contain substantial amounts of filling, satisfying, unprocessed, unrefined carbohydrates that keep our insulin response low with low glycemic index foods and provide satisfaction as well as sustenance.

Low-carbohydrate diets may work for short-term weight loss, but I do not recommend them as an everyday way to eat. I am concerned about how much and what kinds of carbohydrates belong in our diet and how current patterns of refined carbohydrate consumption negatively affect our well-being. Complex bioenergetic carbohydrates with low glycemic index scores are the body's highest-quality fuel and increase the efficiency of both our digestion and metabolism.

I do support the theories and nutritional philosophies of Dr. Robert Atkins, Montignac and Barry Sears, Ph.D., for long-term nutritional strategies. I have been a guest on Dr. Robert Atkins's radio talk show on three separate occasions. Most of the above nutritional researchers agree that at least 40 percent, but I recommend 55 percent, of our daily calories should come from complex, natural very low-density carbohydrates, such as fresh vegetables and fresh fruit, that provide satisfaction but are also moderate to low on the glycemic index. This would mean that for every 1,000 calories we eat daily, 100 to 125 grams should come from complex carbohydrates such as colorful vegetables, salads, fresh organic fruit and berries, whole grains, herbs, seeds or nuts (some soaked), legumes, peas and beans.

THE RIGHT CARBOHYDRATES CURB OUR HUNGER AND MAINTAIN OUR ANABOLIC CAPACITY

Top 20 Refined, Catabolic, High-Glycemic Carbohydrates in Our Average Diets Today	Replace with These Anabolic, Unprocessed, High-Satiety, Low-Glycemic Carbohydrates
French fries	Colorful salads, steamed "crunchy tender" vegetables, baked yam and sweet potato "fries"
Potatoes (baked or mashed)	Yams or sweet potatoes
White bread	Sourdough, whole-grain breads, especially rye, spelt, amaranth, millet and quinoa
Boxed breakfast cereals	Organic oatmeal, seven-grain cereals
Pizza (white crust)	Whole-grain pizza dough, with soy cheese, low fat cheese or feta cheese
Pasta	Whole-wheat, spelt or kamut pasta al dente

Muffins	Whole grain muffins with whole nuts and seeds
White rice	Brown rice or North American basmati rice
Orange juice	Organic whole orange or pink grapefruit
Bananas	Blueberries, raspberries and other berries
Soft drinks	Water, with a dash of lemon or lime juice
Waxed apples	Colorful organic apples
Fruit punch drinks	Real unsweetened fruit juices or, better still, a piece of whole fruit
Skim milk	Rice milk, fat-free organic milk, hemp milk
Peanut butter	Almond butter (unsweetened, unsalted)
Jam	Unsweetened, whole-fruit jams
Pancakes	Multigrain pancakes
Table sugar	Stevia, unsulphured molasses, unprocessed honey, malted barley, brown rice syrup
Pastries, donuts, cakes	An anabolic revitalizing "green drink"
Candy	Celery or carrot sticks, seeds, unsalted raw nuts

If we can successfully make the dietary adjustment from hormone-unbalancing, declining catabolic foods on the left of the table above to the hormone-balancing, revitalizing, bioenergetic anabolic foods on the right, we will have more than accomplished our goal!

12

PROTEIN: THE BUILDING BLOCKS OF LIFE

Half of the dry weight of a lean body is protein. The structures of our hormones, neurotransmitters, muscles, brain cells, immune system and organs are made of protein. The thousands of enzymes that control all of our biochemical interactions are proteins, every one. The very hemoglobin that carries our life-sustaining oxygen from the lungs to all of the 100 trillion cells that make up our body is composed of protein.

We use protein daily for building, repair and energy. Therefore we must consume adequate amounts of protein to keep our body supplied with this critical nutrient. If we eat too little protein, we lose muscle strength, weaken our body's ability to fight off disease and, most importantly, sharply decrease our lifespan. I call this "protein malnutrition."

Almost every North American woman does not eat enough highly bioavailable protein on a daily basis, and may be suffering from "protein malnutrition." On the other hand, if we consume too much protein we lose calcium, develop osteoporosis and lose our hair. When we over-consume protein, we feel sluggish and lethargic.

Our body has limited "short-term" storage facilities for unused carbohydrates in muscle and liver cells, and almost unlimited "long-term" storage for unused fat in adipose cells. But it has no storage system for protein. Consequently, to develop and maintain our existing muscle mass, we have to eat the right amount of protein every day. If we miss our daily quota for even one day, then our body will break down lean tissue to make up the shortage of amino acids to keep our system going.

The proteins we consume from foods are made up of sub-units called amino acids. These amino acids form into protein structures. About 70 percent of the 300 to 400 grams of protein our body restructures each day is recycled, as amino acids, to rebuild new protein. The other 30 percent must come from our diet daily.

THE CASE AGAINST RED MEAT

One popular argument against vegetarianism points to the fact that primal man ate wild game—and lots of it, so we are going against our biological inheritance by avoiding all meat products today. Yes, it's true our ancestors benefited immensely from eating meat. However, the wild game they ate grazed on EFA-rich natural green grasses and roamed freely and actively. As a result, the meat was only 3 to 4 percent fat and contained six times more long-chain Omega-3 fatty acids than today's grain-fed beef. Today we put meat animals such as cows and pigs, for our convenience, into feed lots of grain, not grass, so they "fatten up" to 33 to 40 percent body fat, weigh more and provide a greater financial return for the rancher. They have no EFAs such as Omega-3 DHA and EPA, only enormous amounts of extremely unhealthy saturated fats. Almost all of the benefits of eating meat are now gone.

The fat in beef is the worst animal fat in terms of chemical composition. It contains 51 percent saturated fatty acids, 44 percent monounsaturated fatty acids and only a trace of polyunsaturated fatty acids. The drawbacks from eating animal flesh now stem in part from the large amounts of saturated fat present. There are continual findings that point to a direct correlation between saturated animal fat consumption and degenerative diseases like coronary heart disease, diabetes, arteriosclerosis and cancer.

Of all the saturated animal fats, the fats in red meats cause the greatest problems. Since fat carries flavor, those steaks and roast beefs that are highly "marbled" with white streaks of fat running through the meat, are the tastiest. "If the meat is 'hung' or 'aged' to improve the taste, the fats are thoroughly peroxidized and loaded with free radicals, ready to turn our normal, healthy cells into abnormal, premalignant ones. Such altered cells only need another little push from one cancer-promoting factor or another—say, an environmental pollutant—to turn into full-blown cancer," write Eberhard and Phyllis Kronhausen, Ed.D., in *Formula for Life*.

The safest meat is from wild game that are not deliberately fattened and fed antibiotics, as domesticated cattle are. Hamburger, on the other hand, may be one of the most unsafe meats. The grinding of the meat exposes more surface to the air and promotes oxidation and the generation of free radicals. The grinding also breaks up red blood cells in the meat, releasing iron and copper ions that catalyze the production of still more cancer-initiating free radicals. Finally, the grilling, barbecuing or frying of the hamburger creates carcinogenic pyrolytic compounds.

Red meat is rich in the amino acid methionine, from which our body makes another amino acid called homocysteine, which builds up in the bloodstream.

Homocysteine is one of the worst compounds to have at high levels in our body because it hardens our arteries (arteriosclerosis) and is also a powerful factor in the buildup of arterial plaque—leading to heart disease, heart attack and stroke.

> B-vitamins, specifically folic acid and vitamin B6, along with 97 percent oil-free lecithin, which can be found in quality "green drinks," act as potent methyl donors and can break down dangerous homocysteine.

Red meat consumption has been associated with prostate cancer. A similar link has now been found between red meat consumption and breast cancer, colon cancer and stomach cancer.

There is no need to eat red meat. There are many good alternatives such as fish, chicken, turkey, seafood, low-fat dairy products (especially fat-free organic yogurt)—and the richest source of high-BV protein in the world—undenatured whey protein isolate powder and soy protein isolate powder.

Doctors, nutritionists and many researchers warn us not to eat organ meats such as liver, kidneys and the like. These organs tend to have heavy concentrations of environmental toxins, heavy metals, saturated fat and infectious agents.

BSE: I will admit that the possibility of infection from animal organs or meat may be small at the moment, but it is growing. My real concern for our well-being stems from the outbreak of bovine spongiform encephalopathy (BSE)—"mad cow disease"—in England in the 1990s, and in both Germany and France in early 2001. Human cases of this fatal brain disease, called Creutzfeld-Jakob disease (CJD), resulted from eating the meat of infected cows.

"Mad cow disease" occurs in many animals and humans. It can be transmitted from one species to another by consumption of infected tissue. The disease in beef cattle became widespread in England as a result of the practice of feeding them carcasses of other animals for feed, especially sheep infected with scrapie, the sheep's variation of bovine spongiform encephalopathy. The infectious agents are called prions, a newly recognized pathogen that carries information but is not living. Prions are very small proteins that totally disrupt cellular hormone and neurotransmitter information systems. Prions are remarkably resistant to antibiotics and antiviral agents used to destroy more complex and familiar disease agents like bacteria, viruses and parasites. They cause incurable brain degeneration that is always fatal.

I do not write about spongiform encephalopathies for any other reason than to alert you and make you aware of the hazards of animal products.

Bonemeal, a euphemism for ground-up animal parts, is a meat byproduct fed widely to livestock in North America, such as cows, chickens, turkeys and sheep. To be cautious, do not use bonemeal in your garden and eat only meats from livestock guaranteed not to be fed with bonemeal. Your best choice is to eat organically raised animal products from local farmers.

E. coli and Hormones: Slaughterhouses may have sloppy practices that contaminate meat with deadly forms of E. coli. Another concern I have has to do both with the environmental contamination in large animals like cows and with our methods of raising animals. One modern practice in commercially raised animals is to feed them estrogenic hormones to make them gain weight faster, and antibiotics to support a faster growth rate. These hormones may promote the development of prostate cancer in men, since there is a higher incidence of prostate cancer in men who consume the most red meat. These hormones add to the "total load" of estrogenic pressure on women from many sources, increasing the risk of breast cancer, cancers of the reproductive system, uterine fibroid cysts and fibrocysts in breasts. Furthermore, antibiotics in meat certainly contribute to the ever-growing problem of antibiotic-resistant bacteria.

Since 1995, recombinant bovine somatotropin (BST), also known as bovine growth hormone (BGH), a synthetic hormone, has been used in the United States to make dairy cows produce significantly more milk. I remain very suspicious of BGH. Farmers using BGH note an increase in the inflammation of udders—requiring antibiotic use. Residues of antibiotics in milk contribute to the development of antibiotic-resistant bacteria in people.

Red Meat Alternatives

Large animals live at the top of the food chain. These animals live the longest and accumulate agrichemicals and environmental toxins in their organs and fatty tissues. If you do eat animal foods, consume those that have shorter lives such as fish, chicken, turkey and lamb.

If you eat fish, be wise. Fresh fish has virtually no smell. As soon as it starts to go bad, fish produces a chemical called tri-methylamine, which is a definite sign of spoilage and a fishy odor. If it smells fishy, don't buy it. Canned, white, water-packed, low-sodium albacore tuna has less than 1 gram of fat per 100 grams (3¼ oz), but has 24 grams of superior protein.

Poultry differs from the meat of larger animals because its fat is external to muscle instead of being distributed throughout it, so that it can easily be removed before cooking. Chicken fat has a healthier composition than the fat of sheep, pigs or cows, with only 30 percent saturated fatty acids. Hormones and antibiotics are used full-scale in commercially raised chicken, but there still is a risk of infection, especially from salmonella, because of unsanitary methods used in slaughter and butchering.

There are farmers who specialize in organically raised, free-range, drug-free, hormone-free chickens that run around naturally, not caged and force-fed. We may pay a higher price, but if I ate chicken, this would be the only kind I would buy.

Other farmers are raising wild game that graze on grasses and are organically certified to be free of hormones and antibiotics. These animals have a much better fatty acid profile and contain the valuable Omega-3 long-chain fatty acids. Deer, buffalo, pheasant, quail and ostriches are all a healthful alternative to beef. If I ate meat, which I don't, I would pay more and purchase these meats.

We must all consider the ethics of raising animals for food and causing them to suffer. This may appear radical but it should be part of humanity's compassion toward other living creatures.

Also, raising animals for meat wastes valuable natural resources. The huge amounts of wastes produced by animals raised for meat create a worrisome problem for disposal. In the spring of 2000, seven people died and about 2,000 became ill in Walkerton, Ontario, when the urine and manure run-off from cattle got into an underground spring and then into the water supply. Animals' waste products, full of drugs, hormones and agrichemicals, also find their way into groundwater. The methane gas produced from cow feces is now a significant factor in depleting the earth's atmospheric, protective ozone layer. Andrew Weil, M.D., writes in *Eating Well for Optimum Health:* "Some experts say that cows and cars do almost equal damage to the atmosphere and the environment in general."

A RETURN TO THE BASE OF THE FOOD CHAIN

For the reasons already mentioned, I strongly suggest we consume at least 60 percent of our protein from plant-based sources, while lacto-ovo vegetarians consume 80 percent of their protein from plant-based sources and vegetarians and vegans get 100 percent of their protein from plant-based sources.

Getting our protein from vegetable rather than animal foods has a number of advantages:

- Vegetable protein is cheaper than meat.
- Vegetable protein is less perishable.
- Vegetable protein contains fewer environmental toxins.
- Vegetable protein contains fiber that animal protein does not.
- Vegetable protein is much lower in saturated fatty acids.

- Vegetable protein contains micronutrients that animal protein does not.
- Vegetable protein contains protective phytonutrients that animal protein does not contain.
- Vegetable protein does not have the drugs, infection and hormones found in meat.
- Vegetable protein can be used to create exquisite, ingenious and delicious meals.
- It requires a lot of food to feed cattle to be butchered for meat, whereas that same amount of food, fed directly to people, would significantly reduce starvation and hunger worldwide.

There are some problems with the absorption of plant protein that we should be aware of, however:

- While 95 to 99 percent of animal protein is absorbed, only 75 to 90 percent of plant-based protein is absorbed well.
- Some plant foods contain "blockers" that inhibit the absorption of both iron and zinc from non-meat sources.
- Vegetable protein does not contain the readily bioavailable vitamin B12 of animal protein, but we can use a B12 supplement taken sublingually.

THE PROTEIN CONTENT OF RED MEAT ALTERNATIVES

Food	Amount	Protein in Grams
• Whey protein isolate powder	2 heaping tbsp	30
• Cross-flow, microfiltered whey concentrate	2 heaping tbsp	25
• Fat-free, dry cottage cheese	1 cup (250 mL)	26
• Soy protein isolate powder	2 heaping tbsp	25
• Soy beans, cooked	1 cup (250 mL)	22
• Extra-firm tofu or tempeh	1 cup (250 mL)	22
• Fish (sole or salmon, broiled or baked)	3 oz (85 g)	21
• Chicken breast (roasted, boneless, no skin)	3 oz (85 g)	21
• Turkey	3 oz (85 g)	21
• Cheese, low-fat	3 oz (85 g)	21
• Lentils, boiled	1 cup (250 mL)	18
• Black beans, boiled	1 cup (250 mL)	16
• Pinto beans, boiled	1 cup (250 mL)	14
• Whole eggs (boiled)	2 large	14
• Fat-free, plain, organic yogurt	8 oz (250 mL)	13
• Rice milk	1 cup (250 mL)	8
• Peanuts, dry roasted	1 oz (28 g)	7
• Almond butter	2 tbsp	7
• Sunflower seeds	2 tbsp	3
• Almonds	1 oz (28 g)	3

If we eat a variety of proteins, we are guaranteed to receive lots of the nine essential amino acids we must eat each day, and lots of the 11 nonessential amino acids our body can manufacture from the nine essential amino acids.

Protein Absorption

It is not only the level of protein intake, but the amount of it that is usable or available to our body that must be carefully considered. Vegetable protein sources have a high fiber content, and much of the protein is embedded in this fiber. As a result, only 75 to 80 percent of the actual protein in lentils, soy beans, almonds, sunflower seeds, whole rye, whole grain cereal, beans, peas or legumes, for example, is absorbed.

Legumes, beans and peas, except for soy beans, have higher ratios of carbohydrates to protein and do cause insulin secretion. Soy beans differ from all other legumes, peas and beans because they contain high amounts of both protein and fat relative to carbohydrates. Unlike other beans, peas and legumes, soy beans actually contain more protein than carbohydrate, and therefore should become our primary bean of choice. I calculate that about 80 to 85 percent of the protein in soy beans is absorbed and utilized by our body.

Minimally processed, highly recommended soy foods like extra-firm tofu, tempeh and soy meat substitutes, on the other hand, contain virtually no fiber, and 92 percent of their protein is absorbed.

Protein Source	Biological Value
• Undenatured, whey protein isolate powder	158–170
• Cross-flow ultrafiltration, microfiltered protein concentrate	150–155
• Soy protein isolate powder	140–145
• Whole egg	100
• Cow's milk and dairy products	90
• Egg white	89
• Extra-firm tofu or tempeh	85
• Fish	85
• Beef	80
• Chicken	77
• Milk casein	77
• Soy beans	75
• Rice	60
• Wheat, spelt, rye, amaranth (grains)	55
• Legumes, peas, beans, nuts, seeds	49

Keep the biological value in mind when choosing your protein sources at each meal.

Biological Value of Proteins: Biological value (BV) is the measure of the amount of protein retained in the human body per gram of protein absorbed. Eating the highest-BV proteins daily gives us the absolute best and most absorbed protein. Look at the preceding chart and you'll understand why I so strongly recommend we use undenatured whey protein isolate powder for our breakfast protein power shake. Some researchers may not prefer the BV standard, but prefer another way to judge protein absorption rates. Nevertheless, the BV is excellent and as a comparison we can say that whey protein isolate powder has twice the biological value compared to milk protein, chicken or beef, and three times the biological value of legumes.

PROTEIN STIMULATES GLUCAGON HORMONES

The higher the biological value, the more a protein is absorbed into our system and able to supply a steady flow of necessary amino acids. If we have protein at three meals a day, the supply meets the ongoing, constant demands of our body.

The higher the biological value, the more the protein stimulates the release of the hormone glucagon. Glucagon is the counter-regulatory hormone to insulin that is stimulated by dietary protein. Its primary job is to release stored carbohydrates from the liver to maintain adequate levels of blood sugar for the brain. Glucagon ensures the brain a steady supply of its primary fuel mix, glucose, for optimal mental performance, especially while we sleep.

Whey protein isolates, soy protein isolates and minimally processed soy products high in protein simultaneously reduce insulin secretion and increase glucagon secretion. This decreases our excess cholesterol synthesis and improves our cardiovascular health.

"What's more, glucagon acts like a hormonal brake that inhibits insulin secretion. So by maintaining relatively constant levels of glucagon, we will control insulin levels with far greater ease," writes Barry Sears, Ph.D., author of *The Soy Zone*.

By eating a balanced, but fluctuating, amount of protein throughout the day at each of our three meals, we will constantly produce an adequate, but not excessive, amount of glucagon. At the same time, we will never eat too much protein at any one meal. This is important because any excess protein at a meal can't be stored as protein, but is immediately converted to fat. Excess protein also stimulates the release of insulin—but our goal is to always balance insulin at every meal with the correct protein to carbohydrate ratio, emphasizing very low-density carbohydrates.

Remember that our main carbohydrate sources should be very low-density carbohydrates such as vegetables, along with medium-density carbohydrates such as ripe fruit. We should also be voluntarily reducing high-density carbohydrates such as pastries, breads, pasta, cereals and starches, which we should only use in moderation at our dinner.

Remember, the highest-BV protein is the best protein source for you. Secondly, we should spread out our protein among our three meals, with extra-low-density carbohydrates from vegetables and salads. By supplementing this dietary strategy with two servings of low-density carbohydrates from fruits, we will maintain our protein-to-carbohydrate ratio and promote hormonal balance with our hormones—insulin, glucagon, galanin, neuropeptide Y, serotonin, mela-tonin, dopamine, cortisol and human growth hormone.

Vitamin B12 is only available from animal products. It is one of the most significant nutrients typically missing from the diets of vegans. Fortunately, the body needs only very tiny daily amounts of this vitamin that is used in the manufacture of red blood cells and nerves. Even so, a deficiency is serious, potentially causing irre-versible nerve damage. Fermented foods, such as the soy bean products miso and tempeh, supply some vitamin B12 from the bacterial culture that causes fermentation, but generally not enough. If you are a vegan, please eat B12-fortified foods and use a B12 sublingual supplement daily.

I take B12 sublingual supplementation each morning.

VEGETABLE PROTEIN AND ABSORPTION RATES

It may have surprised you to discover beans, wheat, rice and soy are at the bottom of the biological values, which means our body has a slightly hard time converting vegetable proteins into lean muscle tissues. Legumes, peas and beans contain an abundant amount of two sugars, strachyose and raffinose. We do not digest them well so they ferment in our intestines, causing a lot of flatulence. Beano® is the trade name of a product that contains the sugar-digestive enzyme alpha-glactosidase, which is equally as effective with sugars in cruciferous vegetables such as broccoli, cauliflower and Brussels sprouts.

After the age of 30, we begin to have more and more difficulty digesting proteins. Three whole-food, natural supplements work wonders. The first is to use two broad-range, plant-based digestive enzyme capsules at the beginning of our three meals each day. The second really successful method is to put just 1 tablespoon of certified organically grown apple cider vinegar into 4 oz of room-temperature water and sip this brew 15 minutes before each of our meals. This raises the hydrochloric acid in our stomach for excellent protein digestion and absorption. The third method is to eat red beets—steamed, marinated, boiled or shredded raw into our salads or on top of our protein source for added visual appeal. Red beets contain large storehouses of hydrochloric acid to help in protein digestion and absorption. The highest quality of undenatured, pure, whey protein isolate powders, such as Alphapure™ whey protein isolates, have all the necessary broad-spectrum, plant-based digestive enzymes added to them to ensure our complete absorption and utilization of these extremely elevated biological value proteins.

Absorption Alert: Iron

The body cannot eliminate iron except through blood loss. Other than women who menstruate heavily, there is no need for iron supplements. Iron is an oxidizing agent and too much of it in our body can promote unhealthy chemical reactions in our cells, increasing risks of cardiovascular disease and cancer. Iron stores increase with age and ignite the release of glutamate, which triggers biochemical reactions that lead to strokes and neurological deterioration. Never take iron supplements unless conclusive blood tests show that you have iron-deficiency anemia (both high ferritin levels and high glutamate concentration)— when the body makes fewer and smaller red blood cells, with consequent reduced capacity to transport and use oxygen. The incidence of cancer related to iron supplementation in men, and also in women after they stop menstruating, is very significant. Lactoferrin, extracted from milk, is not only anti-viral and anti-bacterial, but scavenges excess iron to protect against damaging free radicals. Make sure that your multivitamin supplement contains no iron. Animals have plenty of easily assimilable iron in their muscles, so meat eaters have sufficient iron. Vegetarians may not get enough iron and may have a harder time absorbing and using what they do eat. Since I so strongly recommend that we decrease our consumption of meat, we must find iron-rich foods from bioenergetic, whole foods. Iron is plentiful in dark, leafy vegetables such as kale, beet tops, Swiss chard and in leafy lettuces other than iceberg lettuce. It is also concentrated in molasses, beans, free-range organic eggs, sea vegetables, organic fat-free yogurt, nuts, seeds, peas, legumes and in two dried fruits—figs and prunes.

There are two types of iron, heme iron and non-heme iron. Heme iron is derived from meat and accumulates in the body; it can be dangerous at high concentrations, especially for those with heart disease, artery disease or strokes. The beneficial non-heme iron from plants, sea vegetables, legumes, seeds, nuts, whole grains, spirulina, nutritional yeast, fat-free dairy products and organic, free-range eggs does not accumulate in the body. Until recently, the unsubstantiated belief was that "good" non-heme iron from non-meat sources is not absorbed well. It was argued that phytates, polyphenols, tannins and oxalates would bind to non-heme iron and reduce its absorption. The iron status of vegetarian Asians and vegetarian Westerners (their hemoglobin, plasma ferritin and plasma iron-binding capacity) has shown "no particular iron mineral deficiencies." If you choose to take an iron supplement, use a vegetarian non-heme source such as Floradix Iron + Herbs® from Flora. My strongest recommendation is to use the antioxidant alpha lipoic acid, which chelates (binds)excess iron from the brain and eliminates it from the system.

Absorption Alert: Zinc and Copper

Zinc is an essential mineral for maintaining a healthy immune system. Some foods contain phytates, oxalates or other substances that block the absorption of zinc and iron from the proteins we eat, once in the intestine. Coffee and green tea (regular or decaffeinated), whole grains, bran, legumes, soy products, nuts, seeds and spinach are a few examples of foods that contain these blockers. When we eat these foods, we should also supplement with vitamin C, as an ascorbate mixture, to help our body absorb more zinc and iron.

Vegetarians and vegans can become zinc-deficient because their diet contains a large proportion of blockers. To combat this problem, soak seeds, legumes and nuts overnight, discarding the water in the morning. Soaking leaches out 90 percent of the blockers. In addition, use only fermented soy products, as fermentation eliminates these blockers. Also consider using a 30 mg zinc supplement every day.

Zinc and copper are a double-edged sword: too little and our immune system malfunctions; too much and our cells become toxic, as the zinc or copper ions interact with hydrogen peroxide to produce highly neurotoxic hydroxyl radicals. A minute amount of copper is all it takes to perform its meticulous tasks that are so essential to our health. Nuts, seeds, all soy products, beer, legumes, rice, chocolate and seafood contain copper that in overabundance suppresses our adrenal and thyroid glands. Use a zinc supplement daily to balance copper.

Copper and zinc are also neurological double-edged swords. While the body cannot live without them, new research from Florida State University confirms that they can also be neurotoxic (Horning M.S. et al., *The Life Extension Magazine*, April 2001). Abnormal copper-zinc metabolism is implicated in Alzheimer's disease, stroke, seizures and many other diseases with neurological components—where the copper and zinc help to form "gooey" amyloid-beta plaques that cover the brain's neurons, so hormone and neurotransmitter transmission grinds to a halt and we become senile, as in Alzheimer's disease.

Copper and zinc modulate neurotransmitters across those synaptic gaps or intersections, but become neurotoxins at the concentrations reached when they are released from synaptic terminals. The brain must buffer these metals so that they can perform their functions without neurotoxicity. The dipeptide protein molecule carnosine or the product A•G•E inhibitors™ provide that buffering action, plus offer a pH buffering, and are potent antioxidants, neutralizing or "quenching" hydroxyl radical action.

The first recommendation is to use 20 to 30 mg of a zinc supplement daily to balance the copper in our diet. We do need 3 to 4 mg of natural copper daily, which is in the dietary strategy I have presented. The second recommendation is

not to use any supplement with copper in it. The brain must constantly
the zinc and copper metals so that they can perform their functions wi
neurotoxicity, which destroys neurons. The third recommendation is to use
1,000 mg of the dipeptide protein supplement carnosine daily or three capsules
daily of the anti-glycating formula A•G•E inhibitors™ in or with a power protein
shake—from the age of 35 to 40 onwards—to buffer these metals and neutralize
the destructive hydroxyl radical. Carnosine is not available in Canada but is
available in the United States.

PROTEIN: NUTS AND SEEDS

Eat only peanuts or peanut butters that are organically grown and certified to be
aflatoxin-free. Aflatoxin is a potent, natural carcinogen produced by a mold that
commonly grows on peanuts. In addition, many commercial brands of peanut
butter contain partially hydrogenated oils. Read labels carefully. I personally use
organic almond butter. Almond butter is a healthy alternative to peanut butter,
which has a higher percentage of saturated fat.

Nuts in general are a healthy addition to our diet. Recent research confirms
that eating a small handful of various nuts, such as almonds, sunflower seeds,
pumpkin seeds, walnuts, hemp seeds and flax seeds, can lower LDL cholesterol
and reduce serum triglycerides. Nuts are also a good source of fiber, minerals, and
vitamin E. Buy raw, organically grown, natural, unsalted nuts or seeds and keep
them in the refrigerator until needed, to protect their oils from going rancid.

I personally like to dry-roast sunflower seeds and hemp seeds and then add
them to salads, stews, chili, and soups, or just eat as a wonderful snack. Hemp,
used throughout the world as a source of high-quality fiber for clothing and
paper, contains edible seeds and superior oil. The seeds and oil contain no intox-
icating properties.

To dry-roast any seeds or nuts, put a layer of them in a dry skillet and stir them
over medium heat for three to five minutes, until they begin to lightly brown.
Do not use any oil.

13

FATS: NOT ALL BAD

We need a certain amount of beneficial fat as a regular part of our diet. Fats play an important role in our well-being. They boost the functioning of the brain and stimulate the development of the immune system. As part of "The World's Best Diet," I recommend that 20 percent of our daily calories come from fats.

The problem is, most North Americans can't seem to get enough. As Sarah Leibowitz, Ph.D., of Rockefeller University has found, the reason for that is that the body actually has a built-in appetite system for fat. And, our body is hard-wired to store fat. Galanin, the hormone that encourages us to eat fat, starts to rise at noontime as the hormone leptin turns "on" the release of galanin so the body can store some fat for the overnight fast.

But fats are not created equal, and most of the fats we're consuming are providing us with nothing but calories. A gram of fat is more than twice as calorie-dense as a gram of pure carbohydrate or protein.

Fat is made to be stored, requiring only about 3 percent of its calories to convert it into belly, hip or thigh fat. In contrast, the body uses up almost 25 percent of its calories converting excess carbohydrates and protein into body fat.

Often, removing excess fat from the diet means we can eat more bioenergetic foods for superior nutrition for fewer calories. Substituting a baked chicken breast for a fried chicken breast can save us 125 calories, with no loss of taste or amount of food. If we choose a tempeh or tofu entrée, we save another 100 calories, or 225 in total.

THE FAT HAZARDS OF DAIRY

Butterfat, the fat in whole milk that becomes highly concentrated in cream, ice cream, cheese and butter, is the most saturated of the animal fats, delivering a whopping 54 percent as saturated fat.

Clearly, high-fat dairy products, especially ice cream, butter and fatty cheeses, can do you harm. Even 2 percent milk is about 35 percent fat. Even more worrisome is that dairy fat is made up of 66 percent from the destructive saturated fats. The dairy lobby has successfully bypassed the normal food labeling process.

It counts fat by weight, not by percent of calories. Since most of the weight in milk is water, this results in a deceptively low percentage.

If you opt to consume dairy fat, use fat-free, plain organic yogurt or fat-free cottage cheese, and limit butter to 1 teaspoon a day, since it is 100 percent fat.

A CALORIE IS NOT JUST A CALORIE / QUICK PICKS

Food	Calories	Fat (g)	Savings
McDonald's Sausage McMuffin® (2)	870	48	735 calories
vs.			
Whey protein isolate power shake	135	4	44 grams of fat
Subway Italian sub (6 inches)	450	21	170 calories
vs.			
Turkey breast sub (w/o mayo or oil)	280	4	17 grams of fat
Pizza Hut pepperoni stuffed pizza (2 slices)	1,058	52	590 calories
vs.			
Veggie pizza, thin crust (2 slices)	468	15	37 grams of fat
Full-fat plain yogurt (1 cup)	220	16	110 calories
vs.			
Fat-free plain organic yogurt (1 cup)	110	2	14 grams of fat

DAIRY FAT COMPARISON BY PERCENTAGE OF FAT

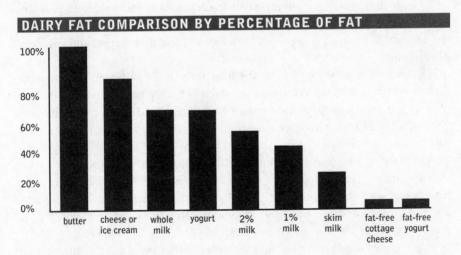

Of all the dairy products, fat-free, plain organic yogurt is the healthiest. Yogurt is loaded with the "friendly" bacteria called lactobacilli. These "friendly" bacteria consume the lactose sugar in milk, and convert milk to yogurt. As the lactobacilli increase, the lactose sugar disappears. Medical treatments with antibiotics often decrease the amount of lactobacillus bacteria in your intestines and cause severe intestinal problems. Non-pasteurized (live) yogurt can be used to treat intestinal problems, as these microscopic-sized living lactobacilli restore the healthy intestinal tract environment.

Lactose is the primary sugar in milk and dairy products. To digest lactose in dairy products, we need the enzyme, lactase. Approximately 60 percent of North Americans are deficient in lactase. (I am.) Yogurt from organic fat-free milk with live "friendly" bacteria or cultures contains no lactose, or only a smidgen of it.

Not only do we need to limit our intake of fat, we need to make smart choices regarding the fat that we do eat. First, we need to understand that not all fats and oils are bad for us.

A NOTE ABOUT CHOLESTEROL

Cholesterol, while typically called a fat, is really a steroid. Cholesterol passes through a chemically defined pathway to become the precursor for making all the critical steroid hormones in the body; hormones such as cortisol, DHEA, testosterone, progesterone and estrogens. DHEA is referred to as the "mother" hormone. In reality, the "mother" of all steroid hormones is cholesterol. In fact, without cholesterol, there would be no estrogens or testosterone!

Cholesterol is a critical structural molecule in every cell membrane, especially in brain cells, which are made up of close to 60 percent fat. Too much cholesterol can stimulate excess hormone production; too little cholesterol causes too little hormone production, especially of testosterone and estrogen.

As with all hormones, a unique balancing act must be maintained to generate wellness. An imbalance in opposing hormones, especially sex hormones such as testosterone and estrogen usually signals biochemical dysfunction and degenerative disease.

Cholesterol is waxy, which means it is not soluble in water. To transport cholesterol around in the bloodstream, which is mostly water, the body coats it with a protein. These protein-bearing cholesterol particles are called lipoproteins—*lipos* is a Greek derivative meaning "a fat." The more protein a cholesterol particle carries, the denser it is. About 60 percent of the circulating lipoprotein in our blood is low-density lipoprotein (LDL). LDLs carry cholesterol to your cells and are the "bad" cholesterol. About 25 percent of your circulating lipoproteins is high-density lipoprotein (HDL). These denser, smaller cholesterol particles pick up cholesterol from our cells and carry it to the liver for proper processing. HDLs are the "good" cholesterols.

Triglycerides are very small, light fat particles that have only a little protein attached to them. The body uses some of the triglycerides in our muscles for energy but stores most of it as body fat. Triglycerides are converted into very low-density lipoproteins (VLDL). These particles get denser as they circulate in the bloodstream until they turn into "bad" LDL cholesterol.

Most health professionals use the following guidelines to evaluate the risk of heart disease when checking blood cholesterol and LDL levels.

Blood Fat	Risk Factor Desirable (mg/100 cc)	Borderline High Risk (mg/100 cc)	High Risk (mg/100 cc)
Cholesterol	less than 200	201–240	241+
HDL cholesterols	65 or more	50	35 or less
LDL cholesterols	130 or less	131–160	160 or more
Triglyceride/HDL	less than 2	3	more than 4

Source: Adapted from the National Cholesterol Education Program (Ottawa; Washington, D.C.).

ESSENTIAL FATTY ACIDS: THE KEY TO HEALTH

Our body can make fat from any food—sugar, protein or fat. But there are two fats we cannot make: linoleic acid (Omega-6) and alpha-linolenic acid (Omega-3), called essential fatty acids (EFAs).

These two fats are essential fats used to make all the special fats in our eyes, brain, ears, adrenal glands and the membranes that surround and protect our 100 trillion cells.

All fats and oils are made of fatty acids. Udo Erasmus, my friend and an expert on fats, in his highly acclaimed book *Fats That Heal, Fats That Kill*, describes each fat molecule as looking like a caterpillar. The fatty part is the head and body, while it has an acid tail. It's a chemical made up of carbon atoms, with hydrogen atoms attached.

Fats differ from each other in the length of their carbon chains, and the number and arrangements of hydrogen atoms.

These shapes are chemical keys that absolutely determine whether a particular fat fits a particular lock in the human body to make a hormone or neurotransmitter.

SATURATED FATS

A saturated fat has all of its carbon atoms filled (saturated) with hydrogen atoms. They are straight and lack the twist and turns needed to fit most of our body's fat locks. We do use some saturated fat, but left in the bloodstream it gets into our brain, heart and liver, oxidizing into fatty deposits that block up and shut down our arteries.

Our body takes all the excess saturated fat (90 percent of the fat we consume) and stuffs it into adipose cells. These fat storage cells can swell up to 1,000 times their size, so we can store an almost endless amount of fat. Saturated fats, being flat like pancakes, stack up easily in our cells and arteries, causing all kinds of physiological problems and making us fat.

UNSATURATED FATS

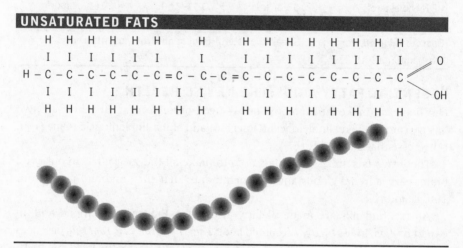

Unsaturated fats have no hydrogens on some sides and thus the carbons are not saturated. An unsaturated fat bends toward its unsaturated side, toward the empty spaces, because the hydrogens on the other side repel each other with electromagnetic charges.

The more empty spaces an unsaturated fat has, the more it bends. These empty spaces are called double bonds and create the cis configuration. This cis configuration is a key that fits our fat locks and turns "on" healthy fat metabolism in the body. The curves and electromagnetic charges created by their double bonds prevent them from clumping in our bloodstream, where they remain liquid.

OMEGA-3 UNSATURATED FATS

cis Fat Configuration

Fish oils and the long-chain fats in our brain have 20 to 24 carbons. These fatty acids are critical for maintaining optimal performance in our brain, cardiovascular system and immune system. Unless you are eating one fish meal a day of either salmon, tuna, sardines or mackerel, you're probably not getting enough long-chain Omega-3 fatty acids.

Finding Good Fats

Alpha-linolenic acid (Omega-3 EFA) from your diet converts after eight enzymatic interactions into DHA and then into EPA. DHA is vital because our brain is made of it. If we eat fish, especially oily fish like salmon, mackerel and sardines, we are getting preformed DHA, saving our body a lot of hard work to try to make it from perilla oil, flax, hemp, walnuts or pumpkin seeds or their oils.

GOOD FATS	
Fat Type	**Food Source**
Monounsaturated fats	Extra-virgin olive oil, canola oil, almonds, pumpkin seeds, sunflower seeds, hazelnuts, avocados
Omega-3 long-chain fats	Fish oils (cod liver oil, salmon, sardines, krill, anchovy, mackerel), flax seeds and oils, hemp seeds and oils, perilla oil, soy products, green leafy vegetables

Omega-3 essential fatty acids act in the body to produce beneficial hormone-like messengers called prostaglandins 1 and 3 (PGE1 and PGE3). Studies show that prostaglandins PGE1 and PGE3 can destroy breast, prostate and lung cancer cells. Prostaglandin-2 (PGE2) in overabundance is a destructive pro-inflammatory hormone-like messenger formed from arachidonic acid (AA) found in red meat, organ meats, egg yolks and full-fat dairy. Imbalances in prostaglandins underlie many common illnesses, from arthritis to heart attacks and strokes.

DHA and EPA, long-chain Omega-3 fatty acids, comprise up to 50 percent of the total fat in the brain and central nervous system and are as critical to the healthy functioning of nerve membranes as they are to arteries. Joseph R. Hibbelin, M.D., chief of the outpatient clinic at the National Institute of Alcohol Abuse and Alcoholism at the National Institutes of Health, suggested that the patients most likely to suffer from depression along with coronary heart disease, alcoholism, multiple sclerosis and postpartum depression may be the ones with low concentrations of Omega-3 fatty acids in nerve membranes. He theorized that deficient levels of the Omega-3s in the nervous system may increase a patient's vulnerability to depression, just as a deficient level in the circulation may increase vulnerability to heart disease. Low blood Omega-3 levels and low markers for serotonin appear together. According to Dr. Hibbelin, "This suggests that dietary intake of these fatty acids might influence the serotonin process and that altering this process may possibly reduce depressive, suicidal, and violent behavior."

We should eat fish three to four times a week or use supplements of fish, or algae oils high in DHA/EPA, organic cold-pressed flax or hemp seed oil or perilla oil (1 tablespoon daily) and extra-virgin olive oil (1 to 2 tablespoons daily).

Serving of Fish (5 oz; 140 g)	Omega-3 EFAs
Sardines in oil	5.6 grams
Mackerel	4.2 grams
Trout	2.8 grams
Salmon	2.3 grams
Tuna	0.9 grams

Omega-3 and Omega-6 Essential Fatty Acid Sources

Allowable Fats at Breakfast

- EPA- and DHA-rich, long-chain Omega-3 essential fatty acids (EFAs) from supplementation from one of three sources:
  (a) fish oil softgels, such as sardine, krill, anchovy, mackerel, salmon oils;
  (b) cod liver oil high in DHA/EPA;
  (c) oil-filled softgels of algae extract (DHA-rich ocean plankton—the DHA can produce EPA in your body), suitable for vegans and lacto-ovo vegetarians.

The goal is to supplement daily with 1,000 mg of EPA (eicosapentaenoic acid) and 650 mg of DHA (docosahexaenoic acid) with each breakfast. If the label does not guarantee how much EPA or DHA is in a serving of two softgels or a tablespoon of liquid fish oils, do not purchase that brand.

If you do use either (a) or (b) polyunsaturated fish oils, be completely sure that they are purified by molecular distillation. No other method will do. If you use (a), sardine or salmon oil, the superior absorbable fish oils are glyceride fish oils. If you use (b), cod liver oil (plain or with a natural flavor), the superior quality oils are emulsified for much better absorption. To maintain their freshness and prevent the oils from oxidizing, both (a) and (b) should contain at least 5 to 10 IU of natural vitamin E per serving of two softgel capsules or per tablespoon of oil.

Allowable Fats at Lunch and Dinner or Before Bed

- Almonds (6), avocado (3 tablespoons), almond butter (1 tablespoon)

- Cashews (6)
- Flax seeds, hemp seeds (2 tablespoons, ground in a coffee grinder), organic flax or hemp seed oil (1 tablespoon)
- Guacamole (4 tablespoons)
- Olives, black or green (5), extra virgin olive oil (1 to 2 table-spoons)
- Peanuts, peanut butter (1 tablespoon)
- Tahini (1 tablespoon)
- Omega-6, GLA-rich borage oil, black currant or evening primrose oil (1/2 teaspoon)

BAD FATS

To make essential fats and oils more stable, the oil industry takes the fat and puts it through a process called hydrogenation, or partial hydrogenation, so the hydrogens lose their electromagnetic repulsion—and so their shape straightens up and now they do not fit the fat locks in our body. Processing and refining turns the biologically active cis fats into aberrant trans-fats. Our body now takes these trans-fats in and tries to make use of them. Unfortunately, it causes chaos and our cellular biochemical interactions go "haywire" and we deteriorate quickly—mentally, emotionally and physically.

Processed foods are jam-packed with these dangerous trans-fats. Vegetable salad dressings and cooking oils, as well as both the French fries and onion rings cooked in them, are a worrisome 42 percent trans-fatty acids. Regular salad oils in restaurants or on grocery shelves are 20 percent trans-fats. Commercial baked goods like cookies, cakes, crackers, muffins, pies and croissants contain up to 35 percent trans-fats. The average North American diet today contains 3 to 4 percent of total calories as these processed, dangerous trans-fats. Recent animal studies have found gross cell abnormalities with diets of only 4.4 percent trans-fats. Most vegetable oils we buy in the grocery store are extracted from hard seeds using excessive heat, pressure, chemical solvents and bleach to mask their harsh flavor. Such extraction methods turn healthy cis fatty acids into unhealthy trans-fatty acids. They are created in huge abundance when an oil is hydrogenated or partially hydrogenated. It is clear that trans-fatty acids are bad for hearts and arteries. Avoid the tropical oil, palm oil; it is high in saturated fat. I furthermore do not recommend that you use peanut oil, as it can contain carcinogenic aflatoxin, a mold that can grow on peanuts.

Our brain is largely composed of fat. What is more, the cells of the brain utilize fat from our diet. If too much of the wrong kind of fat is eaten, it can induce the lipid-rich parts of the brain to oxidize or break down, similar to the rancidity reaction that occurs when we leave French fries out on the counter too long.

Hydrogenated or partially hydrogenated oils promote the inflammation and deterioration of brain cells—food for thought before we eat any more French fries!

Hydrogenated or semi-hydrogenated oils from palm oil, safflower oil, sunflower seed oil, cotton seed oil and corn oil are pro-oxidative and interfere with key metabolic processes because they are highly reactive and produce accelerated ageing free radicals quickly. Look for them carefully on labels and avoid them. They are virulent promotes of the sludging of our metabolic system and play havoc with the normal functioning or our cells.

Most margarines, as are other foods with hydrogenated or semi-hydrogenated oils, are full of trans-fatty acids. They are the outcome of the processing of these oils and are dangerous. A Harvard study found that women eating 4 teaspoons a day of margarine had two-thirds higher risk of heart disease than those eating almost none.

BAD FATS

Fat Type	Food Source
Polyunsaturated fats	Corn oil, peanut oil, grain oils, processed foods
Saturated fats	Animal fats, dairy fats, palm oil
Trans-fatty acids	Processed foods

THE FAT SUMMARY
Fats to Use Daily

1. One tablespoon of organic flax, perilla or hemp oil, half on your vegetables at dinner and half with garlic and yogurt before you go to sleep. This is an exception to the no eating after 7:30 p.m. rule. Better still, grind 2 tablespoons of organic flax or hemp seeds and add it to your protein power shake. The seeds give you fresh oil and lots of fiber that increase stool bulk.

2. Oils containing EFAs such as flax, perilla or hemp oil are very temperature sensitive and unsuitable for cooking. Olive oil, unprocessed coconut butter and ghee (the fat of butter without the milk solids) are the preferred oils to cook with. Coconut oil is suitable for vegans as a dairy-free alternative to butter.

3. One or two tablespoons of extra-virgin "green" organic olive oil on your salads daily. Not only is olive oil slow to oxidize (go rancid), but it may actually fight the effects of free radicals. Extra-virgin olive oil is the monounsaturated oil from the first pressing of the olives and contains beneficial oleic acid. Most often, these olives are superior in quality and the oil maintains a superior quality and flavor. Virgin olive oil is made from the second or third pressing of the olives and is more acidic than extra-virgin. Regular or pure olive oil is often processed with solvents and high heat, which creates an inferior oil, both in flavor and also nutritionally. Avoid it always.

All these oils generally have a four-month shelf life. Check the date of pressing or "best-used-by" dates on the bottle. I highly recommend that you purchase all organic oils in small quantities in non-reactive, opaque bottles. These oils should be low-temperature, expeller-pressed in the absence of light and flushed with an inert gas such as nitrogen to expel all oxygen. Replenish them every week or two with fresh oils. Open one 400 IU softgel of vitamin E and squeeze it into the oil to protect the oil from oxidizing once the bottle is opened.

4. Unless we eat broiled fish like salmon, tuna, sardines or mackerel three times a week, it is wise for us to supplement with fish oils rich in DHA and EPA. Take high DHA/EPA cod liver oil or two to four fish oil or nine algae extract oil capsules on a daily basis. Vegetarians can eat more sea vegetables, such as chlorella, Nova Scotia dulse and spirulina, and can also supplement with extracted algae oil capsules rich in DHA and EPA, which are necessary for optimal neurological and cardiovascular health.

5. Take 1/2 teaspoon of organic borage oil, an Omega-6 EFA rich in gamma linolenic acid (GLA); each 1/2 teaspoon contains 500 mg of GLA. You can purchase high-lignan flax seed oil already mixed with borage oil.

Fats to Avoid

Avoid unhealthy trans-fatty acids in all refined or processed foods that greatly reduce the transmission of hormonal cascades. Most foods, however, don't currently provide information on the label as to the amount of trans-fatty acids. Your best bet for avoiding trans-fats is to choose products that don't list hydrogenated or partially hydrogenated oils in the ingredient list. Hydrogenated oils in any amount are your tip-off to the presence of "bad" LDL cholesterol-raising trans-fatty acids.

Recommended Ratio of EFAs

Most North Americans fail to obtain the optimal balance of essential fatty acids (EFAs) from their diet. That is why dietary supplements such as flax, hemp, fish, primrose and borage oils have become so popular among health-conscious people. Fatty acids serve as building blocks of nerve cells and all cell membranes.

Without adequate levels of the friendly fats, dangerous trans-fatty acids and saturated fats will replace EFAs within all membranes, reducing membrane fluidity and efficiency and thereby starting a process of premature aging and degenerative disease. By taking the right proportions of EFAs, we can maximize the production of beneficial hormone-like prostaglandins PGE1 and PGE3, while minimizing the production of harmful PGE2 series.

Deficiencies in the correct balance of EFAs have recently been linked to cardiovascular disease, hypertension, elevated LDL ("bad") cholesterol, insulin resistance leading to Type II diabetes, mental dementia and memory loss.

A Quick Comparison

PERCENTAGE OF FATS IN ORGANIC, UNREFINED VEGETABLE OILS				
Oil	Omega-3 Alpha-Linolenic Acid	Omega-6 Linoleic Acid	Omega-9 Mono-unsaturated Fats	Saturated Fats
Flax seed	54	15	23	9
Hemp seed	42	18	28	12
Pumpkin seed	12	45	32	8
Canola	8	26	57	9
Borage oil	10	52 (GLA)	23	25
Extra virgin olive oil	—	12	72	16
Cottonseed	—	48	28	25
Peanut	—	29	56	15
Palm kernel	—	2	18	80

The first six oils (Flax seed through Extra virgin olive oil) are labelled **USE**; the last three (Cottonseed, Peanut, Palm kernel) are labelled **AVOID**.

There are two particularly beneficial EFAs you must consume daily and in the right proportion. They are the Omega-6 EFA derivative, gamma linolenic acid (GLA), and the Omega-3 EFA derivative, DHA/EPA. GLA supplementation helps to reverse the effects of aging on fatty acid metabolism, while DHA/EPA is essential for the development and maintenance of superior brain functions and cardiovascular health.

Experts disagree on the exact ideal ratio, but most agree that it lies somewhere between 1:1 or 4:1; that is, 1 part Omega-6 to 1 part Omega-3 or 4 parts Omega-6 to 1 part Omega-3. I highly recommend a 2:1 ratio; that is, 2 parts Omega-6 to 1 part Omega-3, but of the actual derivatives, 2 parts GLA and 1 part DHA/EPA.

The highest source of GLA is the borage seed (23 percent), followed by black currant seeds (15–18 percent) and evening primrose seed (8–12 percent). I prefer the borage source as it is a large seed and the oil can be extracted without chemicals or refining.

I highly recommend that you use 1/2 teaspoon of organic borage oil daily to maintain your GLA levels; and 1 tablespoon of cod liver oil or two to four fish oil capsules or algae extract. In addition, I encourage you to consume 1 tablespoon of organic flax or hemp oil and 1 tablespoon of extra virgin olive oil daily.

The first step in both EFAs' conversion process is controlled by the enzyme D-6-D (delta-6-desaturase). Unfortunately, D-6-D activity declines with stress and age beginning at about age 25. Supplementing with GLA and DHA/EPA actually increases D-6-D activity and improves the metabolism on both Omega-3 and Omega-6 EFAs.

14

17 BIOENERGETIC FOODS TO EAT DAILY

(THEN ADD WATER)

1. GREEN TEA

Both green and black teas come from the leaves of the plant Camellia sinensis. Green tea, however, undergoes less processing than black tea, thus preserving more of the protective phytonutrients called polyphenols, known cancer cell suppressors, and the powerful antioxidant quercetin. In fact, it contains 350 to 400 mg of biologically active polyphenols (the most powerful being epigallocat-echin-gallate or EGCG), compared to only 150 to 200 mg per cup of black tea.

According to Lester A. Mitscher, Ph.D., of the University of Kansas, green tea also lowers levels of bad LDL cholesterol and prevents its oxidation, protects the heart and arteries from oxidative stress, has an overall blood pressure-lowering effect, inhibits blood clotting and significantly reduces a person's risk of heart disease and stroke if 2 to 3 cups are consumed daily.

Dr. Junshi Chen, of the Chinese Academy of Preventive Medicine in Beijing, agrees that the benefits of green tea are dose-dependent. In other words, the more green tea we drink, the greater the protective effect we experience—especially against cancer.

His research concludes that green tea can: inhibit the binding of certain carcinogens to the DNA—especially in the liver, the lungs and the stomach; boost the body's glutathione S-transferase system, which acts to detoxify cancer-promoting chemicals; increase the beneficial enzyme activity of superoxide dismutase (SOD); and enhance immunity by activating several immune system components, such as B cells, T cells and NK (natural killer) cells.

Several U.S. studies confirm Chen's findings. Researchers at the Skin Diseases Research Center, at the University Hospital of Cleveland, found that skin tumors artificially induced in mice by various cancer-causing chemicals were prevented by the addition of epigallocatechin-gallate (the active ingredient in green tea) to the drinking water of mice. They also cite several other studies that demonstrated positive results in a variety of laboratory animals against induced lung, stomach, colon, duodenum and esophageal cancers, simply by substituting green tea for the usual drinking water.

Green tea is especially rich in vitamin K, which allows calcium to be formed into the matrix of your bones and supports mental acuity.

Green tea needs to steep for one full hour to allow all of the epigallocatechin-gallate to be released into the warm liquid. The green tea becomes slightly bitter if left steeping for one hour. You can add a little ginger root to the green tea and this successfully removes the bitter flavor.

Although green tea contains one-third less caffeine than black tea and coffee, it is still a stimulant. If you "get the jitters" from caffeine, you can purchase decaffeinated green tea brands or take caffeine-free green tea extracts as a dietary supplement.

2. "GREEN DRINKS"

Green drinks are the most complete bioenergetic food available. High-quality versions are low in calories and contain no sugars, sweeteners or fats. This makes it a perfect low-glycemic food. Berries are the only fruit to mix in a "green drink."

If they are made from organic ingredients, they are a near-perfect food providing anabolic life insurance.

Green drinks are green because they contain chlorophyll, the green component in every living plant, which is made during the process of photosynthesis. When the sun's energy enters a plant, the plant takes in carbon dioxide, gives off pure oxygen, makes organic vitamins, minerals and protein from inorganic materials in the soil and produces this green color of life. Chlorophyll activates the enzymes that produce vitamins E, A and K in the plant. Vitamin K is the only vitamin shown to keep calcium out of your arteries and glands, thereby lessening arterial calcification and lowering both coronary artery and cardiovascular disease. Vitamin K has been found to be essential to the formation of "osteocalcin," a protein that attracts calcium and helps to build it into strong bones.

Chlorophyll is an antiviral, antibacterial cellular cleanser.

Green drinks are generally powdered, highly nutritious, alkaline-forming, land-based and ocean-grown foods that you conveniently and affordably mix in pure water, fresh vegetable juice or unsweetened fruit juice. Once opened, store green drinks in the refrigerator to maximize the vitality and lifespan of the billions of probiotic "friendly bacteria" they contain from non-dairy sources.

The following are some of the ingredients you'll find in a high-quality green drink:

- Non-genetically modified, organically grown, 97 percent oil-free lecithin that gives you 1,200 mg of phosphatidyl choline (PC) for superior neurological transmissions and 60 mg of phosphatidyl serine (PS) for high-quality mental enhancement. Soy lecithin is also a superior methyl donor that keeps your brain youthful longer and helps to prevent the formation of excess homocysteine, which can cause oxidized cholesterol to block your arteries.
- Organically grown grasses such as alfalfa, barley and wheatgrass. Buffalo and wild horses, as an example, grow strong, lean and fast on a diet primarily comprised of these wild, nutrient-rich grasses. These grasses are a treasure trove of all known vitamins, minerals, phytonutrients, chlorophyll, fiber, Omega-3 EFAs and protein. They contain a powerful antioxidant that prevents the build up of hydrogen peroxide in fat tissues and cells, especially in the brain, where it is extremely destructive.
- Ocean-grown algae or vegetables such as chlorella, spirulina and Nova Scotia dulse. These increase serum albumin levels, the main carrier molecule of nutrients to your 100 trillion cells. Higher albumin levels are necessary for a long and healthy life.
- Soluble and insoluble fibers from brown rice germ and bran, as well as apple pectin, which soak up excess estrogen and heavy metals such as cadmium, aluminum, lead and mercury from the intestinal tract.
- Dairy-free probiotic cultures ("friendly" bacteria) and FOS (fructo-oligo-saccharides, a special non-digestive sugar that feeds these "friendly" bacteria and keeps them alive) combine to keep your intestinal tract healthy and vibrant with vital, living, life-sustaining "good bacteria."
- Organically grown or wild-crafted herbs (picked in the wild) that:
  - protect the brain and connective tissue from aging;
  - are very strong antiviral, antibacterial and anticarcinogenic compounds for immune support;
  - act as adaptagens (biochemical stress modifiers) to help balance the physical, mental or biochemical stresses in the body;
  - increase the cholinergic (nerve impulses) mechanism linked to learning, memory and fluid, coordinated movements of your arms and legs; and
  - contain resveratrol, a powerful cancer-inhibiting phytochemical clinically shown to block the development of precancerous and cancerous growths.

I highly recommend that you make a green drink part of your daily dietary strategy. Take your green drink 15 minutes before a meal on an empty stomach, or two hours after a meal so all the nutrient-rich foods will be quickly absorbed.

People who use green drinks daily notice an increase in their cognitive abilities, as well as an increase in their general levels of energy and well-being. This is because green drinks are abundant in the amino acids called peptides, which can be transformed in your body to neuropeptides. Neuropeptides, such as beta endorphins, are one of the primary links between mind and body. Green drinks are also rich in the nine essential amino acids, especially tryptophan and phenyl-alanine—the primary "building blocks" for your important neurotransmitter hormones serotonin and norepinephrine (adrenaline).

Green drinks sustain the natural human cycle at optimum with plant-based foods steeped in the sunlight and infused with the abundant energy of the soil and rain—pure life energy crucial to maintaining your anabolic drive and the most fundamental way to successfully support your hormonal development, control and fidelity.

3. WHEY PROTEIN ISOLATE

Whey protein isolate—derived from the curd-free portion of cow's milk—is so similar to human breast milk in its amino acid profile that its nutritional value to humans is virtually identical. It is a premium bioenergetic fuel for humans.

Even more remarkable, if whey protein isolate has not been denatured by high pasteurization temperatures or certain processing techniques like aeration, vacuum evaporation and spray drying, the whey protein isolates are enormously effective in boosting human immunity.

The only two 100 percent whey protein isolate powders that my personal research accepts as 99 percent biologically active (undenatured) and meets my strict standards are Enhanced Life Extension Protein (ELEP) and Alphapure™. Both of these protein isolate powders are a product of premium-source cheddar cheese making, while almost all other whey proteins are inferior products from cottage cheese production. Only these two sources are made with low-tempera-ture, cross-flow microfiltration (CFM), ceramic-filtered techniques, which produce an isolate 99 percent undenatured and retaining all of the important subfractions in their natural ratios, with no fat and only 1 percent lactose to make it easily digested and absorbed by lactose-intolerant people.

Low-temperature, cross-flow microfiltration, ceramic-filtered techniques produce a whey protein isolate that is greater than 90 percent protein. Whey concentrates are only 70 to 80 percent protein.

ELEP and Alphapure™ use a crucial manufacturing process that does not degrade or damage the delicate protein subfractions (peptides), such as alpha-lactalbumin, lactoferrin, lactoglobulin, serum albumin and the immunoglobu-lins. For example, mother's milk contains up to 15 percent of the powerful anti-microbial lactoferrin, undenatured whey contains 5 percent lactoferrin and regular whey contains only 0.5 to 1 percent.

Neither of these whey protein isolates contains the ever-popular sugar substitutes such as acesulfane potassium, or Nutra Sweet® (aspartame).

Alphapure™ and ELEP protein isolate powders:

- raise levels of the antioxidant glutathione significantly and safely in your cells and tissues;
- improve exercise tolerance and maintain an anabolic drive;
- increase net muscle protein synthesis;
- restore youthful anabolic metabolism at the cellular level;
- boost immune functions and bioenergetics;
- inhibit cancer cell proliferation;
- protect against free-radical damage;
- protect against catabolic wasting syndrome in cancer patients; and
- raise albumin serum levels, a blood protein molecule that carries 60 percent of all nutrients in the blood and equally distributes them to each 100 trillion cells.

Cancer generally appears when blood albumin levels drop below 4.5 grams per litre of blood. Low levels are 4.2 and excellent levels are 5.8. North Americans average 4.2 and Japanese people average 4.5. There is a well-established correlation between low albumin levels and mortality. *The Lancet*, a British medical journal, published a 1989 British study that followed 7,735 middle-aged men for 9.2 years. Men with the lowest albumin levels had the highest rates of premature death from many different causes.

Alphapure™ and ELEP are two to four times more abundant with the amino acid cysteine than any other whey protein powders I have researched. Stable cysteine, as found in whole foods, produces an enormous amount of glutathione and its antioxidant enzymes glutathione peroxidase and glutathione-S-transferase in your cells, tissues and liver naturally and efficiently.

Whey is one of two major proteins found in milk, the other being casein. Casein is an inferior protein and causes allergic reactions in people and I do not recommend it as a protein source. Be forewarned and read labels carefully.

Each of the subfractions found in whey has its own unique biological properties. These critical subfractions of whey isolate powder have documented antiviral, antimicrobial, anticancer and immune-modulating/enhancing effects.

Whey protein isolate, with the highest biological value (BV) of any protein, is absorbed, utilized and retained in the body better than other proteins. One recent study by C.M. Molker, D. Kalman, W.D. Brink and L.G. Maharan, in *Medical Science in Sports in Exercise* in 1998, found that whey protein isolates corrected the immune suppression often seen in athletes suffering from over-training.

When you make a protein shake using Alphapure™ or ELEP whey protein peptide powders, mix them in a hand-held tumbler. *Do not* blend them in a blender, as the heat and agitation of the blender will denature these remarkable proteins. You will still absorb the protein, but by denaturing either of these two exceptional protein sources, you will destroy their critical immune-boosting capabilities. You can also hand mix them into your oatmeal, cereals, legumes, soups, yogurts and warm miso broths to raise the protein-to-carbohydrate ratios of these foods, making them more nutritionally dynamic.

The Anabolic Power of a Protein Shake

A protein power shake as a meal should supply 27 grams of protein for the average female and 35 grams for the average male.

The ideal mixture of protein is half ELEP or Alphapure™ undenatured whey protein isolates and half from water-extracted, non-GMO soy protein isolates, as in the product transform+.

The whey isolates fix nitrogen in muscle tissue quickly but do not have long staying power. To compensate for this, most whey protein manufacturers add the casein protein from milk that extends whey's staying power. But as we already discussed, casein is highly allergenic and an inferior protein. Preferable to this is getting half your protein from non-GMO soy protein isolates that are not as quickly absorbed as whey protein isolates and give you high-quality protein sustaining capability naturally.

After the age of 30, most of us have difficulty digesting and absorbing proteins. Generally you may experience flatulence, an energy decline and an uncomfortable stomach. You can use broad spectrum, plant-derived digestive enzymes to help you digest these proteins completely.

> Soy protein isolates generally contain from 150 to 300 mg per 10 oz (280 g) of protein of the vitally important phytonutrient isoflavonoids—genistein, daidzein and glycitein—that significantly protect you from breast or prostate cancer initiation and promotion.

Over the past decade, whey protein powders have evolved through several generations. The first generation was considered "concentrates" and was as little as 30 to 40 percent protein with large amounts of lactose. The second generation is inferior whey concentrates with the superior whey isolates added to them to increase their protein content per serving. They are put through an "ion exchange" process that sounds impressive, but chemicals such as hydrochloric acid and sodium hydroxide are used. Whey protein concentrates contain only 70 to 80 percent protein—and all the immune-building subfractions are destroyed. The third generation whey protein 100 percent isolates I recommend are made in a process known as cross-flow microfiltration (CFM), which uses no chemicals. CFM uses high-tech ceramic filters to produce 100 percent isolates that are 99 percent undenatured, with no fat or lactose but over 90 percent protein. No chemicals or heat are used.

4. GOURMET GREENS

Lettuce is North America's favorite green. Lettuce is green because it contains the potent antioxidant and phytochemical chlorophyll. But that beautiful vibrant green color isn't the only good news. Lettuce is a source of healing organic water, fibers, beta- and alpha-carotene, B-complex vitamins, vitamins A, C and E, calcium, iron, potassium, magnesium and manganese, and the dark green varieties also contain co-enzyme Q10, which is necessary for a strong heart. The darker the leaf, the more abundant the vitamin A content. The tips of a lettuce generally contain more of these nutrients than the fibrous rib.

I encourage you to try the wide variety of greens available in most grocery stores and produce markets. Say goodbye to iceberg lettuce and hello to luscious spinach, arugula, endive, leaf lettuce, oak lettuce, romaine lettuce, mesclun, mizuna, mustard greens, bibb, endive, kale, chard, dandelion greens, watercress and parsley. All are full of vitamins that contribute to the growth and vibrant health of nails, hair, and skin. Mustard greens have 600 percent more vitamin C and 500 percent more calcium than iceberg lettuce. Dandelion greens have 20 percent more beta-carotene, 600 percent more iron, 400 percent more vitamin B12 and 300 percent more vitamin C than iceberg lettuce. Watercress is high in sulfur (responsible for the vegetable's strong flavor), which cleans the bloodstream and supports pancreatic health, while iceberg has none.

Whenever possible, buy organically grown produce. Greens should be served at room temperature, immediately after tossing. The younger the green leaf, the tastier it is. Store all greens loosely wrapped in a cotton cloth in the vegetable crisper. Do not store apples with tender greens, as the ethylene produced by apples will cause leaf browning. Environmentally safe storage bags called Ever-Fresh bags also keep fruits and vegetables in the refrigerator fresher and more flavorful, three to ten times longer than conventional storage methods.

Lettuce Get Acquainted

Arugula: The emerald-green leaves have a delicate texture and a sharp, peppery flavor.

Bibb: Medium green leaves have a velvety texture and a mild flavor. The heads are small with curved flat, delicate leaves.

Curly Endive: This frilly-leafed lettuce has a bittersweet taste and pale green color.

Green or Red Looseleaf: Large fan-shaped heads are either light green or tipped in reddish-purple with a mild-sweet flavor.

Mesclun: This lettuce is a widely available, but pricey, mixture of young tender greens and colorful herbs of many flavors, containing red looseleaf, arugula, mizuna, pansy heads, and curly endive.

Mizuna: This lettuce has long, dark green jagged leaves with a mild mustard-like taste.

Watercress: Often mixed with mild-flavored greens like leaf lettuce and bibb, watercress has a distinct peppery flavor, crunchy stems, and deep green, round leaves.

Eating colorful salads is a wonderful way to include raw "live foods" in your daily diet. And remember, presentation is everything. Present your food with a multitude of colors from a wide range of unheated lettuces in salads or as garnishes.

5. GARLIC

Garlic has been used both as food and medicine for a very long time. It figures prominently in cuisine around the world and in both traditional Chinese and Ayurvedic herbal medicines. Today, there is a great deal known about garlic's medicinal benefits and how these benefits are achieved.

Garlic is antibacterial, antifungal and antiviral. It also prevents blood clotting, is an antioxidant and neutralizes free radicals. It helps prevent cancer by blocking both the initiation and promotion of cancer cells.

Garlic, as well as onions, shallots, leeks, scallions and chives, contains the active compound alliin. Alliin is the main compound, but must be acted on by a garlic enzyme called alliinase found in raw garlic to turn it into the active allicin, which your body can use. This only happens when you chop or mash garlic, exposing it to the air for five minutes so the enzyme alliinase is released. Allicin is very unstable when heated. So, if you cook garlic you get the flavor but no medicinal or antibacterial effects. Baked whole garlic, a favorite of gourmet chefs, cannot deliver this potent phytonutrient.

It is allicin that imparts garlic's characteristic odor and flavor. While allicin is the main active ingredient in garlic, it is really a chemical precursor of several other active compounds such as sulfides and sulfide-containing peptides. Garlic also contains amino acids, glycosides, minerals, phospholipids, vitamins and the rare but necessary trace minerals selenium and tellurium.

Antibacterial and Antiviral Activity

Garlic extracts have been found effective against certain strains of bacteria, including some antibiotic-resistant organisms. It has been shown to be effective against the bacterial stomach parasite Helicobacter pylori, which many researchers feel is the cause of peptic ulcers. And it is equally effective against several resilient strains of bacteria, such as Mycobacterium avium, which has been isolated from AIDS patients.

Garlic, in one form or another—preferably crushed, raw, organic garlic or aged garlic capsules—might be useful as an adjunct to standard antibiotic therapy.

Garlic also has antifungal properties, according to Dr. Robert Nagourney in his article "Garlic: Medicinal Food or Nutritious Medicine?" in the *Journal of Medicinal Food*. He states that "garlic can be as effective as, and in many cases, even more effective than, standard antifungal drugs which have unpleasant side effects. Fungus-caused skin problems such as athlete's foot or an internal yeast infection such as Candida albicans, or fungal ear infections caused by Aspergillus, may well be treated by either raw or capsuled aged garlic, or liquid aged garlic taken internally, as well as applied directly to the problem area."

In test tube experiments against herpes simplex types I and II, stomatitis (a viral infection of the mouth) and so critically important, against human rhinoviruses (a class of viruses that cause the common cold), garlic has given "broad antiviral activity."

Garlic Helps the Heart and Circulation

Garlic has a well-documented ability to inhibit blood platelet aggregation and thromboxane formation. Thromboxane is a prostaglandin-like compound that encourages the clumping together of blood platelets—clot formation—that can lead to heart attack or stroke. Garlic, therefore, seems to have the potential to help prevent heart attack and stroke. Garlic's proven ability to scavenge and inhibit free radicals is also a protection against cancer, for all cancers are, at least partially, free radical driven.

Anticancer Effects

There are several recent laboratory studies showing that the active ingredients in garlic—allicin and ajoene—might block both the initiation and promotion of cancer. Dr. Nagourney states that several animal studies have "clearly established the ability of garlic's water- and lipid-soluble fractions to directly inhibit tumor initiation." Furthermore, selenium-enriched garlic was more potent in preventing tumor initiation than regular garlic alone. It would be advisable therefore to take a selenium supplement of 200 mcg, if garlic, either raw or as aged supplemental garlic capsules, is used for cancer prevention.

The Memorial Sloan-Kettering Cancer Center in New York has found that garlic inhibits the growth of cancer cells in the laboratory. In a recent study of colon cancer conducted at the M.D. Anderson Hospital in Houston, Dr. Michael Wargovich determined that diallyl sulfide, a major component of garlic, reduced the growth of colon cancer in mice. Other related experiments showed that diallyl sulfide may prevent cancer of the esophagus and prostate cancer.

Garlic is not metabolized. It is absorbed through the stomach lining, the way alcohol is. This may make some individuals feel slightly sick after consuming garlic. If you cannot eat ordinary garlic, try aged garlic capsules that are deodorized, as a supplement.

Use Fresh Whole Garlic Daily

Do what I do! Just before you retire at night, finely chop two cloves of fresh garlic with a sharp knife and let it sit exposed to the air for five minutes. This chopping releases the phytonutrient enzyme alliinase. Put the chopped garlic on a tablespoon and swallow it with water. The garlic will roam your entire gastrointestinal tract all night long, acting as a toxic garbage cop, literally destroying harmful bacteria, viruses, fungi, parasites, yeast, chemical intruders and carcinogens before they can harm you. Your first bowel movement of the morning will have a strong garlic odor, but you will have absolutely no garlic odor on or about you. Do not chew the minced garlic, just simply swallow it. Garlic only gives off its odor from your skin or breath when you chew it. Practice makes perfect.

Graduate school procedure: This procedure is to swallow your two cloves of finely chopped garlic with water, also swallow one of your 1/2 tablespoons of flax seed oil, and then immediately eat 1/2 cup of fat-free, organic, unsweetened, plain white yogurt or quark. Read in the next section under "Flax Seed Oil" why Johanna Budwig, M.D. and a double Ph.D., put together the combination of flax seed oil and yogurt or quark cheese. This is a highly recommended exception to my basic rule of not eating past 7:30 p.m.

Postgraduate school procedure: With the above recipe, also take two capsules of a synergistic antioxidant formula containing beta-carotene, vitamins C and E as a succinate, selenium, alpha lipoic acid, N-acetyl cysteine, CoQ10, lycopene, bilberry, bioflavonoids and full-spectrum grape extract.

6. ESSENTIAL FATTY ACIDS

The primary reason for human beings' dominance on earth is their brain. The brain is the richest source of long-chain Omega-3 fatty acids (EFAs) in the body.

Dr. Ralph Moss, in his book *Cancer Therapy*, notes that radiologists at the University of California at Los Angeles have found high concentrations of linoleic acid (flax seed oil) in the small intestines of mice. Researchers had puzzled over why cancer rarely develops in the small intestines of mice.

Scientists at the University of Toronto point to lignans in flax seeds as the anticancer agent, especially with colon cancer. In the colon, these plant lignans are acted upon by bacteria and turned into mammalian lignans, which scientists credit with the anticancer effect of this oil. Flax seeds ground or high "lignan" flax seed oil raise alpha-linolenic and long-chain Omega-3 fatty acid levels in both blood plasma and erythrocytes (red blood cells).

There are a total of eight essential fatty acids (EFAs), which fall into two classes—Omega-3 and Omega-6 fatty acids. Omega-3s are abundant in ocean algae, flax seeds, hemp seeds, perilla oil, walnuts, pumpkin seeds and dark meat of fatty fish. Alpha linolenic acid (ALA) is the name of the Omega-3 essential fatty acid found in these bioenergetic whole foods. But like anything else in life, too much of a good thing is bad. Adequate amounts of Omega-3 EFAs are critical for our well-being, but too much ALA literally shuts "off" the delta-6-desaturase enzyme that controls the body's ability to convert (or activate) Omega-6 EFAs in our diet to a more metabolically activated fatty acid known as gamma linolenic acid (GLA).

Unlike ALA (that I want you to limit in your dietary strategy), which is found in virtually every food, GLA is rarely found in food except in small amounts in oatmeal, borage seeds, black currant seeds and evening primrose seeds.

We want GLA but the delta-6-desaturase enzyme to make GLA from ALA is easily incapacitated by stress, a high-density carbohydrate diet, high insulin levels, exhaustion, accumulated sleep-debt, illness and aging. We can take GLA directly in borage, black currant and evening primrose oil, but must limit any of them to 1/2 teaspoon a day. Borage oil is the least processed of them.

The metabolism of Omega-6 essential fatty acids in the body is critically necessary to make good prostaglandins (eicosanoids) that stimulate the synthesis (production) of our hormones. Researchers call these messengers "prostaglandins" because they were originally discovered in the prostate gland. We now know that prostaglandins are made throughout the body.

CoQ10, alpha lipoic acid, DHEA or any male supplemental hormone (such as testosterone) or female hormone (such as estrogen), as a replacement therapy, should be taken with fat at breakfast. They are all best absorbed with some kind of lipid (fatty substance).

Moreover, progesterone and prescription, natural estrogens used for hormone replacement therapy (estradiol, estriol and estrone) should also be taken with flax seed oil at breakfast.

You want to take a maximum of 1/2 teaspoon of organic borage oil daily. Borage oil is the best source of the Omega-6 EFA derivative, gamma linolenic acid (GLA). The body converts GLA into two good prostaglandins E1 and E3 (PGE1 and PGE3), which regulate all other good prostaglandins necessary for arterial muscle tone, sodium excretion and preventing blood platelets from becoming "sticky" and forming dangerous blood clots in your arteries. They also improve clinical symptoms of several inflammatory disorders and suppress the pro-inflammatory prostaglandin E2 (PGE2).

SOURCES OF SMART FATS

Omega-6 EFAs	Omega-3 EFAs
Evening primrose oil	Flax oil
Hemp oil	Hemp oil
Borage oil	Salmon
Safflower oil	Sardines
Sunflower oil	Mackerel
Sesame oil	Tuna
Corn oil	Trout
Meat	Cod liver oil
Black currant seed oil	Soy beans
Egg yolks	Green leafy vegetables
Seeds	Walnuts
Nuts	Herring
Legumes	Perilla oil

We take flax seed oil, hemp seed oil, or perilla oil (seeds of the plant perilla frutescen, also called the beefsteak plant), which contain short-chain Omega-3 fatty acids, so our body can make critical long-chain Omega-3 fats, such as docosahexaenoic acid (DHA) and eicosapentaenoic acid (EPA). Our body has difficulty doing this critical conversion. This is why vegetarians always have lower levels of DHA and EPA in their blood than non-vegetarians do. Once we understand how hard it is for our body to manufacture DHA or EPA from the seeds of flax, hemp, walnut or pumpkin, we can see why we should supplement with DHA- and EPA-rich fish oil capsules or sea algae oil capsules rich in DHA and EPA.

DHA is obtained only from the diet, and our diets are sorely lacking in this fat compared to the amounts our bodies grew accustomed to during evolution. The meat from wild game that our ancestors ate, or even wild game today, contains nearly six times more long-chain Omega-3 fatty acids full of DHA and EPA than today's grain-fed beef. Grain-fed domestic animals raised for human consumption average 30 to 40 percent body fat, full of unhealthy saturated fat. DHA will make EPA. To add insult to injury, we further deplete levels of Omega-3 fatty acids in the brain by smoking and drinking alcoholic beverages.

Low DHA levels in children seriously affect their learning and behavior. A study at Purdue University in Indiana assessed learning, behavior and health problems in boys aged six to 12, and compared this to blood levels of Omega-3 fatty acids. Low levels of Omega-3 essential fatty acid levels were associated with behavioral problems, sleep problems and temper tantrums. Furthermore, boys with low Omega-3 levels were more likely to develop learning difficulties.

There is also some evidence linking low DHA levels in brain tissue to serious mental disorders, such as schizophrenia and bipolar disorders.

When researchers monitor eating habits across countries, they find that as fish consumption goes up, depression rates go down. There is a sixty-fold difference in depression rates across countries from those with the highest depression rates, such as North America and Europe where Omega-3 fat consumption is lowest—to the lowest depression rates in Japan and Taiwan, where Omega-3 fat consumption is highest. A great number of neurological conditions, such as depression, attention deficit disorders and learning difficulties have a high correlation with deficient levels of DHA in the bloodstream.

Researchers conclusively have found that patients with bipolar depression (the most difficult form of depression to treat) often respond dramatically to very high-dose supplementation with oils rich in DHA and EPA.

A growing body of research indicates that infants who are deficient in levels of Omega-3 fatty acids have less than optimal neurological responses, especially intelligence.

Our best bet is to omit or intelligently restrict red meat consumption to two extra-lean servings a week and to eat more fish, especially Omega-3-rich fish, such as salmon, mackerel, sardines and canned, low-salt, water-packed white albacore tuna or salmon.

If you are a vegetarian and do not eat fish, eat more sea vegetables such as Nova Scotia dulse, spirulina and chlorella. Use 2 tablespoons of organic flax or hemp seeds ground in a coffee grinder or 1 tablespoon of their refrigerated oils daily. I strongly recommend and encourage you to use 1 to 3 grams a day of oil-filled softgels, liquid or extracts from algae rich in DHA and EPA. These are not very "glamorous" prescriptions for superior mental and physical health, but they really work!

Excessive levels of insulin cause a corresponding overproduction of one particular polyunsaturated fatty acid called arachidonic acid (AA). Your body needs some arachidonic acid for hormone balance, but excessive levels (as is the case with a majority of North Americans) of this hormone-like fatty acid in your diet are dangerous. Excessive levels of AA trigger the overproduction of toxic cytokines, tumor necrosis factor alpha (TNF-a) and interleukin one beta (IL1B).

Cytokines, TNF-a and IL1B have been shown to play a major role in cartilage destruction and the pro-inflammation process. Furthermore, arachidonic acid is the precursor to a fourth powerful pro-inflammatory initiator, prostaglandin-2 (PGE2), a fatty acid. When TNF-a, cytokines, IL1B and PGE2 attack the linings of joints, the result is inflammation, pain, distorted joints, tissue destruction and eventually immobility. This escalates into rheumatoid arthritis, osteoarthritis and a wide variety of age-related diseases like cardiovascular disease (our number one killer), congestive heart failure, Type 2 diabetes and immune dysfunction.

Excessive levels of arachidonic acid (AA) cause severe inflammation. It is found in fatty red meat, organ meats and egg yolks. Therefore keep consumption of these dietary sources of AA to moderate levels. Many chronic diseases such as cancer, heart disease, diabetes and arthritis are a consequence of elevated levels of arachidonic acid.

We should also avoid consuming too much of another kind of polyunsaturated fat, known as Omega-6 essential fatty acids, found in virtually every food—protein, vegetables and grains (primarily linoleic acid, as found in safflower, sunflower, corn and soybean oils), dairy, poultry, meat, nuts, seeds and legumes. The higher the fat content of a food, the higher the linoleic acid content. Excessive levels of Omega-6 fatty acids, especially true with high levels of insulin, can eventually increase the levels of arachidonic acid and cause a negative hormonal cascade. The good Omega-6 EFA I recommend is borage oil.

Look for the words "hydrogenated" or "partially hydrogenated vegetable oil" on packages of any prepared, processed food. If it is there, you know it contains dangerous trans-fatty acids that act as "anti"-essential fatty acids and are implicated in heart disease. Trans-fatty acids do not exist in nature. They are essential fatty acids that have been dangerously transformed, by commercial processing (known as hydrogenation) into a new spatial configuration that is more stable at room temperature to prevent oxidation. The increased stability of these fatty acids makes them ideal for processed foods but a dangerous fat in your body. Trans-fatty acids occupy the active site of the delta-6-desaturase enzyme, effectively preventing proper hormone synthesis and instead, turning the fat into excessive and destructive arachidonic acid (AA). DHA shuts the delta-6-desaturase enzyme "off."

Biochemists know that only naturally occurring cis-fatty acids work in the human body, not the trans configuration that happens when modern processing procedures heat, bleach, deodorize and hydrogenate fats and oils. Trans-fatty acids are insidious and ubiquitous, yet the amounts in processed "foods" aren't required to be listed on the labels. Many fast foods are practically nothing but trans-fatty acids, sugar and salt. A large order of French fries, for instance, could easily

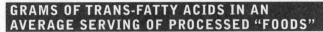

GRAMS OF TRANS-FATTY ACIDS IN AN AVERAGE SERVING OF PROCESSED "FOODS"

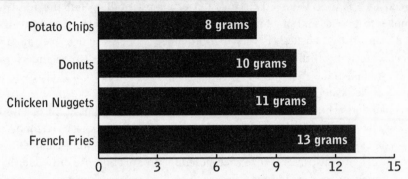

Potato Chips — 8 grams
Donuts — 10 grams
Chicken Nuggets — 11 grams
French Fries — 13 grams

0   3   6   9   12   15

contain nearly 13 grams of trans-fatty acids. Seven grams equals about 1 teaspoon. Use common sense to do everything possible you can to avoid getting sick. Avoid trans-fatty acids. Sounds easy and logical, right? The U.S. Department of Agriculture says that among teens 13 to 19 years old, French fries make up 31 percent of their total vegetable consumption. These eating habits don't improve much with age. Among adults aged 19 to 30, French fries make up 25 percent of total vegetable consumption. Be forewarned and be wise!

The British medical journal *The Lancet* reports that the majority of plaque buildup that blocks arteries is made up of mostly trans-fatty acids, accumulated from the diet—and not saturated fat. This is a startling new discovery signifying the destructive nature of trans-fatty acids in processed foods.

Use only organic high-"lignan" flax seeds or flax seed oil, perilla oil (a vegetable oil), or organic hemp seeds or hemp seed oil that you purchase refrigerated and preferably in small opaque bottles. Use 1 tablespoon of either cold-pressed flax seed, hemp seed or perilla oil daily. Check the pressing date on the bottle. Purchase oils pressed in the last three months. Grind 2 tablespoons of flax seeds or hemp seeds in a coffee grinder daily and add uncooked to your prepared oatmeal or protein power shake if you do not want to use pre-made oils.

Johanna Budwig, M.D., a double Ph.D. in chemistry and physics and two-time Nobel Prize nominee, suggests taking flax seed oil with yogurt, quark cheese or fat-free cottage cheese. She says fat-free dairy foods contain certain sulfur-bearing amino acids, which combine with super unsaturated oils, like flax seed oil or primrose oil, to make them more water soluble and hence more easily absorbed.

The most powerful demonstration of the effectiveness of EFAs came when the *American Journal of Clinical Nutrition* reported the unique case of native

Greenlanders. In 1908, researchers noted that heart disease was unknown among Greenland natives, whose diet consisted of almost nothing but the meat and blubber from seals and small whales. Because these mammals feed exclusively on cold-water fish, their flesh is very high in Omega-3 EFAs, which in turn confer their protection on the people who eat them. These native Greenlanders were again studied in the 1930s and 1970s. In the decade from 1970 to 1980, there was not a single death from heart disease among a group of 3,000. However, native Greenlanders who move to Denmark and begin eating a typical European diet quickly develop levels of heart disease comparable to their Danish neighbors.

Whatever source you use for supplemental DHA and EPA long-chain Omega-3 essential fatty acids, scrutinize each potential product and use only one that is guaranteed to be purified by a sophisticated engineering process known as molecular distillation, which removes PCBs, mercury, heavy metals and other ocean contaminants without affecting the DHA or EPA.

The reason I stress this point is for you to understand the exceptionally complicated biochemical pathway for you to make DHA or EPA, whereas eating DHA in a supplement is easy. You can use 1/2 to 1 tablespoon of flax or hemp seed oil in Johanna Budwig's recipe before you go to sleep, but you are far better off taking additional supplemental oils rich in long-chain Omega-3 fats from fish or algae oil to successfully increase the neurological enhancement you will receive from preformed DHA and EPA, than trying to make DHA and EPA in your body from short-chain perilla oil, flax seeds, hemp seeds or their oils.

Nine-Step Synthesis of DHA from Flax Seed or Hemp Seed Oil and the Enzymes Required

Alpha Linolenic acid (ALA)
  • Delta-6 Desaturase
Stearidonic acid
  • Elongase
Eicosatetraenoic acid
  • Delta-5 Desaturase
Eicosapentaenoic acid
  • Elongase
Docosapentaenoic acid
  • Elongase
Tetrapentaenoic acid
  • Delta-6 Desaturase
Tetrahexaenoic acid
  • Peroxisome beta oxidation
Docosahexaenoic acid (DHA)
  • Peroxisome beta oxidation
Eicosapentaenoic acid (EPA)

7. POWERFUL SEA VEGETABLES

In the Orient, sea vegetables are highly esteemed for their medicinal and nutritional qualities. Sea vegetables are nutrient dense, being full of vitamins, minerals and trace minerals such as chromium and selenium, which are rarely found in modern-day soils and contain special forms of absorbable organic iron and organic iodine vital to proper thyroid functioning. They are also rich sources of absorbable, organic calcium.

Arame, kombu, spirulina and chlorella contain a number of complex types of sugars called polysaccharides, which research shows to be effective against many types of cancer. There is also research from McGill University scientists presented at a medical symposium in 1967 indicating that alginates in brown sea vegetables like Nova Scotia dulse are capable of "preventing absorption of radioactive products of atomic fission," which means they would protect you from the radiation of an X-ray or radiation therapy for cancer patients.

You might have to acquire a taste for sea vegetables, but once you include them in your diet, you will be hooked. I like to add Nova Scotia dulse or arame to my miso soups. Other versatile sea vegetables are agar, alaria, hijiki, kanten, kelp, nori, sea palm and wakame. Some "green drinks" conveniently contain sea vegetables.

Arame: This is a sea vegetable with a delicate and sweet flavor. Dry-roast it, then sprinkle it on tofu, beans, salads or vegetables.

Nova Scotia Dulse: Soak it for three minutes then dry-roast it in a frying pan for five minutes. Or buy it prepared in a small bottle and use as a salt substitute.

Spirulina: This is a blue-green algae that is a virtual treasure trove of nutrients. It is available in capsules or as a powder that can be mixed with water. Or drink it as part of a high-quality "green drink."

Kombu: This sea vegetable has a natural, mild flavor. Soak it for three minutes in cold water, then cook for 35 to 40 minutes as a base or stock for beans or soups. Kombu aids digestion.

Japanese Chlorella: This green single-celled algae is a powerhouse of macro- and micronutrients. This is also available in capsule form or can be consumed as part of a high-quality "green drink." Chlorella absorbs heavy metals in our body, such as mercury, and eliminates them before they cause damage.

8. EXOTIC SPICES AND BIOENERGETIC HERBS

Colorful and pungent spices from around the world are phytonutrient powerhouses. Use them daily and enjoy their flavors while benefiting from their health-promoting properties.

Get acquainted with such spices as cardamom, cinnamon, cloves, ginger, mustard seed and turmeric. And with condiments such as chili peppers and horseradish root. Use common herbs like basil, fennel seeds, lemon balm, marjoram, mint, parsley, rosemary, sage, tarragon, thyme and watercress liberally as color and taste enhancers on all main-course dishes. Use edible flowers for decoration.

The spices and herbs that I like to use to give food regional flair in different dishes are:
- Chinese: garlic, anise, ginger, parsley and watercress.
- French: garlic, bay leaves, rosemary, tarragon, parsley, thyme and watercress.
- Greek: garlic, cinnamon, parsley, mint and oregano.
- Indian: coriander seeds, cumin, curry, ginger, cardamom, fenugreek, parsley, mustard seeds, chili, turmeric and horseradish.
- Italian: bay leaves, basil, garlic, fennel seeds, marjoram, oregano, rosemary, parsley, red pepper flakes, watercress, sage and tarragon.
- Mexican: cilantro, chili, cumin and oregano.
- Middle Eastern: garlic, cumin, mint, parsley, oregano, cinnamon and watercress.

Each herb and spice has its own unique properties. Turmeric, for example, contains the active component curcumin. It is the ingredient that gives turmeric its vibrant, sun-yellow color. Turmeric has been used in the ancient Ayurvedic system of Indian medicine for thousands of years to treat indigestion, flatulence, skin diseases, urinary tract infections and stomach problems, and to keep dishes cooked with oils from going rancid or spoiling.

Curcumin is a very powerful antioxidant that is an extremely effective inhibitor of the most destructive free radicals, the corrosive superoxide anion and hydroxyl radicals. Most antioxidants quench oxygen-free radicals directly in a head-on collision. The three "curcuminoids" in curcumin merge with free radicals and scavenge, as well as absorb, many of the free radicals' destructive characteristics before they even become active.

Powerful Herbs

All herbs have unique healing properties, as well as an array of delightful flavors. Medicinal herbs have been the focus of recent medical research, much of it in Japan, Europe and at the University of Toronto. This research has documented the remarkable therapeutic properties and components of medicinal herbs as phytonutrients, antioxidants, enzymes, an immune-enhanced increase in natural resistance and self-defense, anti-inflammatory properties, analgesic effects and the ability to confer resistance to stress of all origins within cells, tissues and organs.

Medicinal herbs, as bioenergetic whole foods, work directly on the healing system, increasing not only immune capability, but also the body's ability to repair itself, replace damaged structures, regenerate new structures and reinvigorate vital energy. They generally do not cause any irritating effects, as compared to synthetic pharmaceutical drugs.

In the year 2000, about 25 percent of all prescription pharmaceuticals came from botanical, herbal sources because the active ingredients are too complex to be synthesized. Trust nature and the Divine Blueprint.

In reviewing the *Holy Bible* I found this statement, "Their fruit will be for food, and their leaves for healing" (Ezekiel 47:12).

Scientists and medical researchers are finally taking this category of natural medicines seriously. Below and on the following page are ten medicinal herbal extract combinations and the active biological results they confer in your body. These combinations are available in leading health food and whole food stores. I personally use many of them.

Herbs such as mint have been used for centuries to aid digestion, clear the palate and ease the stomach, reducing after-meal bloating and gas. Use the following potent herbs in your meals or as an herbal tea after your meal.

- **Mint:** Aids digestion, relieves fatigue and aids headaches. Use as a condiment or soothing tea to benefit from its volatile oil, menthol, which you can inhale.
- **Parsley:** Sweetens the breath and relieves indigestion. Add as a garnish and then be sure to eat it!
- **Rosemary:** Increases the flow of bile to aid digestion, is a tonic for stress and supports neurotransmitter synthesis.
- **Sage:** Helps to balance digestive enzymes and hormones, thereby lessening menstrual cramping and hot flashes.
- **Watercress:** Promotes digestion and the growth of "friendly" bacteria in the intestinal tract; strengthens gums and reduces water retention.

Liver Support	For Sleep	Immune Support	Adrenal Gland Support	For Menopause
Artichoke leaves	Griffonia	Astragalus root	Astragalus root	Black cohosh
Dandelions	Hops	Echinacea	Burdock root	Chaste tree berry
Milk thistle	Kava kava	angustifolia	Jiaogulan	Dandelion
Turmeric	Lemon balm	Echinacea pallida	Licorice root	Dong quai
	Passion flower	Echinacea	Siberian ginseng	Red clover
	Scullcap	purpurea	Suma	
		Grapefruit seed		
		Pau d'Arco		

For Memory	For Prostate	For Joint Mobility	For PMS	For Weight Loss
Ashwagandha	Saw palmetto	Methyl-sulfonyl-methane (MSM)	Chaste tree berry	Garcinia cambogia
Bacopa	Chinese		Burdock root	Citrus aurantium
Gotu kola	licorice	Boswellia	Black haw	Grapefruit juice
Ginkgo biloba	Pygeum	Devil's claw root	Alfalfa seed	powder
Siberian ginseng	Cornsilk	Juniper berries	powder	Coleus forskohlii
	Stinging nettle	Ginger	Red clover	Cayenne
		Turmeric	Ginkgo biloba	Gugulipid
			Black cohosh	Alpha lipoic acid
				Green tea

A wonderful book on how to prepare medicinal teas and tonics is Christopher Hobbs's *Herbal Remedies For Dummies*.

WHEN TO TAKE HERBAL SUPPLEMENTS

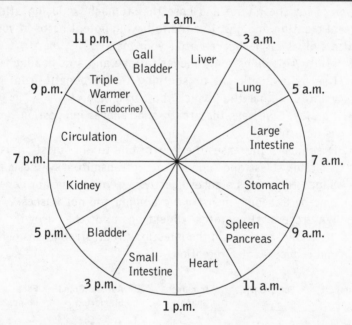

9. INCREDIBLE MISO

Miso is made from concentrated, fermented soybean paste and comes in different types and shades, from dark brown to ochre to red, each with its own distinctive taste. White, yellow and tan misos are generally lighter and sweeter in flavor; they contain less salt and are aged less. Barley miso, known as mugi miso, is made with fermented barley and is mellow and light. Soy bean miso (hatcho miso) has a rich, hearty taste. Brown rice miso (kome miso) is the sweetest of the misos.

Miso has been credited with anti-cancer properties. For one thing, it contains genistein, which inhibits the blood-vessel growth on which tumors depend. It may also be responsible for the lower incidence of breast cancer in Japanese women. Japanese researchers reported that in animal experiments, a diet supplemented with miso reduced the incidence and delayed the appearance of induced breast cancer.

I highly recommend that you consume a bowl of miso soup daily with some sea vegetable. A powerful combination is miso soup, sea vegetables, extra-firm tofu, garlic, green onions, a few lentils or garbanzo beans, and fresh ginger. I simply make miso broth once or twice a week and put it in the refrigerator in a glass jar. You can also use it daily in salad dressings, legume dishes, or combined with tahini as a vegetable topping or as a quick soup base.

When making miso soup or adding miso to any sauce, vegetable or salad dressing, do not expose the miso paste to high temperatures, such as in boiling water. High temperatures will kill the medicinal and "friendly" live bacteria in miso, derived from the fermentation process. Simply add the miso to the water, soup or sauce once it has cooled off enough to be eaten. Miso should only be dissolved in liquids at a temperature that you would eat or drink without burning your mouth.

10. NON-GMO SOYBEANS, SOY SPROUTS, TOFU AND TEMPEH

Soy products have been found to have numerous health benefits. One benefit is lowering cholesterol. *The New England Journal of Medicine* in 1995 found that consuming an average of 50 grams of soy per day lowered cholesterol levels by 9 percent. Such a cholesterol level reduction should lead to a 20 percent reduction in heart disease risk. Furthermore, a study published in 2000 in the *American Journal of Clinical Nutrition* showed that eating just 20 grams of soy a day can reduce levels of cholesterol in as little as nine weeks.

Another benefit of soy products is cancer prevention. Dr. Anne Kennedy of the University of Pennsylvania believes that the bountiful protease inhibitors found in soy foods have a selective toxicity for malignant cancer cells. Dr. William R. Fair, chief of urology at Memorial Sloan-Kettering Cancer Center in New York City, reports that soy protein is almost as protective as a low-fat diet in slowing the progression of prostate cancer.

Tofu: Tofu is probably the soy product people are most familiar with. Also called soybean curd, tofu is made from soybean milk, water and nigari, a natural sea salt coagulant. It is protein-rich and versatile. Depending upon how much liquid is extracted from the curds, the tofu is labeled soft, medium, firm or extra-firm. Use only extra-firm tofu because it is highest in protein and lowest in carbohydrates.

While it is high in protein, tofu has no fiber and must be eaten with vegetables, whole grains, salads, nuts, seeds or fresh sprouts. Always use a sea vegetable, such as Nova Scotia dulse, when you cook tofu, to add organic iodine. Organic iodine supports thyroid function because the goitrogens present in soy products tend to suppress the thyroid.

Only eat extra-firm, organic, non-GMO tofu two to three times a week at most. Once you've opened the container, refrigerate any leftovers in water in a tightly-sealed container. Change the water daily and the tofu will last for about five to six days.

Tempeh: Tempeh is made of whole, cooked soybeans infused with a bacterial culture to form a dense, chewy cake. It can be marinated or grilled or sautéed and added to soups, chili, casseroles or stir-fries, or used as a veggie burger. Do not be concerned if you notice any gray or blackish spots on the surface of the tempeh; this is the health-supportive bacterial culture used in the fermentation process. Tempeh contains E. faecalis THIO, a strain of beneficial lactic acid bacteria that is six times stronger than any other "friendly" bacteria in killing bad bacteria like E. coli, H. pylori and the superbug Staphylococcus aureus. Tempeh, a fermented food, is a better source of protein for you than tofu. It is one of the few vegetarian sources, along with sea vegetables, of absorbable vitamin B12.

Soy Sprouts: Soy sprouts from certified organically grown and non-GMO soy beans are the only uncooked, unheated source of the potent phytonutrients genistein and daidzein. They decrease prostate cancer, heart disease, breast cancer, ovarian cancer and other cancers. You are able to digest these unheated forms of phytonutrient-rich soy sprouts easily and effectively.

Soy Protein Powders: The soy protein powders that I recommend are known as soy protein isolates. They contain more than 90 percent protein. Soy protein powders can be added to virtually any food like oatmeal, cookies, dips or protein shakes to increase the protein-to-carbohydrate ratio.

Soy Milk: Soy milk is a rich, creamy milk of whole soybeans that are simmered in water and strained, then pressed to extract the nutrient-rich beige liquid. Some manufacturers may add a wide range of sweeteners, which I urge you to avoid. Soy milk has become very popular. I do not believe you should drink soy milk since it is not fermented and you may have great difficulty digesting it.

Soy Nuts: Soy nuts are the equivalent of peanuts, and the unsalted, baked varieties make a great snack by themselves.

Edamame: Edamame are fresh green soybeans harvested when they are still young and sweet-tasting. They are served as a snack or a main vegetable dish. Fresh or frozen green soybeans are sold in Asian and natural food stores. They are my favorite way to eat soybeans. Boil the green beans, in the pod, for ten minutes. Pop the beans out of their pods directly into your mouth and discard the pods.

Getting Used to Soy Products

Soy beans and soy products may cause some discomfort, gas and indigestion when you first start using them. You may experience difficulty digesting the complex sugars in them that are not readily absorbed. Bacteria in the large intestine ferment these sugars and produce gas as a byproduct. Within weeks of adding soy to your diet, your body will adjust to them and the uncomfortable symptoms will go away on their own. Until then, try these strategies:

- eat small portions, gradually increasing portion size over a month;
- fortify meals with soy protein isolates, which are almost pure protein; and
- try Beano® to break down the indigestible sugars before they get to the bacteria in your large intestine.

Organic—Again, a Must for Soy

I recommend that you use only certified organically grown soybeans, or products made from them like extra-firm tofu, miso, natto and tempeh, since pesticides are used heavily on soy beans. Do use rice, oat or hemp milk (rather than soy milk—which is not fermented) fortified with calcium, magnesium, zinc and iron as a substitute for cow's milk. Use extra-firm tofu only two to three times a week. Vegetarians and vegans should use more tempeh, natto and miso.

Limit soy consumption in children under six years of age, and do not use soy milk with babies. Always use a little certified organic Nova Scotia dulse when you cook with soy to support your thyroid functions. Familiarize yourself with genuine fermented, organic soy products in natural food stores but strictly avoid processed soy "foods."

There are hundreds of unacceptable soy products made from chemically processed soy full of unhealthful ingredients and additives. If you only purchase organically grown, fermented soy products, made from non-GMO (not genetically modified organisms) soy beans, from small dedicated companies in your area, you will avoid the processed food companies that are cashing in on soy's great reputation with their toxic and chemically laden processing techniques. Remember, these processed foods are one molecule removed from being plastic. Avoid them—be forewarned—and don't give them your hard-earned money to damage your sensitive tissues. They are chief suspects in undermining your natural health and have long-term detrimental effects.

High-tech "food" processing companies purchase high-protein soy chips that are the waste product once soy beans are squeezed to produce oil for margarine, shortenings and salad dressings. Soy beans now cover 87 million acres of North American farmland. They contain haemagglutinin, a clot-promoting substance that causes red blood cells to clump together and trypsin inhibitors that block enzymes needed for protein digestion. Soy also contains goitrogens (substances that tend to depress thyroid function) and phytic acid.

> Fermented soy products that I recommend, such as extra-firm tofu, tempeh and miso that takes the purée of cooked soy beans and ferments it with magnesium sulfate, have the phytic acid, goitrogens, tipsin inhibitors and haemagglutin almost totally removed. Furthermore, I suggest using Nova Scotia dulse when cooking tofu to nullify the remaining goitrogens and support thyroid function. Modern processors do not remove these, plus they acid wash the soy beans in aluminum tanks that leech aluminum into their products. Numerous artificial flavorings, particularly MSG are added to commercial soy protein isolate and textured vegetable protein to mask the "beany" flavor. Nitrites, potent carcinogens, are then formed during spray drying. Avoid commercial soy products, soy-reinforced breads, meat alternatives and soy cereals. They are processed, unhealthful "foods."

11. PURPLE, BLUE AND DARK RED FRUITS

Modern science has confirmed that dark-colored berries, plums, tart cherries, dark-colored cherries, prunes and red, purple and dark-blue grapes contain a wealth of health-giving and possibly even life-extending phenolic compounds, including proanthocyanidins, anthocyanins, quercetin, resveratrol and ellagic acid.

Researchers have now made powerful extracts that provide standardized doses of the active polyphenols in berries and grapes. Full-spectrum grape extract and bilberry extract are the best known and contain 95 percent procyanidolic values, with large amounts of the powerful and protective phytonutrients resveratrol and ellagic acid.

Various authors and researchers use different, and sometimes confusing, terminology. Proanthocyanidins, being short chains of catechin subunits, are also called oligomeric condensed tannins and are sometimes referred to as oligomeric proanthocyanidin complexes, or OPCs. Anthocyanins, which are the largest molecules, are sometimes called polymeric condensed tannins. Both types of compounds, often referred to by the general term such as polyphenols, procyanidolics, polyphenolics or flavonoids, or even simply "plant pigments," are widely distributed in plants, especially the peel, seeds, flowers and bark. (The broad term used by the general public to describe all these compounds is polyphenols, and the research community generally calls them procyanidolics.)

Berries, dark grapes and cherries contain a complex mixture of procyanidolic compounds, which are generally called phenolic compounds and include phenolic acids, quercetin, catechins, tannins, ellagic acid, epicatechins, proanthocyanidins and anthocyanins. Dark, dry red wine contains over 200 phenolic compounds.

It is only recently that we have learned that heart disease is largely inflammatory in nature. Inflammation destabilizes the arterial plaque. Polyphenols inhibit the metabolism of arachidonic acid (AA) and therefore prevent the formation of pro-inflammatory PGE2. Some polyphenols, such as resveratrol, quercetin and ellagic acid, are network antioxidants that reduce glutathione, keeping it active for a longer period of time. In addition, they:

- protect against a nitrogen-based and destructive free radical, peroxynitrite, a mediator molecule in inflammation;
- inhibit cell adhesion molecule proteins, preventing the over-recruitment of immune cells in inflammation;
- help to prevent atherosclerosis and give you cardiovascular protection, as well as cancer protection;
- prevent the formation of advanced glycated end-products, called AGEs; and
- reduce inflammation-causing prostaglandins, leukotrienes and nuclear factor kappa-B.

Epidemiological studies confirm that those who consume plenty of polyphenol-rich foods have a lower risk of cancer. Gary D. Stoner, Ph.D., director of the cancer chemoprevention program at the Ohio State University Comprehensive Cancer Center in Columbus, states, "ellagic acid detoxifies carcinogens."

Blueberries, raspberries, strawberries and dark grapes contain the potent anticarcinogenic compound called ellagic acid. Resveratrol in particular has been studied for its powerful anticarcinogenic properties, and it decreases proliferation of induced apoptosis (programmed cell death). The fact is that polyphenols are network antioxidants that raise glutathione levels, especially in the liver. The liver needs enormous amounts of glutathione to detoxify the endless carcinogens and other toxins you are constantly exposed to. Centenarians have youthful levels of glutathione. Polyphenols lower blood sugar levels and therefore reduce insulin levels, which is what a calorie-restricted diet does.

12. LEGUMES

Beans, peas and lentils should be eaten three to four times weekly by everyone. Legumes are a great source of soluble fiber, especially water-soluble gums that slow down food absorption and inhibit the formation of bile acids—a process that protects us against colon cancer. This gum-like fiber also seems to be responsible for lowering cholesterol and triglycerides.

Another protective compound in legumes is protease inhibitors to protect against skin, breast and liver cancers. Protease inhibitors are compounds that prevent the enzyme protease (protein-digesting enzyme) from breaking down proteins randomly in our body so we don't cannibalize muscle tissue. They also work successfully against tumor formation.

Beans and legumes contain relatively more protein than other plants. Unfortunately, only about 70 percent of the protein will be absorbed by your body, because 30 percent of the protein passes through your intestinal tract bound to the indigestible fiber found in beans and legumes.

Preparing Legumes

Soak beans overnight and discard the water to remove most of the phytic acid which binds to minerals such as zinc, calcium, magnesium and iron to form phytates. Phytates are insoluble so they pass right out of your body, taking the minerals with them. Beans should then be cooked in new water for a few minutes and that water also discarded. Only then are beans ready for final cooking. Adding kombu or Nova Scotia dulse reduces intestinal gas. If you find it necessary, use two capsules of a broad-spectrum plant-based digestive enzyme to properly digest legumes, rather than avoiding them and losing out on their phytonutrient bounty.

PROTEIN AND CARBOHYDRATE CONTENT OF BOILED BEANS		Protein Grams	Carbohydrate Grams
Bean			
Soybeans	(1 cup)	21	18
Lentils	(1 cup)	14	22
Pinto beans	(1 cup)	11	26
Black beans	(1 cup)	11	28
Red kidney beans	(1 cup)	11	28
Navy beans	(1 cup)	10	30
Chick peas	(1 cup)	10	30

Furthermore, beans and legumes (except soy beans) contain larger amounts of carbohydrates relative to their protein content, so add another protein-rich source such as soy protein isolate powder or Alphapure™ whey protein isolate powder, or a hard-boiled egg or a few tablespoons of fresh seeds or nuts ground in a coffee grinder to your cooked beans or legumes. This raises the protein-to-carbohydrate ratio.

I estimate that about 65 percent of North Americans are deficient in the digestive enzyme alpha-galactosidase. If you are one of the 65 percent, just as I am, do what I do. Purchase Beano® (alpha-galactosidase) at your whole food store, health food store or grocery store. It is a liquid and comes in a little opaque bottle. It tastes like soy sauce. Simply add five to eight drops of Beano® to your first spoonful of beans, tofu, peas or cruciferous vegetables (Brussels sprouts, cauliflower, broccoli, etc.). You will have no gas and great digestion. It is that simple! If you require even more digestive help, use two capsules, at the beginning of each meal, of a broad-range digestive plant source enzyme combination.

13. WHOLE CEREAL GRAINS

Michio Kushi, the leading North American proponent and educator of the macrobiotic method of eating, draws attention to the fact that carbohydrates in cereal grains work with other nutrients to form compounds called glycosamino-glycans, which help to detoxify the body. They are also a good source of the fat-soluble antioxidant vitamin E, a potent free radical scavenger.

Grains, seeds and nuts—when combined—create a complete protein, a high concentration of complex carbohydrates and necessary fiber. Put whole, organic sunflower seeds, pumpkin seeds and sesame seeds on your rolled oats. Add five or six almonds and grind 1 to 2 tablespoons of flax seeds in a coffee grinder for five seconds and add them to your prepared oatmeal. Eat half of your daily seeds and nuts raw—eat the other half soaked overnight in water that you discard.

Experiment and avoid wheat products for one month. Try other sprouted organic whole grain combinations in breads, such as rye, millet, spelt, kamut or amaranth. Another healthy addition to these flours is natural sourdough, which removes the phytic acid from the grains. If you're wheat intolerant, as I am, you may just feel 100 percent better by doing this.

Gluten is the gluey collection of proteins found in wheat, rye, barley, oats, spelt, kamut and triticale. Gluten sensitivity or intolerance has a wide variety of reactions; the worst is celiac disease, an autoimmune condition that destroys the lining of the small intestine. *The Journal of Pediatric Gastroenterology and Nutrition* (vol. 31, supplement 3) states that "one in every 111 healthy adults and one in every 167 healthy children suffer from this condition." Also, 10 to 25 percent of North Americans are classified as gluten-sensitive in which hyper-activity, depression, skin conditions, middle-ear infections, bloating, indigestion, diarrhea, abdominal pain and joint pain may result. If you suspect you have trouble with gluten, do two blood-antibody screens called anti-gliadin (IgG and IgA) and antiendomysial antibody (anti-tTG). Try avoiding gluten totally for one month to see how you feel.

Most breads are high on the glycemic index, which means they break down to sugar very fast and provide a burst of energy. But this may be quickly followed by

hunger and moodiness. It is in the processing of wheat that this problem origi-
nates, not in the whole wheat berry itself. Wheat is ground to small particle sizes
that allow digestive enzymes quick access to break them down to sugar.
Furthermore, the leavening action of yeast on ground flour increases the surface
area of the flour molecules even more, providing more access to digestive enzymes
for the quick breakdown to sugar. So it is not wheat, but finely ground flour, that
is a major contributor to obesity and cardiovascular disease in Western cultures.

14. MUSHROOMS

Most common button mushrooms, popular in the West, contain poisonous,
carcinogenic compounds called hydrazines. They are developed by mushrooms
to protect themselves from being eaten by animals. Dr. Beth Toth, a biologist at
the University of Nebraska, states that 66 percent of all European mushroom
varieties contain these dangerous compounds. My advice to you is to not eat raw
button mushrooms. Avoid them always.

Most of these poisonous compounds, but not all, are destroyed by cooking.
One type of hydrazine called agaritine is only partially destroyed by cooking.
Agaritine is converted in the body into a highly reactive, mutagenic metabolite;
at low doses, that substance produces stomach tumors in mice. Even if you only
eat cooked mushrooms, you are still at some risk.

Shiitake, portobello, oyster, morel, coriolus, chanterelle, maitake and reishi
mushrooms are medicinal and good to eat. The best way of using them,
according to time-honored Chinese medicinal tradition, is to prepare a concentrated broth from them and drink the broth between meals to prevent digestive
stomach acids from breaking down some of their immune-supporting phytonutrients to inactive compounds before they can reach the small intestine and be
absorbed.

The primary therapeutic compound in these mushrooms, just as in sea
vegetables, is a complex sugar, polysaccharide. These mushrooms contain one
called lentinan that boosts interleukin-1 and interferon production and acts as a
powerful immune system stimulant. Lentinan has been found effective against
cancer when added to the food of mice.

One way of getting most of the benefits of pure, extracted lentinan from
shiitake mushrooms is to take freeze-dried shiitake or reishi concentrate in
capsule form. Check the label to ensure that it does not contain a lot of corn
starch (dextrose).

If you cannot find fresh shiitake or reishi mushrooms in your food market,
Chinese groceries and most health food stores have dried shiitake or reishi
mushrooms. Soak them overnight in pure water and then add them to salads,
soups or vegetables. I like to sauté them with onions in water and then add some
extra-virgin olive oil at the last minute.

15. FOODS RICH IN PROTEASE ENZYMES AND INHIBITORS

Nature has given you protease enzymes so you can tear down the proteins you eat and rebuild them as your own integral hormones, cell walls, neurotransmitters or muscles. To guard against indiscriminate degradation of your existing protein structure, protease enzymes (in a process called proteolysis) target only the protein you have eaten within protected areas of the stomach or in protected areas of the blood, lymph and extracellular spaces. This way you can "digest" foreign debris, trespassing viruses, bacteria or hydrolyzed protein components of the cell membrane for resynthesis without the fear of cannibalizing your own body.

The second function of protease enzymes is to help modulate cellular pH by allowing entry of anions while dispensing the buildup of volatile acids in the blood and by relieving tissue acid buildup. Protease enzymes stimulate the production of carbonic anhydrase, which transports excess CO_2 to the blood-stream, where the gas can be carried to the lungs as carbonic acid ($H_2 CO_3$), where it is converted to water plus CO_2 and exhaled.

Protease enzymes must be accompanied by protease inhibitors so that proteases can help you without harming you. They are both equally important to initiate protein breakdown and to inhibit protease's random digestion of your body's protein structures. This requires that your diet contain a balance of proteases and corresponding protease inhibitors. Luckily, foods rich in protease enzymes always contain protease inhibitors.

However, the proteolytic enzymes secreted by the pancreas begin to decline after the age of 30 or so, and we find it more and more difficult to fully digest proteins. A simple solution is to eat more red beets, a natural source of stomach acid that aids in digesting proteins.

Protease-rich foods include fresh pineapple, papaya, figs, mango, kiwi, all ripe fruits, vegetables (especially sweet potatoes) and legumes such as peas, beans, lentils, peanuts and soy beans. Other sources include fresh sprouts, eggs, raw nuts and seeds soaked overnight in water.

Protease inhibitor sources include raw nuts or seeds, legumes, eggs, ripe fruit and vegetables.

16. SOY LECITHIN GRANULES

Phyosphatidyl choline (PC), phosphatidyl serine (PS) and glyceryl-phosphoryl-choline (GPC) are all-powerful neurotransmitters. They all provide you with mental acuity, the ability to learn, creativity and an acute memory. PC and PS allow electromagnetic impulses to travel along the neurons in the brain and to carry messages across the many synaptic gaps between neurons.

PC increases growth hormone (GH) synthesis because it stimulates growth hormone-releasing hormone (GHRH).

PS, found in especially high concentrations in the brain, helps brain cells conduct nerve impulses, thereby enhancing communication within the brain. PS also acts as a revolving door in brain cells, allowing nutrients into the cell and providing an exit medium for toxic cellular debris. Your body can use PS to make acetylcholine, the memory-enhancing nerve hormone.

Oil-free soy lecithin granules provide PC and PS to boost nerve hormone activity of dopamine and serotonin, lower levels of the stress hormone cortisol and stir activity in the higher brain centers, especially in the pituitary gland, the cortex and the hypothalamus. Parris Kidd, Ph.D., of PMK Biomedical Nutritional Counseling in El Cerrito, California, presented much of this information at the American College of Nutrition Conference in 1998. His research suggests that consuming more PC and PS can turn back your mental clock by up to 14 years.

Soy lecithin emulsifies and removes the "bad" cholesterol called low-density lipoproteins (LDL), and increases the "good" high-density lipoproteins (HDL) your body needs. LDL is devastating, as it clogs the arteries and increases the chances of heart or coronary disease. Soy lecithin can also reduce high blood pressure, dramatically increase fat-soluble vitamins A, D, and E absorption by as much as 100 percent, give hair added texture and sheen, help to convert dangerous homocysteine (a protein byproduct, especially from animal protein) to non-toxic compounds, allow the skin to retain more moisture and remain elastic, and act as "fat fighters" by emulsifying fats so they can be burned more efficiently in the mitochondria, within each cell.

I believe it is beneficial to supplement your diet daily with 2 tablespoons of oil-free soy lecithin granules—nutty-flavored little golden nuggets—which can be found in your health food store cooler. (Avoid liquid, tablets and capsules that may be rancid or oxidized.) Add them to cooked dishes such as oatmeal or stews or add them to your power protein shake. Only organic soy beans, certified to be non-GMO, should be used. Always store lecithin granules in the refrigerator.

The highest quality "green drinks" are a convenient way of daily consuming non-GMO organic soy lecithin granules in well-balanced proportions. The high-end "green drinks" include large amounts of phosphatidyl choline (1,200 mg) and phosphatidyl serine (60 mg). They are an alkalizing food.

All brain cells need choline to form the neurotransmitter acetylcholine and to function properly. Alzheimer's disease is characterized by an underproduction of acetylcholine. Your body manufactures acetylcholine with the help of phosphatidyl choline (PC), folic acid and vitamin B12 but after the age of 30 it might not produce enough to maintain normal brain functions such as thinking or the proper storage and retrieval of information. Phosphatidyl choline (PC) supplementation during pre- and postnatal development in animals produces marked improvements in memory. People pass memory tests with flying colors when they are given (PC) supplements to raise acetylcholine levels, but flunk these same memory tests when acetylcholine function is intentionally blocked by medication. If your diet has insufficient choline, one popular medical theory states that the cholergenic (memory neurons) will utilize the choline from their own neuron's membranes in a cannibalistic fashion, degrading its actual structure, and thus causing the cells to become hormonally dysfunctional.

I cannot say enough about soy lecithin granules and their contribution to human life and longevity. Try them, and see for yourself.

You can also naturally boost PC and PS levels by including more salmon, sardines, mackerel or tuna in your diet. Or try capsules containing krill oil, salmon oil, cod liver oil or sardine oil, or algae oil capsules rich in DHA and EPA. The long-chain Omega-3 fatty acid DHA, present in fish oil, appears to boost the body's ability to make PS and PC.

17. BOVINE COLOSTRUM

Colostrum is a bioenergetic natural food, and is the substance that a mother's breast produces during the first 72 hours after giving birth. Mothers generally call it a "pre-milk fluid." Research clearly demonstrates that bovine colostrum and human colostrum are nearly identical. After those first 72 hours, the mother produces milk rather than colostrum.

Colostrum contains powerful growth and immune factors that ensure the health of the newborn, whether it is animal or human. Colostrum contains vitamins, minerals, protein and sugars to stimulate new growth. Colostrum also contains immunoglobulins, growth factors, lactoferrin, antibiotic factors and protein subfractions that are specifically designed to protect us from invading toxins, viruses, bacteria, agrichemicals and carcinogens. Colostrum is a concentrated source of the amino acid L-carnitine, known to accelerate the burning of fat in the body for fuel and to support neurological functions.

Bovine (cow's) colostrum is available in such abundance because cows produce up to 30 to 35 liters of colostrum in the first three days after giving birth.

In our youth, our cells divide and produce new cells that are identical. As we age, a senescent factor (SF) becomes involved in cellular duplication. The SF causes cells to duplicate at a slower rate or causes dysfunctional cellular duplication—this is an accelerated aging process. Bovine colostrum contains growth factors that boost oxygen and nutrient supplies to cells so they remain more elastic, vibrant and youthful, and both divide as well as reproduce exactly. These growth factors stimulate cell and tissue growth by initiating DNA and RNA formation. Research demonstrates that bovine colostrum supplementation increases human growth hormone (GH) activity by stimulating the synthesis of IGF-1 and IGF-2 in the liver. IGF-1 and IGF-2 are extremely abundant in colostrum and are the growth factors that control how cells grow and repair themselves. They also burn body fat and build lean muscle tissue. Accelerated aging is generally characterized by lower levels of growth hormone secretion and, therefore, also correspondingly lower levels of IGF-1 and IGF-2 (GH messengers) being synthesized in the liver. Bovine colostrum is the only natural source for IGF-1 and IGF-2. Furthermore, colostrum prevents gastro-intestinal tract (GIT) injury due to medication use. It actually keeps the GIT mucosa lining sealed and impermeable to toxins.

Colostrum is available in both powder form and liquid. If you use the liquid, put 1 teaspoon under your tongue upon rising and let it be absorbed through the epithelial tissue in your mouth. Swallow after one minute. Consider using 1 teaspoon of powdered colostrum daily in your protein power shake. I strongly suggest that you use only colostrum from North American cows.

ADD WATER

After oxygen, water is the second most important nutrient in your body. Women's bodies are comprised of about 63 to 65 percent water and men's bodies are about 68 percent. Water is critical to maintaining an anabolic drive and for your optimum survival.

In North America, the average adult consumes about 2 quarts of water a day, with two-thirds coming from water and other beverages, and one-third from the food we eat.

To know if you are drinking enough water, simply monitor the color of your urine. If your urine is pale yellow to clear throughout the day you are consuming enough water to satisfy your body's requirements. If your urine is strong smelling or dark yellow (unless you are using B vitamins), your kidneys are working too hard and you need to start drinking more water throughout the day.

Do not wait to drink your water quota for the day all at once. Your body's need for water is constant. Prehydrate by drinking water every one to two hours. Do what I do, I carry an enclosed container with a straw in it and leave it both on my desk as I work, and take it in my vehicle.

You should drink a minimum of six 8-oz glasses of water a day, and more if the weather is hot, you perspire more or you exercise for more than 30 minutes.

Several studies indicate that consumption of both caffeinated beverages and alcoholic beverages can lead to water loss because they act as a diuretic. If you consume caffeinated beverages or alcoholic beverages, drink two glasses of water for every caffeinated beverage or alcoholic beverage you consume, and use a high-quality multivitamin-mineral supplement as good insurance.

Each quart of sweat we lose contains approximately 500 to 1,000 mg of sodium, 150 to 250 mg of potassium and about 500 mg of chloride. We can replace these mineral electrolytes by eating lots of bioenergetic colorful vegetables, salads and ripe fruit.

Often we misinterpret thirst signals as hunger signs and eat when we really should be drinking water.

Our skin is 80 percent water. The most important cosmetic help or nutritional support we can give ourselves that will promote a clear, smooth, radiant complexion is to drink, throughout the day, clean, pure water.

WHAT IS YOUR BODY MADE OF?

Your body is made of:

Water	63–70%
Proteins	15–19%
Fat	12–15%
Minerals	3%
Carbohydrates	2%
Vitamins	1%

THE WATER CONTENT IN VARIOUS TISSUES IN YOUR BODY

Digestive juices	86%
Blood	83%
Kidneys	82%
Skin	80%
Brain	74%
Muscles	70–75%
Liver	69%
Bones	22%

The average body contains 95 to 96 pints of water, 65 pints inside your cells and the remainder outside your cells. Our body's water supply is responsible for and involved in regulating every biological process, especially synthesizing hormones, neurotransmitters and maintaining ultimate body balance and super-symmetry—homeostasis.

We should increase our water intake gradually, by adding one 8-oz glass of water on each successive or second day. Increasing water intake too quickly can overwork our unprepared kidneys and digestive system.

Crystal-clean water is one of the sweetest things imaginable. We should drink our water quota, spread out throughout the day. It will pay off in more vigorous and healthy years for life, and enable us to maintain peak performance, both physically and mentally. In *The Power of Superfoods*, I have a detailed chapter on water that examines the pros and cons of bottled water, as well as in-home water purification systems such as reverse osmosis, steam distillation and acid-alkaline electrolysis.

Your household water is probably chlorinated and fluoridated by your municipality. The chlorine and fluoride are added to kill bacteria, which means they kill all bacteria, including the beneficial bacteria in your intestines. In addition, your water may also be picking up copper and lead as it passes through metal pipes on its way to you. Even worse, it may have been contaminated along the way by dangerous pathogens, such as E. coli or cryptosporidium, which chlorine doesn't kill. The serious water contaminations in Walkerton, Ontario in May of 2000 or in North Battleford, Saskatchewan in May of 2001 were caused by these two pathogens.

Pesticides are deadly chemicals used to eliminate weeds, insects and other fungi in crops. More than 60 million pounds of just two pesticides, Atrazine and Simazine, are used in North America annually and they leech into groundwater, rivers and lakes.

They are so toxic the EPA in the U.S. mandated that a maximum level is equivalent to less than one drop in a swimming pool.

Nitrates and nitrites are toxins made when either animal wastes, human wastes or field fertilizers come into contact with water. In 1992 the National Pesticide Survey in the U.S. tested 1,349 communities and detected nitrates in 57 percent of domestic wells, and 52 percent of community wells.

You can purchase in-home water-testing kits that will only take you ten minutes and will accurately test for the above potential contaminants. For more information, check out the web site at www.silverlakeresearch.com.

To protect your family, I strongly recommend that you install household water filters on all taps in your home. My preference is for ceramic filters with a UV (ultraviolet) light to additionally kill bacteria, viruses and parasites. They are reasonably priced, easy to install and last a long time. If you do not filter your water, stick to high-quality bottled water whenever possible.

Many people tell me they are astonished at the increase in energy they feel and the radiant complexion they have after increasing their daily water consumption. I personally drink 12 8-oz glasses of water every day and highly recommend that you slowly, over several weeks, build up to eight, ten or 12 glasses daily.

The most important time to drink water is the moment we first arise in the morning. Our metabolic processes were cleaning our 100 trillion cells and the metabolic waste has been brought to our intestinal tract. Water also washes the metabolic waste safely out of our system before it can accumulate and be reabsorbed (auto-intoxication) by the cleansed tissue. Room temperature, or slightly warm water, with a teaspoon of fresh lemon or lime juice in it, helps to rehydrate our tissues.

15

———

YOUR LIFE-LONG
AND LONG-LIFE
INSURANCE PLAN

———

Whether you're 22 or 72, you can improve your health and happiness in the years to come by making a few simple changes *now*.

Remember, to protect yourself against environmental toxins, agrichemicals, cancer and degenerative diseases, you must eat a variety of natural, bioenergetic whole foods such as vegetables, fruits, sea vegetables, legumes, whole grains, culinary herbs and spices, medicinal mushrooms, medicinal herbs, pure water and, especially high-quality "green drinks" and green tea daily. These foods, as part of a calorie-reduced but nutrient-dense diet, will provide you with most of the micronutrients you need.

You may also find it helpful to add supplements to your diet. See Appendix D for the names of reliable suppliers of the products noted in this chapter.

SUPPLEMENTING WITH VITAMINS, MINERALS AND ANTIOXIDANTS

Since we're all caught up in our 24-7-365, faster-is-better lifestyle, I recommend supplementing your diet with vitamins, minerals and antioxidants that neutralize the destructive free radicals produced every day by your cellular metabolism.

All adults should consider taking the following:
- Vitamin A complex of mixed carotenoids in a softgel that contains:
  - beta-carotene   25,000 IU
  - lycopene   5,000 mcg
  - alpha-carotene   492 mcg
  - cryptoxanthin   115 mcg
  - zeaxanthin   98 mcg
  - lutein   59 mcg

- Vitamin B-complex in a capsule containing 50 mg of each B vitamin, 1 mg of folic acid and 60 mcg of biotin.
- Vitamin C-complex in a capsule containing 250 to 750 mg of a combination of the following:
  - calcium ascorbate
  - manganese ascorbate
  - zinc ascorbate
  - magnesium ascorbate
  - potassium ascorbate

  This should be in a bioflavonoid complex of rosehips, acerola berries, quercitin, rutin and isoflavones.
- Vitamin E in a capsule containing 400 IU of d-alpha tocopherol-succinate and a softgel of d-gamma tocopheryl (or tocopherol). If you are 35 years of age or older, you may absorb your vitamin E better in a dry powder form, not a fatty oil. The dry, white powder form I recommend is called a succinate.
- Four capsules of a comprehensive "network" antioxidant formula such as protect+.
- Vitamin D in a small tablet only in the winter months when you are not exposed to any sunlight. The preferred form is vitamin D-3 at 1,000 IU.
- Some form of probiotic formula with a minimum of six billion live, active cells of "friendly bacteria" per capsule with 200 mg of fructo-oligo-saccharides (FOS) per capsule. Some of the more beneficial strains to take in combination are:
  - L. rhamnosus
  - L. acidophilus
  - L. casei
  - B. longum
- Coenzyme Q10 (CoQ10) with tocotrienols. Softgels of CoQ10 come in 30, 60 and 100 mg strengths. CoQ10 is fat soluble and should always be taken with vitamin E, the mixed tocopherols and a meal containing fat such as olive oil, fish oils, flax seed oil, almond butter, etc.
- Calcium citrate and magnesium citrate, two of the most popular and easily available minerals. You may want a capsule of 200 mg of elemental calcium and a capsule of 150 mg of elemental magnesium. Consider also one capsule containing 30 mg of zinc, a selenium complex of 200 mcg of selenomethionine or HVP chelate, and 200 mcg of chromium. Minerals are taken with dinner and before you go to sleep.
- A high-quality "green drink" containing:
  - A phosphatide complex of 22 percent phosphatidyl choline (1,200 mg per serving) and 3 percent phosphatidyl serine (60 mg per serving).
  - The critical flavonoid-glutathione sub-network of herbal extracts containing milk thistle, Siberian ginseng, ginkgo biloba, Japanese green tea, European bilberry and full-spectrum grape seed and skin extract.

THE ROAD TO HEALTH

Every decade of our life—including those critical months before our birth is characterized by physical growth, development or deterioration, escalating or diminishing hormone levels, lifestyle stages and certain common health concerns. The following are some recommendations for optimizing your health and overcoming the hurdles typical of these different life stages. The herbal remedies, lifestyle advice, vitamin and mineral supplements, and those foods critical to defying the aging process, however, are not meant to be exhaustive, but they could make a huge difference in the way you think, feel and look in the coming years.

When it comes to supplements—more is not always better. It is far better to take smaller amounts of vitamins and antioxidants throughout the day and spread your mineral supplementation between dinner and before going to sleep.

It appears that the "portals of entry" in the small intestine shut down and turn to "off" when a large amount of a vitamin or mineral suddenly appears. Your body is designed to seek, absorb and distribute small amounts of vitamins and minerals constantly, not all at once, to maintain hormone supersymmetry and homeostasis.

Taking small amounts, as in homeopathic medicine, guarantees your ability to absorb or to stimulate certain processes. Too much of a supplement becomes inhibitory. When you reduce supplement dosages and take them more frequently throughout the day, you achieve optimal absorption.

Prenatal to 15 Years of Age

The role of nutrition in a child's health can't be underestimated—even before its life outside the womb begins. Numerous studies have shown that good maternal dietary strategies and optimal nutrition affects the health of infants and can impact their well-being even in adulthood.

The most widely known example of nutritional impact on a developing fetus is the importance of a mother's adequate folic acid intake prior to and into pregnancy in preventing neural tube defects.

Other research from the Birth Defects and Genetics Diseases Branch of the U.S. Centers for Disease Control and Prevention has shown that multivitamin use in women from three months prior to pregnancy through the first trimester reduces the risk of congenital heart defects in babies.

With children, the earlier a pattern of good nutrition is established, the more likely it will continue over the years. A study that tracked 3,714 elementary school children found that healthy habits, such as a lower-fat, lower-processed food diet and vigorous physical activity, that were instilled during elementary school years persisted into adolescence.

Unfortunately, healthy eating is not a reality for many North American children. *Dole's Fruit and Vegetable Update: What America's Children Are Eating* reports dismal dietary habits. Of all foods eaten at lunchtime, only 8 percent are fruit and 7.5 percent are vegetables, while over 50 percent consists of processed foods like cookies, desserts, chips, salty snacks, candy and gum. At home, fruit makes up 3 percent of food eaten, while vegetables add up to 25 percent of the dinner meal. *The Continuing Survey of Food Intakes of Individuals* states that 80 percent of children aged two to 11 fall critically short of getting the recommended daily amounts of calcium, iron, zinc and protein—all of which are essential for growth, development of the immune system and cognitive performance.

Children on restricted diets seem to be particularly at risk for nutritional deficiencies. For example, children who have been on a vegan macrobiotic diet until six typically suffer from vitamin B12 deficiencies as adolescents and related impaired cognitive function, even if they adopted an omnivorous diet later.

Childhood obesity is the most visible consequence of a diet lacking healthy choices. If children gain excess weight before their fifth birthday, they are more than twice as likely to be obese adults. According to the North American Academy of Pediatrics, 10 percent of four- and five-year-olds are too heavy for their age, and 11 percent of children aged six to 17 are overweight.

At the Institute of Cancer Research's Annual Conference in 2000, it was suggested that one's childhood diet may predict breast cancer risk later on in life more strongly than diet during adulthood.

A 1992 ground-breaking Canadian study, which appeared in the medical journal *Lancet* (November 1992), examined the effects of a 12-month daily multivitamin regimen of vitamins A, C, E and beta-carotene, as well as minerals such as iron, zinc, folic acid and calcium on infection-related illness. Children eating a diet of bioenergetic whole foods, fortified with a multivitamin, multimineral supplement, "showed higher numbers of T-cell subsets and natural killer cells, enhanced proliferation response to mutagens, increased interleukin-2 production and higher antibody response."

Besides disease prevention, an adequate intake of proper nutrients can have positive effects on mental health, behavior and cognitive function.

In an experiment using 245 children aged six to 12, those who were given a multivitamin, multimineral supplement for three months showed an average increase of 5 to 9.6 percent in non-verbal intelligence, an ability which is associated with academic performance.

In attention-deficit/hyperactivity disorder (ADHD), while genetics and environmental factors certainly play a major role, nutrient deficiencies are all too commonly found among sufferers. A study of 116 children showed that magnesium deficiency was evident in 95 percent of children with ADHD. Oral supplementation with 200 mg of magnesium per day for six months, on the other hand, has shown a significant decrease in hyperactivity. When magnesium is given with vitamin B6 and fish oils rich in DHA and EPA, improved behavior results.

Research has also shown that an Omega-3 fatty acid deficiency in boys aged six to 13 correlates to a higher frequency of behavioral, learning and health problems.

The bottom line is, as a parent it is important and worthwhile for you to provide solid guidance and foster the right dietary and lifestyle habits early in your child's life to offer him or her protection from a number of diseases and mental and emotional deficiencies from childhood on.

Recommendations

- Daily, give children aged one to six, 1 teaspoon of a "green drink" powder in 8 oz (250 mL) of water or 4 oz (125 mL) of unsweetened juice plus 4 oz (125 mL) of water. Children seven to 12 may have 2 teaspoons of "green drink" powder in the same amount of liquid; for those 12 and older, 3 teaspoons. This will boost their acetylcholine neurotransmitters to support good cognitive functions.
- Give them a protein shake daily with 15 grams of whey protein isolate powder, 8 oz (250 mL) of rice or almond milk, 2 tablespoons of soy lecithin granules, 1/2 cup of blueberries (fresh or frozen) and two heaping tablespoons of fat-free, natural yogurt. If you want to supercharge this tasty shake, empty a multivitamin, multimineral capsule for children into the shake recipe before mixing.
- Make certain your salads and vegetables look and smell appealing.
- Feed them salmon, tuna or mackerel three times a week or give them a supplement of fish oils, cod liver oil or algae extract daily.

15 to 25 Years of Age

During this time, our metabolism is at its peak. Hormone levels are at optimum and lean muscle mass is easily formed. Cognitive levels, our immune responses, cardiovascular health, hair quality and skin texture are also at their best.

This is a critical time to form positive habits—physically, mentally, emotionally and health-wise. Try to avoid or minimize the use of alcohol, tobacco and recreational drugs. The "high" from their use destroys your sensitive dopamine cells and accelerates emotional aging. If you can do just those three things, plus average nine hours of sleep in a totally dark room each night, your immune system will be strengthened for a lifetime.

Aging begins in earnest at 25 years of age. This is the time to begin an exercise program five days a week, combining both anaerobic (weight training) and aerobic (spinning, rowing, biking) exercise. One recent study at the Pennsylvania College of Medicine conducted by Tom Lloyd, Ph.D., and colleagues, studied the calcium intake of 81 girls for six years. Results showed that calcium intake between the ages of 14 and 17 had little to do with bone density. However, the more physically active the girls were, the greater their bone strength was throughout their lives.

Try to avoid fried foods that are full of biologically destructive trans-fatty acids found in hydrogenated or partially hydrogenated oils. Be cool, be natural, eat naturally. Be in rhythm with nature.

I am concerned about the eating habits of children. If they get great satisfaction and become accustomed to the tantalizing taste of unhealthful, processed, fast "foods"—those habits may persist throughout their lives.

This phenomenon is called "programming" and is cleverly achieved through seductive, compelling, billion-dollar advertising. How can our children stand up against this?

Set a healthful example for your children's sake. I advise you to change some of your eating habits to set a good example at the same time as improving your health and avoiding the all-too-familiar midday doldrums. You must adapt wisely and so your children must adapt wisely to survive well. It is that basic.

I personally never eat at fast-food restaurants or take-outs. I am very happy eating healthily and I want you to be also. I stand by that statement.

Recommendations

- Try to eat a salad every day.
- Experiment and find vegetables you really like and try them raw, steamed, grated or roasted.
- Instead of eating red meat, try chicken cooked with the skin off and the fat removed. And have fresh, broiled fish three times a week to keep your brain and nervous system full of DHA and EPA.
- Make a "green drink" the energizing food you have each and every morning.
- Use a multivitamin capsule with breakfast and a multimineral with dinner.
- Eat three meals a day of bioenergetic whole foods to keep yourself fueled with high-octane energy.
- Get a juicer and juice yourself a glass of fresh vegetable juice each day for radiant skin and glowing hair.
- Get buffed by working out hard at the gym five days a week.
- Drink lots of water to keep your skin clear; use a sports container with a plastic straw to minimize the amount of air you take in.

25 to 35 Years of Age

In this decade of our lives, our bone mass is at its peak. We have reached our maximum height. We should stretch daily to loosen and lengthen our body. If you haven't already started, this is the time to do weight-bearing exercises three to four times a week at the gym, to maximize bone density.

Our metabolism begins to slow down and we start to lose a little muscle and gain fat if we are not active.

Hormone levels begin to decline and this is noticed as hair becomes slightly thinner and some men begin to lose their hair.

Sleep patterns are not as deep and if we have children, this can be a decade of sleep deprivation. It can also be a time of financial stress. You must prioritize your time because family, relationship, work, community and environmental commitments stress your schedules.

Take some time for your own renewal, especially to meditate, pray, exercise, go for hikes, write poetry, read inspiring books and gaze at stars.

Recommendations

- Feed your head daily with a morning "green drink" plus fish oil softgels to fuel your central nervous system and boost your cognitive abilities.
- Make one of your meals a power protein shake with fresh or frozen berries with a capsule of probiotic cultures, like acidophilus. A power protein shake made with whey protein isolates gives you 30 to 35 grams of the highest biological value protein in the world. In addition, it is undenatured, so it builds up your immune system—especially the powerful cellular antioxidant glutathione, which cleanses your 100 trillion cells of waste products and cellular debris of regular metabolism, and escorts denatured bacteria, viruses, parasites, fungi and carcinogens out of your delicate cells for removal from your body.
- Be sure to get enough protein and minerals, as this will help to grow new hair. At breakfast supplement with:
  - one capsule of carotenoid complex
  - one capsule of vitamin B-complex
  - one capsule of vitamin C-complex
  - 1,000 mcg of vitamin D in winter
  - one capsule of vitamin E, 400 IU
  - one capsule of gamma vitamin E

  Before going to sleep, take 1 teaspoon of flax seed oil, 1/2 cup of fat-free organic yogurt and three garlic capsules or two cloves of chopped garlic. Also take minerals to include 200 mg of elemental calcium, 150 mg of elemental magnesium, 30 mg of zinc, 25 mg of manganese, 200 mcg of selenium and 200 mcg of chromium.
- Get your blood moving by exercising aerobically for 20 to 30 minutes three to four times a week to improve circulation.
- Learn to say no to people if you're overloaded. The stress in your life from juggling career and family demands produces excess cortisol that wears you down.

- Preventive care is crucial now. Avoid, or seek help, to deal with chronic stress in relationships, at work, in the family or within yourself; join a self-help group.
- Consume enough water. If you aren't hydrated when you exercise, your body won't efficiently absorb protein and other nutrients essential for building muscle.
- Use an herbal combination daily as a supplement to build up the adrenal glands so you can better deal with stress now and throughout your life. This combination should contain:

– licorice	600 mg
– jiaogulan	200 mg
– Siberian ginseng	100 mg
– astragalus root	800 mg
– burdock root	280 mg
– suma	240 mg

35 to 45 Years of Age

This is the "decade of vulnerability" (for some individuals, it may be from age 40 to 50). The average North American woman ages 18.6 years and the average man ages 16.2 years during this time. This is the make or break time. Either you will really do all that I recommend and reap huge rewards—or you'll let it go and lose the survival advantage.

Bone loss begins at this time, and you notice more soreness after physical activity.

Hormone levels in women and men begin to fluctuate, causing men to lose some of their ergogenic drive and for women to experience menstrual irregularities. This makes it difficult for a woman to get pregnant and carry a child to full term. The testosterone level in men decreases, which can lead to benign prostate enlargement.

Sun spots and wrinkles appear from the effects of sunburns or overexposure to sun in earlier years. Your eye lens becomes stiffer resulting in more difficulties with near vision. The first signs of high cholesterol and osteoporosis show themselves.

Recommendations

- Consider using three capsules of A•G•E inhibitors™ or 1,000 mg daily of the amino acid-like supplement carnosine. They protect your protein, neurological processes and cells from wearing out too soon.
- Never eat after 7:30 p.m., especially any sweet or carbohydrate that raises your insulin levels or cortisol levels, and prevents your youthful, regenerative hormone, growth hormone (GH), from being synthesized and secreted.
- Tweak your diet to make sure you are eating 40 grams of fiber daily to soak up any excess cholesterol, estrogen and environmental toxins.
- Use 2 tablespoons of soy lecithin granules plus 1,000 mg of carnosine daily in your power protein shake to help emulsify and eliminate excess cholesterol.

- Consume at least one fermented, organic soy product per day, such as soy protein isolate powder, tofu, miso, tempeh or soy beans, so as to consume the phytonutrients genistein and daidzein that protect your breasts or prostate from cancer.
- It is critical to exercise three to four times a week, doing 30 minutes of aerobic exercise that works up a sweat, and 15 to 30 minutes of intense weight-resistance training.
- Keep moving by walking or riding your bicycle instead of driving whenever possible.
- Stretch to stay flexible. This will also increase blood flow and keep your muscles loose. Soreness occurs when your muscle fibers break down from overuse or lack of flexibility.
- Begin hatha yoga, Tai Chi, aerobics, spinning or water aerobic classes.
- Slowly increase your clean water intake to ten glasses a day. Water will flush out post-exercise pain by washing out excess lactic acid that makes your muscles sore.

  Although the colon of a 55-year-old functions much like that of a 25-year-old, at around 30, the kidneys begin to shrink and are less efficient filters and pumps. As a result, waste products plus medicines and other substances clear the bloodstream more slowly. Drink eight to ten glasses of water daily, through a straw, to help flush out your kidneys and bloodstream.

- Eat more colorful vegetables, especially cruciferous vegetables (such as broccoli, broccoli sprouts, cabbage, mustard greens and watercress), which contain compounds to help prevent breast or prostate cancers.
- Take all the vitamins and minerals suggested for the 25 to 35 group but now add 100 mg of CoQ10.
- At lunch time begin taking your advanced, synergistic, antioxidant supplement to neutralize free radicals; take one capsule at each meal and one before going to sleep.
- Get a complete blood, urine and salivary profile for pro-aging oxidants and for antioxidant capacity.
- Take a second green drink mid-afternoon to give you a natural energy boost without caffeine and to protect your 100 trillion cells with the glutathione-flavonoid sub-network of herbal extracts.
- Before sleep, add another supplement to your regime to build up the quality of the cellular structure in your intestinal tract and to help growth hormone (GH) be synthesized and secreted—use 5 to 10 g of the amino acid L-glutamine, sublingually, and let it dissolve for one minute before swallowing.
- Exfoliate to loosen dead skin and promote circulation, rub a loofah sponge all over your body in the shower once or twice a week. End your shower with a blast of cold water to tighten your skin, improve blood flow and make your blood alkaline.

- Get deep REM (rapid eye movement) sleep, which is when your body releases growth hormone that repairs and regenerates tissue.
- Sleep for at least 8.25 hours a night in a completely dark room.
- If deep sleep is not possible, use 1/3 mg of melatonin sublingually one hour before sleep; use only pharmaceutical-grade melatonin four times a week.
- Smile a lot and say nice things to people. Do good and be good.
- Examine your natural human lifecycle as an integral part of nature.
- This is the age to reconcile who we are, where we came from, why we are here and where we go with our unique life. Begin to meditate, pray earnestly, ponder, watch the stars as a star gazer, write poetry, get closer to your own spriituality, and develop into a loving, compassionate, conscious human being.

45 to 55 Years of Age

Bone loss and hair loss increase for both men and women. In their lifetime, one out of two women and one in eight men over 50 will have an osteoporosis-related fracture. Don't be one of them. Keep exercising to lift your endorphins (feel-good hormones) and continue with your dietary strategy based on bioenergetic whole foods.

The cumulative effects of stress and poor habits start to appear as ailments such as heart disease, hair loss and diabetes. But you can control these conditions by walking briskly for 45 minutes a day and trying to get 100 percent of your protein from plant-based foods, supplemented with fresh Omega-3-rich fish, broiled, three times a week.

Your cortisol hormones rise as stress is encountered. The dilemma is that with each chronological year, your response to the same stress is greater and lasts longer. The elevated cortisol levels are extremely corrosive to your heart tissue and hypothalamus command center in the brain. Reduce your stress with exercise, walking, good nutrition and 8.5 hours of sleep nightly.

Two stress busters I highly recommend are (1) a full-body, deep massage for one hour every two weeks, and (2) a cleansing sauna, infra-red sauna or a steam bath to detoxify and relax once a week. These are a tranquil spiritual exercise.

Your family and career tend to be well-established at this point, allowing you time to devote yourself to community or environmental issues.

By age 52, on average, menopause arrives for most women. Health effects include mood swings, hot flashes, vaginal dryness, weight gain, thinning skin, fatigue and insomnia. You can successfully sidestep 95 percent of all these symptoms. Be conscious of getting the correct protein amount at each of your three meals. High and low levels of glucose can exacerbate hot flashes and mood swings. Avoid refined sugar, sweetened foods and processed foods made from refined wheat.

Eat hormone-friendly foods such as fish oils, pumpkin seeds, sunflower seeds, almonds and walnuts that are all rich in essential fatty acids, which help balance hormones.

CORTISOL RESPONSE TO STRESS WITH AGE

This graph illustrates that as we grow older, the body's response to stress is greater and lasts longer.

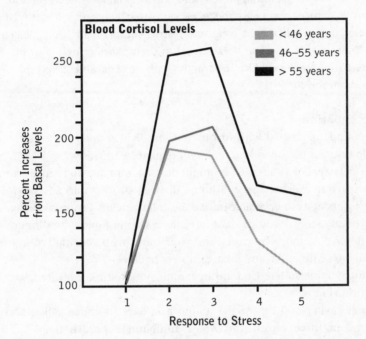

Blood Cortisol Levels

- < 46 years
- 46–55 years
- > 55 years

Percent Increases from Basal Levels

Response to Stress

Begin a new supplement: women should take two capsules of evening primrose oil and a 1/4 teaspoon of borage oil, before sleep, with yogurt, garlic, vitamin C, vitamin E, calcium and magnesium. If osteoporosis has begun, add the mineral supplement silica to your bedtime ritual. Use two capsules of atomized aqueous extract of spring horsetail—or if you are really concerned, use six drops sublingually of stabilized orthosilicic acid, which is the biologically active form of silicon. Silicon is essential for bone formation and strengthens your skin, nails and hair. Your yogurt, garlic and oil combination before sleep is an exception to the rule of not eating after 7:30 p.m., since this does not raise insulin levels.

This is the decade when most heart disease, heart attacks and strokes begin to form. They are caused by arteriosclerosis, or hardening of the arteries, which can result from high cholesterol, diabetes or hypertension. Positive lifestyle changes, like becoming physically active, can decrease your risk. CoQ10 builds strong heart muscles and protects your mitochondria (energy factories in your cells) from early burn-out.

Improve your habits and eliminate unhealthy ones like smoking and excess alcoholic consumption. Limit coffee to 2 cups of black, organic coffee a day, and never after noon. Or better still, switch to organic green tea and boost your immune response to cancer.

A 1999 study found three of the B vitamins—folic acid, B6 and B12—taken together reduce levels of homocysteine, a harmful substance in the blood, which is a byproduct of eating animal protein and is associated with heart disease. Your "green drink" reduces homocysteine levels very effectively and is a methyl donor.

Only eat pasta at one meal a week and restrict eating breads, buns, bagels and muffins. There are no pasta or bread trees! In their place, enrich your diet with more heart-friendly foods like asparagus, leafy greens and a second "green drink" mid-afternoon.

Recommendations

- Take 200 mg of CoQ10 with tocotrienols, in divided doses, with fatty meals to help nourish the heart and maintain regular heartbeat.
- Try a CoQ10 gel or vitamin C serum product on your face to reduce wrinkles.
- Keep up your exercise, get 8.5 hours of sleep in total darkness and try to make a glass of fresh vegetable juice daily, following my formula on page 289.
- Take your synergistic antioxidant formula, a second time, with dinner.
- Protect your memory by exercising your mind with reading, volunteering time to a worthy cause and taking on new hobbies.
- Use glucosamine sulfate (sodium free) and chondroitin for injured, sore, stiff or arthritic joints.
- Consider taking 500 mg of the amino acid-like substance called acetyl-L-carnitine or three capsules of A·G·E inhibitors™ (which helps transport nutrients to the brain) twice a day with food.
- Work through your doctor to block the demise of your dopamine neurons. Dopamine is the hormone that keeps you attentive, alert, bright and motivated. During this decade, dopamine neurons self-destruct and dopamine levels plummet quickly.

55 to 65 Years of Age

If we haven't taken care of ourselves earlier, we really start to see the results at this point. The fastest-growing age of those signing up for health club memberships is 55.

Generally, our senses of smell and taste decrease, as well as our vision and hearing. We may also begin to wake up more often to go to the bathroom. Chances are our family is independent and we are planning to slow down our work responsibilities.

This is a dynamic and exciting time to use your knowledge, age, maturity and insight to really work on yourself, and become a wonderful human being. Make this your goal!

For men, one of the most common causes of frequent night-time urination is benign prostatic hyperplasia (BPH) or enlargement of the prostate. More than 55 percent of men at age 60 experience symptoms. Testosterone is oxidizing into dehydrotestosterone, which slows down your ergogenic drive. The body wants to move dehydrotestosterone away from the testes so it deposits it at the outer extremity of the head where it causes hair roots to get weak, spindly, dry and fall out. You can keep the hair on your head, reduce the enlargement of your prostate, prevent testosterone from turning into dehydrotestosterone, and prevent testosterone from binding to SHBG (Sex-Hormone Binding Globulin) by using the following four herbal extracts daily:

- saw palmetto   450 mg
- pygeum   125 mg
- corn silk   120 mg
- stinging nettle root   30 mg

It is estimated that at age 50, male testosterone levels are 33 to 50 percent less than they were at age 25, and women by 50 produce only 50 percent of their testosterone levels compared to age 25.

You can increase testosterone without hormonal supplementation using bioenergetic whole foods and exercise. As testosterone levels rise, your body reduces any excess body fat.

Maintaining testosterone levels is the key to better strength, better cardiovascular health and a healthy libido. The dietary suggestions in this book are your best and most powerful "drug" to achieve elevated testosterone levels.

Recommendations

- Decrease portions at meals and eat more frequent, smaller calorie meals to stabilize glucose metabolism.
- For deep sleep use three capsules of sleep+ one hour before sleep.
- Take three capsules of A•G•E inhibitors™ or add 1,000 mg daily of carnosine to your power protein shake.

65 Years of Age—and Beyond

Both men and women need to increase dietary fiber to control weight and decrease LDL cholesterol and triglyceride levels, which go up at this age. Since weight gain characterizes this age category, your diet needs to be modified to reduce calories, saturated fat and high-glycemic-index foods.

You may want to work with your physician to consider human growth hormone (GH) injections as well as topical gels to raise and stabilize GH levels. A blood test called somatomedin C (IGF-1) measures growth hormone activity in your body.

Please be forwarned that there is much controversy over GH injections and the possibility that they may promote some types of cancerous growth.

Recommendations

- Emphasize lower- and upper-extremity strength, balance and coordination in your exercise routine. Build flexibility through hatha yoga or Tai Chi.

- Build up the postural muscles of the legs and buttocks and the trunk muscles by doing spine-neutral and abdominal strengthening exercises, such as the Swiss Ball techniques.
- Work with a knowledgeable physician to monitor your hormone levels and replace them with transdermally applied creams, skin patches or gels, and include natural estrogens, natural progesterone, testosterone, DHEA, melatonin, Deprenyl and growth hormone if necessary.
- Take hormones with a great degree of caution and with an awareness of possible adverse or unintended side effects. Take a "hormone holiday" periodically; that is, stop taking them. Their effects can be felt for several days after you stop. After the "holiday" readjustment period, a new therapeutic cycle can be started. DHEA and melatonin are neurohormones because they affect hormonal systems of the brain and body. The best rule of thumb is always take the least amount of a hormone your physician feels is safe.
- Keep the brain juices flowing by learning memory games, doing crossword puzzles, balancing your checkbook without a calculator, writing the alphabet from A to Z using your non-dominant hand, or taking a class that requires you to take notes and complete tests. These neurological exercises will cross-fertilize and foster new ideas that keep a human mind active and vital throughout life, even into the 7th, 8th, 9th, 10th decades and beyond. A rich network of satisfying social interactions and commitments—as well as participating in complex interpersonal exchanges and "bi-directional" communications actually help protect seniors from cognitive decline, dementia, depression, loneliness and mental isolation, and delays or prevents Alzheimer's and mental deterioration.
- Minimize animal proteins and use whey protein isolate powder for your protein at two meals a day and use more plant-based protein. Use 1,000 mg of carnosine daily in your protein shake.
- To keep aging arteries from inflammation and clogging, increase the Omega-3 oils in your diet by eating more fresh deep-ocean fish, mackerel, salmon, tuna and sardines. Take 1/2 teaspoon of GLA-rich borage oil a day.
- Eat prunes daily as an excellent source of fiber and a digestion aid.
- Make a second "green drink" mid-afternoon.
- Drink three cups of green tea daily.
- Increase your daily CoQ10 intake to 300 mg a day.

DIETARY RECOMMENDATIONS FOR COMMON HEALTH CONCERNS

Many common health problems can be treated with bioenergetic foods or herbs alone. But be sure to always work closely with your health professional before self-diagnosing any symptoms you are experiencing.

Allergy-like Symptoms

- Reduce animal protein to three servings of cold-water salmon, tuna, mackerel and sardines a week, and utilize plant-based protein sources.
- Eliminate milk and dairy products.
- Avoid wheat, corn, sugar and artificial sweeteners.
- Eat organically grown fruits and vegetables as much as possible.
- Use three capsules daily of immune-building Moducare.

Anemia Due to Iron Deficiency

- Increase your consumption of dried beans, sea vegetables (like Nova Scotia dulse, spirulina and chlorella), leafy greens, unsulphured molasses, dried fruit, lean wild game and "green drinks."
- Always use 500 to 750 mg of vitamin C as an ascorbate complex with iron-rich meals to aid in the absorption of organic iron.

Asthma

- Eliminate wheat, corn, soy and sugar—one at a time—rotating over several months to see if you get relief when a potential food intolerance is removed.
- Eat ginger, pineapple and the herb turmeric liberally in your food choices for their anti-inflammatory effects. Also use the herbal combination listed under chronic fatigue syndrome on page 252.
- Avoid egg yolks, full-fat dairy and animal products for three months because of their high arachidonic acid (AA) content, which promotes pro-inflammatory PGE2 hormone-like messengers.
- Use full-spectrum grape seed and grape skin extract, which contains 95 percent procyanidolic values, resveratrol and ellagic acid, to reduce histamines.

Bladder Disorders

- Avoid both regular and decaffeinated coffee, caffeinated teas, soft drinks, all alcohol, black pepper and all forms of sugar as a sweetener.
- Do drink two to three glasses of unsweetened cranberry juice daily (cranberry juice inhibits the ability of bacteria to adhere to the cells lining the bladder and urinary tract, thereby making the environment less suitable for those bacteria to colonize and grow).

Body Odor

- Avoid alcohol, coffee and all caffeinated drinks.
- Decrease consumption of all animal products.
- Avoid processed foods with hydrogenated or partially hydrogenated oils.
- Bathe in water fortified with 1 cup of organic apple cider and 1 cup of whey protein isolate powder.
- Have a "green drink" daily to deodorize, and eat lots of green vegetables, especially parsley, watercress, kale and chard.

Cancer Prevention

- Eat plenty of fresh, colorful fruits, salads, vegetables and sea vegetables.
- Eat fresh, ripe pineapple every day to allow its bromelain content to keep your mouth healthy.
- Increase long-chain Omega-3 fatty acids in the diet from fish or algae.
- Minimize or eliminate animal protein and all regular dairy products.
- Use only organically produced, hormone-free lean meat, skinless poultry and fat-free dairy products if you do use animal-based protein.
- Use culinary herbs and spices liberally, including garlic, ginger and turmeric.
- Eat fermented soy foods daily, especially miso.
- Use a "green drink" daily and drink 3 cups of green tea daily.
- Eat enokidake, maitake, shiitake, reishi and coriolus mushrooms or their teas made with magnetically charged water to enhance absorption of the vital nutrients.
- Avoid processed foods, refined wheat products, and fried foods that might contain biologically damaging trans-fatty acids.

Cholesterol (High)

- Increase Omega-3 fatty acids from fish, or take supplements of fish oil or algae.
- Try to eliminate or minimize saturated fat.
- Eat foods low on the glycemic index and minimize refined carbohydrates.
- Eat garlic and cayenne pepper daily.
- Drink plenty of water.
- Eat 40 grams of fiber daily.
- Eat plenty of fresh, colorful fruits and vegetables.

Chronic Fatigue Syndrome

- Use four capsules of acidophilus "friendly bacteria" in your protein shake.
- Eat a wide variety of fruits, vegetables and sea vegetables.
- Eat immune system-enhancing mushrooms (such as shiitake, maitake, reishi and coriolus) regularly, or drink teas made from them.
- Use whey protein isolate powder daily but reduce protein intake to 75 percent of ideal for two months.
- Drink lots of water.
- Sleep nine hours a night in total darkness.
- Take 5 grams of L-glutamine sublingually before sleep.
- Use the medicinal herbal extract combination:

– MSM	750 mg
– boswellia	300 mg
– devil's claw	450 mg
– juniper berries	150 mg
– ginger	225 mg
– turmeric	15 mg

Constipation
- Drink more clean water, up to ten 8-oz glasses a day.
- Drink 2 cups of chamomile tea each evening.
- Increase your fiber consumption by eating more fruits, vegetables and salads, and a moderate amount of nuts, seeds and whole grains.
- Use a "green drink" daily.
- Drink 4 oz (125 mL) of aloe vera gel in a glass of water daily.

Diabetes
- Eat more low-glycemic-index foods.
- Eat six small meals a day, emphasizing protein, salad and vegetables.

Diarrhea
- Avoid sugary foods, processed foods, spices, coffee, alcohol and any dairy products for several days.

Eczema
- Increase Omega-3 essential fatty acids from fish oil or algae oil.
- Avoid dairy products except fat-free organic plain yogurt.
- Eat more fruits and vegetables.
- Avoid trans-fatty acids (from processed foods) that are biologically damaging.
- Avoid alcohol and caffeine.
- Wash the area with ground-up oatmeal, leave 30 minutes, then wash off.

Fibrocystic Breasts
- Eat fermented soy foods daily, especially soy protein isolate powder.
- Eliminate all sources of caffeine and alcohol.
- Eat only organically grown foods or animal proteins.
- Avoid all dairy and red meat, except fat-free organic plain yogurt.
- Have a "green drink" daily.

Hypertension
- Have a "green drink" daily.
- Increase soluble and insoluble fibers by eating more salads, vegetables and prunes.
- Avoid processed foods as much as possible.
- Avoid table salt and salty foods.
- Use two cloves of chopped garlic before bed, with flax oil and yogurt.

Irritable Bowel Syndrome
- Eliminate all caffeine sources.
- Eliminate all soft drinks.
- Avoid all sugars, sweeteners and artificial sweeteners.
- Increase consumption of fiber-rich foods like fruits, vegetables, legumes and whole grains. In particular, eat more pineapple, which is rich in the digestive enzyme bromelain.

- Use an herbal combination designed to cleanse and build up the liver.
- Use 2 teaspoons of immune-stimulating colostrum daily, in divided doses, plus a green drink to set the proper pH in the gastro-intestinal tract.

Premenstrual Syndrome

- Drink a "green drink" daily to set the proper pH in the gastro-intestinal tract.
- Eat more fermented soy foods daily with a sea vegetable.
- Eliminate all sources of caffeine.
- Avoid sugary, sweet and salty foods.
- Eat more protein at each and every meal.
- Eat only organic vegetables, fruits and animal products, which are free of hormones and drugs. Use supplemental diindolylmethane (DIM), an extract from cruciferous vegetables, daily to balance mood-related hormones.
- Use an herbal formula specifically for PMS daily.

Menopause

- Eat fermented soy foods on a daily basis with a sea vegetable.
- Eat organic animal and dairy products, free of hormones and drugs.
- Reduce saturated fat by eating no red meat and only organic fat-free yogurt from dairy.
- Have a "green drink" daily.
- Consume Omega-3 fatty acids high in DHA and EPA.
- Use an herbal formula specifically for menopause daily.
- Use 2 teaspoons of immune-stimulating colostrum daily, in divided doses; use diindolylmethane (DIM) daily if you are on hormone replacement therapy.

Osteoporosis

- Eat fermented soy foods daily with a sea vegetable.
- Eat leafy greens (like chard, kale and lettuce) and "green drinks" for their vitamin K content, which is necessary for the formation of osteocalcin, a protein that builds calcium into bones.
- Reduce saturated fat from all animal sources.
- Eat 2 cups of fat-free, plain organic yogurt daily.

Pain Management

Pain, such as in arthritis, caused by inflammation, is brought on by the release of hormone-like compounds called prostaglandins. Studies show, however, that preventing the release of these compounds can stop or reduce pain. A key to this is inhibiting the enzyme cyclooxygenase-2 (COX-2), one of the triggers, according to *Nutrition Science News* (August 2000).

COX-2 inhibitors were introduced in the mid-1990s and are slowly taking the place of non-steroidal anti-inflammatory drugs (NSAIDs) such as ibuprofen and aspirin, which can cause undesirable side effects. Two prominent drugs, Celebrex and Vioxx are synthetic COX-2 inhibitors available by prescription only.

Natural, very effective COX-2 inhibitors that inhibit the metabolism of arachidonic acid (AA) and therefore prevent the formation of pro-inflammatory PGE2 are:

- Omega-3 long-chain fatty acids from fish oils or algae oils extracts, rich in EPA and DHA;
- polyphenols such as ellagic acid, resveratrol and resorcinol in full-spectrum grape seed extracts;
- lactoferrin (from milk) found in whey protein isolates and supplements; and
- phytonutrients/antioxidants like genistein, quercetin, a vitamin E complex, a vitamin A complex, alpha lipoic acid, N-Acetyl-Cysteine, CoQ10, lycopene, bilberry, selenium, a vitamin C-complex, citrus bioflavonoids and green tea.

Prostate Problems

- Eat fermented soy foods daily with a sea vegetable.
- Eat plenty of fruits and vegetables, especially cooked tomatoes mixed with olive oil, which give you the potent phytonutrient lycopene.
- Eat 2 to 3 tablespoons of raw pumpkin seeds daily.
- Drink 3 cups of green tea daily.
- Use plant-based protein and whey isolates exclusively.
- Use an herbal supplement specifically for the prostate and which contains stinging nettle root, saw palmetto, pygeum and corn silk.
- Use 2 tablespoons of immune-stimulating colostrum daily, in divided doses.

Stomach Upsets

- Eliminate alcohol and smoking.
- Eliminate fried foods and processed foods.
- Eat garlic and ginger daily, and drink ginger tea.
- Eat fresh pineapple, which is rich in the digestive enzyme bromelain.

SLOWING THE AGING PROCESS

Increasing hormonal miscommunication occurs generally with increasing chronological age—but you can, at any age, re-establish hormonal communication through diet, lifestyle and thoughtful supplementation.

Yes, you can slow down the aging process! The four primary markers of accelerated aging can be reversed by eating bioenergetic whole foods and eliminating both processed foods and excess stress. It is really all that simple!

We are then more capable of being mentally clear, emotionally stable and physically robust. With these three qualities maximized—we have the ability to compassionately help, love and support the mental, emotional, physical and ultimately the spiritual welfare of all humanity—one person at a time! Now we develop into a true selfless human being, the quintessence of human evolution. The epitome of human excellence!

We are then in perfect supersymmetry with ourselves, with all other human beings, with all of nature, with our true Self, with our divinity.

16

GUIDELINES FOR SELECTING, PREPARING AND ENJOYING FOOD

Before you take the first step, there are guidelines or tactics I follow when buying, preparing and enjoying my food that I would like to share with you. We've already discussed some of these, but here's a brief summary:

- Go out of your way to incorporate a wide variety of colors in your vegetable and salad choices to ensure a wide variety of phytonutrients. Remember to use some form of sea vegetable daily.
- When cooking vegetables, leave them "crunchy-tender." Also, do not cook raw, live herbs, but use fresh mint, thyme, marjoram, chives, parsley, basil, cilantro and tarragon on top of your food choices.
- Cook with spices such as cardamom, cinnamon, cloves, ginger, mustard seed, cayenne, paprika, peppercorns, saffron, nutmeg, coriander, chili powder and allspice and benefit from their healing properties.
- Do not fry foods in oil or butter. Simply sauté your foods in a little pure water until they are "crunchy-tender," then add fresh extra-virgin olive oil just before serving for the full bouquet of that lovely fragrance without any excess heating to the oil.
- Add miso to gravies, dressings and cooked vegetables for extra flavor and nutrition.
- Make your dishes visually appealing by adding raw, finely chopped vegetables (for easy digestion) such as red peppers, sweet onions, green onions, yams, carrots, beets or turnips and different sprouts to lentil and legume dishes, stir fries, casseroles, lasagnes, baked dishes, pasta dishes, fish, chicken or wild game.
- Consume two pieces of ripe, whole, preferably organic fruit each day. Make

one choice colorful berries and another citrus, eating some of the white pulp and rind. Eat fruits by season as much as possible.

- Spice up salads and vegetables with fresh garlic.
- When you drink your eight to ten 8-oz glasses of pure water a day, add a few drops of freshly squeezed lemon juice per glass. Also drink 1 or 2 cups of herbal tea daily, especially green tea—but don't add any sweeteners.
- Use a variety of plant-based protein sources daily, even if you mainly consume animal-based protein, but check that they are not genetically modified.
- When you use dried legumes, soak them for three to 12 hours, discarding the water and the dissolved phytic acid, then cook them.
- Use organic flax seeds, sunflower seeds, pumpkin seeds, almonds and hulled sesame seeds as snacks and raw in your oatmeal. Use nut butters sparingly. Almond butter is better for you than peanut butter.
- Use a variety of excellent alternatives to cow's milk, such as rice, oat, almond and hemp seed milk.
- Buy as much organic food as possible; that is, food that has not been exposed to pesticides, herbicides, fungicides, waxes and ripening-retardant chemicals.
- When using bread, avoid wheat. Try unleavened breads that contain no flour, yeast, sugars or oils. Generally they are called Essene breads and date back to the time of Christ.
- When using rice, choose whole brown rice or North American basmati rice. Basmati rice from India may contain agri-chemicals—avoid it.
- Be alert to the new wave of bio-engineered, genetically modified (GMO) foods that I am highly suspicious of, and personally avoid.
- Avoid chemical-laden and overly processed foods containing monosodium glutamate (MSG), a chemical taste enhancer that is added to many prepackaged foods and often used in Asian cooking. MSG can legally be listed as "natural flavors," "vegetable protein," "hydrolyzed food protein" and "hydrolyzed plant protein."
- Avoid saturated fats in full-fat dairy and red meats. Avoid trans-fatty acids.
- Stop several times a day to be grateful to your body, as well as nature, and thank them both with sincere appreciation. Giving thanks before the eating or sharing of food generates a feeling of healthy cohesiveness between us and the food that generally extends to the rest of the day. Be exceedingly grateful for your food.

FOOD-BUYING TACTICS

Buyer beware! Stay on the periphery of a grocery store where you will find the produce section full of vegetables and fruits; the dairy and dairy alternative sections; the bins of grains, peas, legumes, seeds and nuts; lean meats; fresh fish; and soy products such as extra-firm tofu, tempeh and miso.

Once you enter the aisles, you encounter mostly processed, packaged, canned and frozen foods. You will require a few selections from these interior aisles—but realize that generally 40 percent of the cost for foods in the aisles is for their colorful and attractive packaging. In fact, according to the *Tufts University Newsletter* (August 1997), one out of every four packaged foods charges you *more* for the container than the contents.

I shop at both my local grocery stores and at the natural food store, which stocks organic produce. They carry all the soy foods; good prepared foods; a full line of high-quality dietary supplements; whey protein isolate powder; soy protein isolate powder; "green drinks"; and a large selection of bioenergetic whole foods such as nuts, seeds, legumes, peas, beans, sea vegetables, culinary herbs, organic fat-free plain yogurt, medicinal herbs, organic cold-pressed oils and genuine wheat-free pastas, breads and noodles.

Please have some sense of the importance of reading labels on food products you are thinking of buying. My experience and advice to you is:

- Avoid products that contain ingredients you cannot pronounce or are unknown to you.
- Vigilantly watch for bad ingredients like partially hydrogenated or hydrogenated oils.
- Avoid or minimize consumption of products containing chemical additives and synthetic food enhancers like monosodium glutamate (MSG), aluminum and the preservatives BHA, BHT and TBHQ.
- Avoid products containing artificial sweeteners; artificial colors; fructose, high-fructose corn syrup, maltose, dextrose, sucrose, sorbitol and sugar; nitrites, nitrates and sulfites.
- Avoid products with refined flour.
- Try to purchase foods that are organically grown, non-irradiated, not genetically modified, locally grown and in season.
- Whenever possible, buy dairy products, poultry, meats and eggs from animals bred and raised free of antibiotics and growth hormones. If you eat dairy, only eat fat-free dairy.
- Only purchase organic fat-free yogurt or cottage cheese.
- Purchase all oils in small bottles that have been cold pressed and not chemically treated, close to the pressing date, then refrigerate them when not in use. Oils can go rancid quickly, even after you have eaten them, so squeeze one capsule of vitamin E oil in each bottle, once opened, to prevent oxidation of the oil and excessive, corrosive, free radical proliferation.
- Avoid chemical food coloring agents like blue 1, blue 2, yellow 3 and yellow 6. I do not object to natural coloring agents like beet (red-purple), carotene (orange-yellow), chlorella or spirulina (green) and annatto (yellow-orange).

GIVING YOURSELF A HEALTHY PLACE TO COOK

If you really want to make positive, lifestyle changes for better health, purchase and prepare bioenergetic whole foods in an appealing, attractive fashion.

You will spend several hours a day in your kitchen so make it a healing place. If working in your kitchen is stressful, that stress will be transmitted through your food and weaken the immune systems of those who consume it.

Simplify your storage spaces. Give yourself good lighting and fresh air. The kind of light bulb you use affects how you feel. Full-spectrum lighting, which is close to natural sunlight, is health-enhancing. The rays of natural light, including small quantities of ultra-violet light, stimulate your cryptochrome, (the skin's light meter cells) and positively stimulate a myriad of body functions. You can find full-spectrum light bulbs in all natural food stores.

Full-spectrum light, which includes ultra-violet light, activates the synthesis of vitamin D, needed for the absorption of calcium. Furthermore, in recent studies the UV component of sunlight has been shown to reduce both blood pressure and cholesterol, and to treat symptoms of psoriasis. Being exposed to large amounts of UV light is thought to increase the risk of cancer, but UV light in small amounts is essential.

Regular light bulbs give off a predominance of yellow, red and infrared light. Research demonstrates that animals do not do well in this light and only domesticated animals experience cancer—not animals living in nature and exposed to daylight and night darkness. Fluorescent bulbs lack the blue-violet portion of the spectrum. If you are constantly exposed to fluorescent light, you will feel fatigue and your stress hormone cortisol will become elevated. Fluorescent light is now banned in many hospitals in Europe.

Choose Healthy Cookware and Cooking Methods

The kind of cookware you use to prepare food can make a difference in the food's nutritional value. Slowly build up a collection of pots and pans that are stainless steel, with double-or triple-sealed bottoms. Avoid all aluminum cookware, as the aluminum leeches into your food and interferes with calcium absorption into your bones and can cause kidney disease. You should also use a stainless steel steamer with one or two inner baskets so you can start off some vegetables steaming (like yams) and then add others in the top basket for only a few minutes (like kale, chard and asparagus).

The ideal kitchen would also have a juicer, a good glass blender and an electric coffee grinder for nuts and seeds. A hot air popper sure makes for fun in the kitchen.

How you cook bioenergetic whole foods affects their nutritional value. Here are the techniques I use:

- **Steaming** over a pot with just one-half inch of water is great for vegetables. Vitamins and minerals are better preserved than if the vegetables are cooked in water.
- **Boiling** vegetables results in a majority of the nutrients escaping into the boiling water. But you can boil legumes, peas and beans because you discard the water that contains gaseous compounds.
- **Baking** allows for nutritious juices that escape, creating a gravy for the vegetables. Baking works for root vegetables like garlic, yams, onions, sweet potatoes, potatoes, carrots and beets.
- **Poaching** foods such as eggs, vegetables, fruit, tofu and fish in a small amount of water collects nutrients into a small amount of liquid used to keep foods moist.
- **Water sautéing** allows you to easily control temperatures when cooking stir-fries, vegetables, tofu, tempeh, seafood and chicken. Gently cook your food in a little water and add extra-virgin olive oil only at the last minute. Try adding miso to your dish before serving.
- **Stewing** allows you to break down foods so you can easily digest and absorb the nutrients. All the juices become the broth, to which you can add miso before serving.
- **Stir-frying** in a wok is a method of quick cooking that preserves nutrients and keeps seafood, vegetables, chicken, tofu, and tempeh colorful and "crunchy-tender." Start with a small amount of water and add canola oil or extra-virgin olive oil at the last minute of stir-frying. You can add miso to stir-fries just before serving.
- **Roasting** is great for root vegetables like carrots, small turnips, potatoes, garlic, parsnips, ginger root, yams, sweet potatoes, onions, garlic and beets.
- **Pressure cooking** in a stainless steel, double- or triple-bottom pressure cooker is the method I prefer to cook presoaked legumes.

Cleaning Your Kitchen

Plastic cutting boards were once thought to be more sanitary than wood cutting boards. New research now shows that plastic surfaces harbor germs after they are washed, but a wood cutting board shows no signs of bacteria after being washed well. If you prepare meat on your counter top or cutting board, wash it well before any other food comes into contact with that surface.

Everyone likes a sparkling-clean kitchen that inspires creativity. Visually, it looks wonderful to leave stainless steel or copper-bottom pots and pans out or conveniently hanging. Unfortunately, most of the polishes, cleansers, disinfectants, degreasers and deodorizers sold commercially contain a wide assortment of biotoxic chemicals that build up in your system with constant use. They include carbon-based compounds (VOCs) that are released from cleaning agents as gases, xylene, benzene, naphthalene, phenol and many more that are not even listed on the labels. Collectively, over time, they will cause you headaches, fatigue, nausea, dizziness and skin irritations. Long-term exposure could be a contributing factor in cancer. They add to your total toxic load. As you make efforts to prepare and eat healthier, bioenergetic whole foods—why not clean your kitchen with non-toxic cleaning agents? Many companies offer safe, non-polluting cleaning products that are non-chlorinated and biodegradable. They are widely available in natural food stores and in your favorite grocery store. Look for them! You can also make your own high-quality cleaners that do not sacrifice human safety and environmental responsibility. Be an alchemist and make sensible, eco-friendly, non-toxic cleaners. Finally, don't simply pour your present chemical cleaners down the drain; take them to your local toxic waste depot.

Sandalwood Laundry Alternative

For an average size load pre-mix:

1.5 oz liquid castile soap
1 cup baking soda
1 cup white vinegar
1 cup washing soda
1/2 cup hydrogen peroxide
10 drops tea tree oil
10 drops essential oil of sandalwood

Lavender-Tea Tree Scrub for Pots and Pans

Mix ingredients together and add enough water to make a smooth paste and then put in a small, recycled squirt bottle:

4 tbsp finely ground oatmeal
3/4 cup baking soda
2 tsp liquid castile soap
10 drops lavender essential oil
10 drops tea tree oil

Eucalyptus Bath and Kitchen Cleaner

Mix ingredients into a large recycled spray bottle and shake before using each time:

1 cup water
1/2 cup white vinegar
2 lemons, juiced
2 tsp liquid castile soap
10 drops tea tree oil
10 drops grapefruit seed extract
10 drops essential oil of eucalyptus
10 drops essential oil of lavender

Three of the worst breeding grounds for bacteria are the sponges, the kitchen dishcloth and your toothbrush. At the end of each day, put the used dishcloth in your laundry basket. Do not dry it out and reuse it the next day. Every day, start with a fresh, clean dishcloth. Do not use sponges that breed bacteria; rather, use recycled paper towel. Every day, put six drops of hydrogen peroxide on your toothbrush bristles for 10 seconds, then rinse off with hot water before you use it.

WASHING PRODUCE

I always wash produce before using it, in spite of the fact that I purchase organically grown produce, grains and legumes. If you use conventionally grown fruits and vegetables, it is especially important to wash them carefully and peel them when appropriate. Recent research tested 17 different fruits and vegetables and found that washing and peeling them removed 100 percent of all pesticides from 60 percent of the produce, with significantly lower signs of pesticide residues in the rest of them.

The simple and successful washing method used by the researchers is to swirl tomatoes, berries, green beans, grapes, cherries, sprouts, lettuces, peas, broccoli or leafy vegetables in a diluted solution of biodegradable dish detergent and room-temperature water, for ten seconds, then rinse them with warm water. They also scrubbed sturdier fruits and vegetables, using a vegetable brush, with this solution for ten seconds. Scrubbing, rinsing and peeling removed all residue from carrots, potatoes, squash and bananas. Peel cucumbers and apples that are waxed to remove fungicides.

I highly recommend that you use a more powerful cleaning solution by purchasing bottles of prepared fruit and vegetable wash. They are generally made from water, fatty polyglycosides (from corn starch), sodium citrate (a salt of citric acid) and cellulose collides (from cotton and wood). A 700 mL (24 oz) bottle may cost $7.00 and last you three full months. The results are even much better than using dish detergent. These washes are widely available in natural food stores and grocery stores.

You can also make your own wash of freshly squeezed lemon juice, 4 table-spoons of baking soda and six drops of grapefruit or citrus-seed extract.

Wash produce before you store it in the refrigerator so as not to contaminate other food.

STORING NUTS, SEEDS AND OILS

Store nuts and seeds in the refrigerator or freezer to prevent their oils from going rancid. Keep all oils in the refrigerator when not using them. Genuine extra-virgin olive oil will solidify. This does not affect its nutritional value in any way. Simply run hot water over the bottle for 30 seconds to render it back to a useable liquid.

Keep any colostrums, all fish oils, all softgels of vitamin E and vitamin A as carotenoids, all CoQ10 and tocotrienols and any capsules of acidophilus-type supplements you have in the refrigerator once they have been opened.

SOAKING SEEDS, NUTS AND GRAINS

One problem with whole grains, seeds, nuts and beans is that their fibers contain phytic acid. In your intestines, phytic acid combines with zinc, calcium, magnesium and iron to form phytates. The phytates are insoluble, so they pass out of your body, carrying minerals with them. Over the long run, eating a diet high in whole grains, beans, nuts and seeds, as many vegans and vegetarians do, can lead to an outright mineral deficiency.

The phytic acid in nuts, seeds, beans and whole grains can be almost totally eliminated quite easily. In the case of grains made into breads, for example, natural fermentation, if real sourdough is used, removes almost all of the phytic acid. An alternative to whole wheat bread is bread or wrap-ups made from any sprouted grain—as the sprouting process removes most of the phytic acid.

If you are going to cook whole grains such as wheat berries, spelt, buckwheat, rye, whole oats, quinoa, millet, brown rice, amaranth and kamut—soak them for several hours in buttermilk, which greatly reduces the phytic acid. The lactic acid in the buttermilk breaks down the phytic acid in the bran. This is what happens when you soak uncooked beans in water for several hours before cooking; the soaking and rinsing removes most of the phytic acid from the skins and greatly improves digestibility.

You want to consume a small amount of phytic acid, which acts, in small doses, as an antioxidant and inhibitor of the destructive hydroxyl free radical, which is corrosive to brain cells. Bacteria in your intestine liberates inositol, a B vitamin, from the fiber-phytic acid. Inositol is necessary in synthesizing both serotonin and acetylcholine.

FOLLOWING THROUGH AWAY FROM HOME

Dining out has become a way of life for North Americans, who eat two out of every five meals away from home. Often we view dining out as a time to splurge, a "time out" when good nutrition doesn't count. Use the suggestions below and you can easily maintain "The World's Best Diet" at any type of eatery:

- A dish can only be as good as its worst ingredient.
- Balance your meal with a salad, fish, a vegetarian entrée, or a small portion of lean meat. Skip the bread and the dessert.
- Look over the entire menu. Restaurants frequently feature healthful dishes low in fat and salt to meet the demands of a growing number of health-conscious patrons.
- Avoid fried foods.
- Ask your server how a food is prepared, and if it is not to your expectations, request it made-to-order. You can also request changes or substitutions.
- Ask for your sauces on the side. Most of an entrée's fat and calories come from the sauce.

- Rather than fat-laden creamy dressings, ask for extra-virgin olive oil and put tablespoon on your salad with a little fresh lemon.
- Ask for a medley of steamed vegetables and add a dash of lemon, mustard, or an herb such as dill or oregano to liven up the dish.
- Request a double order of steamed vegetables or salad.
- Avoid buffets. The mere sight of large quantities of food attractively presented, most often encourages overeating.
- Order non-carbonated, bottled water with a wedge of lemon.

We do not live by nutrients alone. Eating is not only an important influence on health, but also a major source of pleasure, and a primary focus of social interaction. I firmly believe there are huge differences in the "nutritional vibrations" between the same foods cooked or prepared by various people. The intent, love, concern and energy of the food preparer can affect the state of consciousness of those who consume it. Think of this carefully when you select restaurants in which to eat. Consider the aesthetic appearance of their foods—their freshness, color and odor. What type of people work there and what their attitude is about cleanliness, food preparation and serving.

17

LIVING SEVEN DAYS ON
THE WORLD'S BEST DIET

Congratulations! You have read this book, are now aware of the connection between your health and what you eat, have made the decision to take a positive step forward with all that you've learned, and you're about to reap the rewards.

Create a new paradigm in your kitchen and in your revised dietary strategy today. It is the foods you fuel your body with today that dictate your peak performance level and optimum self-healing capability tomorrow. The bioenergetic whole foods you eat today will give you vitality and mental acuity—or the processed, chemically treated partial foods you eat today that rob your vitality and mental acuity will show up on the balance sheets of your wellness and health.

There is no time that is too early or too late to begin. The time is now. Be wise for your own sake! Your body is governed by a complex network of neurotransmitters and hormones. The way they interrelate, the body's metabolism for energy, its biomechanical system for movement, and, indeed, even how you conduct your life are unique to each individual. To be successful you don't need to be obsessive with your new dietary strategy. You can be consistent and deliberate in incorporating the following dietary strategies one week at a time, then one day at a time, then one meal and one snack at a time. It is all that easy! It is a conscientious return to the base of the food chain so you can eat high-octane fuels that are in harmony with your longstanding genetic predisposition to bioenergetic, low-calorie whole foods. This gives you the necessary edge to survive!

In this chapter you will find all that you need to create your own seven days of menus:

- a recommended daily schedule for meals, snacks, protein shakes, minerals and supplements, and other health-enhancing actions and activities;
- charts to help you select foods according to their nutritional benefits;
- guides to understand portion size; and
- recipes to get you started.

When creating menus and cooking these or other recipes, remember and employ the "Four Principles of Eating Right": adaptability, variety, moderation and balance. These principles of a superior dietary strategy have not only rendered stunning results in leading research laboratories (such as the University of Toronto, UCLA, the University of Wisconsin, McMaster University, the University of British Columbia and Harvard) but, even more excitingly, have entered another stage and are already in use in tens of thousands of kitchens from coast to coast.

Aside from this, you can modify and tailor these suggestions to your own special needs and time limits. But it is important that you make an effort to slowly or quickly (either you are a "tip-toer" or a "plunger") plan your weekly and daily menu on paper. When you put something down on paper, you have demonstrated your commitment. This will encourage you to make a basic shift in progressively monitoring and purchasing your food supplies from nature's bioenergetic whole foods. Never impulse buy! High-tech synthetic food manufacturers know how to package foods for irresistible eye appeal and make their products look good, smell good and taste good. Don't be fooled!

Eating a wide range of bioenergetic whole foods, from readily available traditional North American foods to delicious ethnic foods, can be both nutritious and stimulating to your brain and body.

The recipes are not meant to be followed to the letter or in the exact order given. They offer an idea of the many healthful and enjoyable possibilities available to you. You may interchange any protein and vegetable dishes. Use garlic, onions, leeks, shallots, scallions, salsa, parsley, cilantro, watercress, oregano, basil, thyme and rosemary as liberally as you can. Use natural dried spices and herbs in abundance to suit your taste, as well as fresh herbs to decorate your main entrée for visual appeal.

Look at this chapter as an educational tool as well. The elite athletes that I've worked with did not set records or win gold medals without a specific dietary strategy and daily training log. Your lifestyle regimen becomes your daily training log needed to promote youthful vigor and vitality, no matter what your current chronological or biological age.

THE DAILY SCHEDULE

Each meal suggestion is approximately 500 calories; 55 percent low-density carbohydrates (69 grams); 25 percent protein (30 grams); 20 percent fat (12 grams); and 10 to 15 grams of soluble and insoluble fiber.

My recommendations balance your fat, protein and carbohydrates with moderate amounts of calories and allow you to adapt to food preferences, tastes and seasonal availability. As you become more comfortable with this dietary strategy, branch out from these food groupings and adapt the guidelines to include your favorite foods.

These meals are designed to keep you in hormonal balance, satiate your appetite and keep you feeling full for three to four hours. Consider food a blessed gift. Bless it while you chop, cook and serve food. You're not only giving yourself and your loved ones true, bioenergetic whole foods, in a home-cooked fashion but, more importantly, you are giving the lasting gift of optimal good health. Bravo! Please consider saying, singing or quietly thinking a grace or thanksgiving over, and with, your food before you begin to eat. Bon appétit.

Remember, make sure the food you eat adheres to the dietary strategy outlined in this book, satisfies your hunger and gives you pleasure. Bioenergetic whole foods have their own rewards, pleasures and powerful healing response. Value these dynamic foods for their health-promoting properties as much as for their flavours.

Be a conscious alchemist in your kitchen by preparing foods that are utterly nutritious, with dazzling eye appeal, and satisfying aroma, texture and taste.

TIMING OF MEALS, SNACKS, CLEANSERS AND SLEEP

Meal	What	When	Approximate Time
1. Morning anabolic cleanser	−8–32 oz (125 mL–1 L) room-temperature water with $\frac{1}{2}$ teaspoon of fresh lemon	Upon waking	6:00–6:30 a.m.
2. Alkaline booster	−"Green drink" in 6 oz (90 mL) of water or unsweetened juice −35–100 calories	Within 15–45 minutes of waking	6:45 a.m.
3. Breakfast **Sample:** − Power Protein Shake	−60% complex carbs −30% protein −10% fat, high in EPA and DHA −*500 calories total	Within 30–60 minutes of waking	7:00 a.m.
4. Snack 1	−Carrots, celery, zucchini sticks; sunflower sprouts or broccoli sprouts; red pepper, cucumber, turnip, sweet yam rounds −*100 calories	Three hours after breakfast	10:00 a.m.
5. Green tea	−2–3 cups of unsweetened green tea		11:45 a.m.

6. Lunch	−35% complex carbs	Two hours	12:00 p.m.
Samples:	−45% protein	after snack	
−Flat Bread Pizza	−20% fat as flax oil		
−Three Bean Salad with Tempeh	and borage oil		
−Yummy Peaches-n-Cream	−* 500 calories total		
Yogurt Sundae			
−Black Bean Rollups			
−Zesty Cottage Cheese Salad			
−Open-Faced Savory			
West Coast Veggie Burger			
7. Snack 2	−Piece of colorful fruit,	Three hours	3:00 p.m.
	berries or melon	after lunch	
	−*150 calories		
8. Dinner	−60% complex carbs	Three hours	6:00 p.m.
Samples:	−20% protein	after snack	
−Tarragon-Lemon Chicken	−20% fat as olive oil		
with Steamed Vegetables	−*500 calories total		
−Chunky Miso Soup			
−Baked Lemon-Ginger Salmon			
with Grated Root Salad			
−Marinara Sauce on Kamut			
−Roast Turkey with Herb Rub,			
Wild Rice and Roasted Vegetables			
9. Evening herbal tea	−Unsweetened chamomile	Two hours	8:00 p.m.
	and ginger tea	after dinner	
	*50 calories		
10. Evening catabolic cleanser	−1–2 cloves of finely	Before bed	10:00 p.m.
	chopped garlic or four capsules		
	−½ tablespoon of organic		
	flax seed oil		
	−½ cup of fat-free		
	organic plain yogurt		
	−*100 calories		
	Optional		
	−400 IU vitamin E		
	−500 mg vitamin C as mixed ascorbates		
	−1 protect+		
	−3–5 grams of L-glutamine, taken sublingually		
	−1,000 mg of calcium and 1,000 mg of magnesium		
	as taurates, aspartates or citrates with silica		

DIETARY STRATEGY

The following charts list groups of foods based on their nutrient and calorie content. This is just a sampling, but it provides initial structure and specific examples for you to begin to follow "The World's Best Diet."

Vegetables and Fruits

All servings in the table below are cooked unless marked raw.

VEGETABLE	SERVING SIZE
Beans, green	2 cups
Beets	2 cups
Broccoli	2 cups
Brussels sprouts	2 cups
Cabbage, raw	3 cups
cooked	1½ cups
Carrots	2 medium
Carrot juice	½ cup
Cauliflower	2 cups
Chard	2 cups
Collards	2 cups
Dandelion greens	2 cups
Eggplant	2 cups
Kale	2 cups
Lettuce, raw, all types	4 cups
Mustard greens	2 cups
Okra	¾ cup
Onions, raw	¾ cup
cooked	⅔ cup
Parsnips	⅓ cup
Peas in pod	1 cup
Peas, green	½ cup
Rutabaga	2 cups
Tomato, fresh	2 medium
Tomato paste	1 cup
Tomato plum	2 medium
Tomato sauce	¾ cup
Turnip green	2 cups
Sea vegetables	
Nova Scotia dulse	1 tablespoon
Kombu	1 tablespoon
Arame	1 tablespoon

All servings in the table below are raw unless marked cooked.

FRUIT	SERVING SIZE
Apple	1 medium
Apple sauce	1 cup
Apricots, fresh	6
Apricots canned, no sweetener	8 halves
Banana	1 medium
Berries, fresh or frozen:	
blackberries	2 cups
blueberries	2 cups
boysenberries	2 cups
raspberries	2 cups
strawberries	2 cups
Cantaloupe	2 cups
Cherries	2 cups
Dates	4
Figs	3 dried
Fruit rollups	2 rolls
Grapefruit	1 medium
Grapes	1 cup
Kiwi	2 small
Honeydew melon	2 cups
Papaya	½ medium
Peach	1 large
Pear	1 large
Plum	4 medium
Pineapple	1 cup packed
Pomegranate	1 medium
Prunes	6 medium
Tangerine	2 large
Watermelon	3 cups

Counting Antioxidants and Phytonutrients

We have long known how to measure carbohydrates; now, we also know how to measure the two main phytonutrients—antioxidant and carotenoid levels—in bioenergetic whole foods. Some very recent studies have used a sophisticated evaluation technique that can accurately measure the total antioxidant and carotenoid capacity of foods, so we now have the tools to analyze exactly which vegetables and fruits can boast being low in carbohydrates but high in antioxidants and carotenoids.

The Atkins Center for Complementary Medicine in New York City, founded and run by cardiologist Robert C. Atkins, M.D., has been able to determine the ratio of both antioxidant value and carotenoid values to carbohydrates in grams. The higher the ratio, the more antioxidant and phytonutrient protection you get per gram of carbohydrate. With these ratios, you now have a scientifically accurate way to choose the foods that are best for you.

The charts of vegetables and fruits on pages 271 to 273 rank popular vegetables and fruits in descending order of antioxidant and phytonutrient protection and give their score. The score is based on a complex formula (known as the Trolox equivalent) that compares the antioxidant or phytonutrient capacity of the vegetable or fruit. The charts also list the carbohydrate content of a typical serving of the vegetable or fruit and give you either an antioxidant-to-carbohydrate ratio or a phytonutrient-to-carbohydrate ratio.

The charts show that you get some of the best protection per serving from kale, garlic, chard, spinach, broccoli, red peppers, lettuce, beets, tomatoes, all berries—and the least protection from cucumbers, celery, corn, pears and honeydew melon. You see that some foods that are high on the antioxidant or phytonutrient scale are also high in carbohydrates; they therefore have a low ratio. Research in this area is still in the early stages, and only a small number of fruits and vegetables have been analyzed.

The starchier the vegetable or fruit, the lower its ratio of antioxidant or phytonutrient protection to carbohydrate. For instance, sweet potatoes are touted as a substitute for regular potatoes and considered particularly healthy because of their beta-carotene content. You can easily see from the first table that sweet potatoes aren't particularly high in antioxidants relative to other vegetables. They are, however, very high in carbohydrates—an average-sized baked sweet potato contains 55.4 grams of carbs—giving the sweet potatoes an antioxidant/carbohydrate ratio of only 0.15. If you are eating only a restricted number of carbohydrates, you might think twice about sweet potatoes; you'd be much better off using your carb allowance on chard, greens, broccoli, kale, spinach, beets, red peppers or Brussels sprouts.

TOTAL ANTIOXIDANT PROTECTION OF SOME VEGETABLES

Vegetable	Antioxidant Score per Serving	Carbohydrates in Grams	Antioxidant-to-Carbohydrate Ratio
Kale	48.2	7.4	6.5
Swiss chard	48.2	7.4	6.5
Garlic (2 cloves)	46.4	2.0	23.2
Spinach	34.0	6.8	5.0
Watercress	34.0	6.8	5.0
Parsley	34.0	6.8	5.0

Brussels sprouts	31.6	13.6	2.3
Broccoli	25.8	8.0	3.2
Beets	23.4	11.4	2.1
Red peppers (raw)	16.2	6.4	2.5
Corn	14.4	41.2	0.3
Onion (1 tablespoon)	11.2	1.8	6.2
Eggplant	10.2	6.4	1.6
Cauliflower	10.2	5.8	1.8
Cabbage	9.6	8.0	1.2
Potato (1 whole)	9.2	102.0	0.09
Sweet potato (1 whole)	8.6	55.4	0.15
Leaf lettuce (2 leaves)	8.2	1.0	8.2
Green beans	7.8	9.8	0.8
Carrots	6.4	16.4	0.4
Squash	5.6	7.8	0.7
Iceberg lettuce (2 leaves)	4.6	0.8	5.8
Celery (raw)	2.2	1.5	1.5
Cucumber (raw)	2.2	3.0	0.7

Servings are 1 full cup cooked unless otherwise indicated.

Adapted from the following sources:
Cao G., E. Sofic and R.L. Prior, "Antioxidant Capacity of Tea and Common Vegetables,"*Journal of Agriculture and Food Chemistry 44* (1996): pp. 3426–3431; Pennington, Jean A.T., ed., *Bowes and Church's Food Values of Portions Commonly Used*, 16th ed., Philadelphia: Lippincolt, 1994; Atkins, R., and S. Buff, *Dr. Atkins' Age-Defying Diet*, New York: St. Martin's Paperbacks, 2001.

TOTAL CAROTENOIDS IN VEGETABLES

Food	Carotenoid Content in mcg per Gram	Carbohydrates in Grams	Carotenoid-to-Carbohydrate Ratio
Kale	440.0	7.4	59.5
Swiss chard	280.0	7.4	30.0
Turnip greens	260.4	3.2	81.4
Collards	254.4	7.8	32.4
Spinach	245.8	6.8	36.1
Watercress	189.6	6.8	31.2
Parsley	189.6	6.8	31.2
Sweet potato	187.5	55.4	3.4
Carrots	95.0	16.4	11.3
Butternut squash	114.0	21.4	5.3
Red pepper (raw)	52.8	6.4	14.5

Romaine lettuce (raw)	80.0	1.4	55.8
Tomato (raw)	73.2	5.8	12.6
Broccoli	65.4	8.0	8.2
Apricots (raw)	52.0	15.8	3.2
Zucchini	51.4	6.9	7.3
Brussels sprouts	41.0	13.6	3.0
Green beans	26.8	9.6	2.7
Endive (raw)	19.2	1.6	12.0
Corn	19.0	41.2	0.5

Portions are 1 full cup, cooked, unless otherwise indicated.

Adapted from the following sources:

USDA-NCC Carotenoid Database for U.S. Foods, 1998; Pennington, Jean A.T., ed., *Bowes and Church's Food Values of Portions Commonly Used*, 16th ed., Philadelphia: Lippincott, 1994; Atkins, R., and S. Buff, *Dr. Atkins' Age-Defying Diet*, New York: St. Martin's Paperbacks, 2001.

Fruit

TOTAL ANTIOXIDANT CAPACITY OF FRUITS

Fruit	Antioxidant Score per Serving	Carbohydrates in Grams	Antioxidant-to-Carbohydrate Ratio
Blueberries	48.0	20.6	2.3
Blackberries	40.0	18.4	2.2
Strawberries	24.8	10.6	2.3
Plums and prunes	16.8	17.2	1.0
Orange	13.6	16.4	0.8
Kiwi	11.0	22.6	0.5
Pink grapefruit	9.0	19.0	0.5
Red grapes	7.8	15.8	0.5
Green grapes	5.8	15.8	0.4
Banana	4.2	26.8	0.2
Apple	3.8	21.0	0.2
Tomato	3.2	5.8	0.5
Pear	2.4	25.0	0.1
Honeydew melon	1.8	15.6	0.1

Servings are 1 full cup and raw.

Adapted from the following sources:

Wang, H., G. Cao, and R.L. Prior, "Total Antioxidant Capacity of Fruits," *Journal of Agriculture and Food Chemistry* 44 (1996): pp. 701–705; Prior, R.L., et al., "Antioxidant

Capacity as Influenced by Total Phenolic and Anthocyanin Content, Maturity, and Variety of Vaccinium Species," *Journal of Agriculture and Food Chemistry* 46 (1998): pp. 2686–2693; Pennington, Jean A.T., ed., *Bowes and Church's Food Values of Portions Commonly Used*, 16th ed., Philadelphia: Lippincott, 1994; Atkins, R., and S. Buff, *Dr. Atkins' Age-Defying Diet*, New York: St. Martin's Paperbacks, 2001.

Grains and Starchy Vegetables

Each cereal, bread, pasta, rice or starchy vegetable and its amount stated below is equal to approximately 35 grams of carbohydrate, 150 calories, and 6 grams of protein.

GRAIN OR STARCH	SERVING SIZE
Bagel	1 medium
Bread:	
rye	2 slices
whole wheat	2 slices
rice	2 slices
spelt	2 slices
Cereal, cooked:	
oatmeal	2 cups
barley	2 cups
kasha	2 cups
7-grain	2 cups
cream of rice	2 cups
Corn on the cob	1 medium
Crackers:	
graham	4
brown rice	6
Dinner roll	1 medium
Hamburger bun	1
Hot dog bun	1
Noodles or pasta	1 cup
Pancake	1, 6"
Pita bread	1, 6"
Popcorn, air-popped	4 cups
Potato: baked	1 medium
mashed	¾ cup
Rice	½ cup
Squash	1 cup packed
Sweet potato, yam	1 medium
Tortilla, corn or sprouted wheat	2

Legumes and Meat

Each of the following cooked protein sources supplies 25 grams of protein, 175 calories and 30 grams of carbohydrate on average.

PROTEIN	SERVING SIZE
Veggie burgers	2 patties
Whey protein isolate powder	1½ heaping tablespoons
Soy protein isolate powder	2 heaping tablespoons
Cooked peas and beans:	
soybeans	2 cups
lentils	2 cups
pinto beans	2 cups
black beans	2 cups
red kidney beans	2 cups
navy beans	2 cups
chick peas	2 cups
Beef, fat removed	4 oz (115 g)
Veal	4 oz (115 g)
Chicken, no skin or fat	4 oz (115 g)
Fish	5 oz (140 g)
Shellfish: clams	5 oz (140 g)
crabs	5 oz (140 g)
shrimp	5 oz (140 g)
scallops	5 oz (140 g)
Soy foods: soy burger	6 oz (170 g)
tempeh	6 oz (170 g)
extra-firm tofu	6 oz (170 g)
Tuna, albacore, solid, low-sodium, water-packed	6 oz (170 g)
Turkey, no skin	4 oz (115 g)
Eggs, free-range, organic	2
Egg substitute	½ cup
Chicken or turkey luncheon meat, 95% fat-free	6 slices

Fats and Oils

The following servings of fats provide approximately 120 calories and 10+ grams of fat.

FATS AND OILS	SELECTION SIZE
Butter (or ghee—clarified butter)	1 tablespoon
Chocolate, semi-sweet, dark Belgium	1 square, 1 oz (28 g)
Coconut	½ oz
Cream cheese, low-fat	4 tablespoons
Cream, sour, low-fat	4 tablespoons
Mayonnaise	1 tablespoon
Oils: canola	1 tablespoon
flax seed	1 tablespoon
hemp seed	1 tablespoon
extra-virgin olive oil	1 tablespoon
Olives, black or green	10
Fish oils: cod liver oil	1 tablespoon
salmon oil	1 tablespoon
sardine oil or other fish oils	2 softgels

GOOD FATTY FOODS	SERVING SIZE
Avocado	½ medium
Cheeses: soy cheese	1 oz (28 g)
low-fat, cow	3 oz (85 g)
Ice cream, low-fat	1 cup
Nuts and seeds: almonds	2 tablespoons
cashews	2 tablespoons
flax seeds	2 tablespoons
sunflower seeds	2 tablespoons
macadamias	6 medium
peanuts, Spanish	2 tablespoons
almonds	2 tablespoons
walnuts	8 halves
pumpkin seeds	½ cup
sesame seeds	2 tablespoons
almond butter	1 heaping tablespoon
peanut butter	1 heaping tablespoon

Dairy and Dairy-Substitute Products

Each food listed below provides approximately 130 calories, 10 grams of protein and 15 grams of carbohydrate.

ITEM	SERVING SIZE
Buttermilk, fat-free	1 cup
Powdered, fat-free milk	2/3 cup
Fat-free organic yogurt, plain	3/4 cup
Fat-free organic milk	1 cup
Lactaid (lactose-reduced low-fat milk)	1 cup
Low-fat milk	2/3 cup
Low-fat yogurt	2/3 cup
Cheese: cottage cheese, creamed	3/4 cup
cottage cheese, fat-free, dry curd	1 cup
grated Parmesan	1/3 cup
grated Sapsago	1/2 cup
low-fat cheese	1/3 cup
Goat milk	1 cup
Soy milk	1 cup
Rice milk	1 cup
Grain milks	1 cup
Almond milk	1 cup
Hemp milk	1 cup

Freebies

The following foods contain negligible calories but do supply many vitamins, minerals, antioxidants, phytonutrients and fiber:

Celery

Cucumbers

Endive

Escarole

Green onions

Lettuce

Parsley

Peppers—green, orange, yellow, red, chili

Radishes

Spinach

Summer squash

Zucchini

Herbs and spices

Lemon juice

Mustard

RECIPES

Trying out a new recipe is like taking yourself on a real adventure. You can always try out a recipe and then decide it's not for you—or try it again with slight modifications that please you and your loved ones. Variety is the spice of life so use lots of variety to satisfy even the pickiest of palates.

POWER PROTEIN SHAKE

    8 oz (250 mL) unsweetened rice milk, almond milk, fat-free milk
    2 level scoops (30 grams) whey or soy protein isolate powder
    2 tablespoons organic flax seeds
    5 almonds (soaked overnight)
    1 tablespoon pumpkin seeds
    1 tablespoon sunflower seeds
    2 heaping tablespoons organic, fat-free yogurt or 1 BioK+ yogurt
    1 cup fresh or frozen blueberries or other berry
    Optional: 1 to 2 tablespoons of bee pollen
               2 tablespoons of soy lecithin granules
               1 tablespoon Engivita yeast

Blend the rice or almond milk, yogurt and blueberries in a blender for ten seconds. In a coffee grinder, finely grind the flax seeds, almonds, pumpkin seeds and sunflower seeds for ten seconds. Add the finely ground nuts and seeds to the blender liquid.

Pour from blender into a hand-held tumbler with a secure lid. Add the protein powder to the tumbler and shake vigorously for six seconds.

Any optional ingredients can be added to the tumbler, except bee pollen, which should be ground in the coffee grinder.

You should take your supplements with this power protein shake. As a supplement supplying your long-chain, Omega-3 essential fatty acids, you must take 1 tablespoon of an emulsified, molecularly distilled, cod liver oil or two capsules of salmon oil or sardine oil or six to nine capsules of algae extract oil to supply your brain and nervous system with EPA and DHA.

Vegetable Sticks and Rounds

For vegetable sticks, slice carrots, celery, zucchini and summer squash. For vegetable rounds, slice radishes, cucumbers, red or green peppers, tomatoes, turnips, yams, sweet potatoes, parsnips and rutabagas. You may add parsley, watercress and cilantro to any of the vegetable slices. Try adding a few pieces of raw Nova Scotia dulse for a real tasty surprise.

The most suitable sprouts to add are broccoli sprouts and sunflower seed sprouts.

SALAD DRESSING

    1 to 1 1/2 tablespoons extra-virgin olive oil
    1 teaspoon fresh lemon juice
    1 teaspoon of salt-free herbal seasoning such as Spike or Mrs. Dash
    Chopped fresh dill, basil, parsley and watercress
    Dash of non-irradiated black pepper
    1/2 teaspoon Nova Scotia dulse
    1 teaspoon seaweed gomasio (Japanese sesame seeds)

For your vegetables, use lemon juice, salt-free herbal combinations, miso and 1/2 tablespoon of organic, cold-pressed flax seed oil.

FLAT BREAD PIZZAS FOR TWO
2 6-inch (15 cm) diameter multigrain pita breads, cut in half horizontally
2 teaspoons olive oil
1 tablespoon minced garlic
2 large tomatoes, chopped
1 cup red onion, thinly chopped
2 cups fresh spinach, washed and chopped
8 halves of walnuts
1 teaspoon dried basil
1 teaspoon dried oregano
1/2 cup crumbled low-salt feta cheese or white chicken breast diced

Preheat oven to 400°F (200°C). Bake four pita halves for four minutes. Cool. Combine oil, garlic, tomatoes, spinach, onions, walnuts and seasonings in a large bowl and mix thoroughly. Divide vegetable mixture evenly and heap onto pita halves. Sprinkle with feta cheese or diced chicken breast and bake for five minutes only.

CHUNKY MISO SOUP FOR TWO
1 red pepper, diced
1 large carrot, finely grated
4 cups water
1 1/2 teaspoons of toasted sesame seeds
1 small red onion, chopped
2 medium stalks of celery, coarsely chopped
2 medium carrots, chopped
2 medium shiitake mushrooms, stems removed and sliced
2 tablespoons of fresh ginger, peeled and coarsely chopped
1 cup of frozen or fresh green peas
1/2 cup of red kidney beans cooked (from can)
5 tablespoons red barley or yellow rice miso paste
10 oz (285 g) extra-firm tofu
4 scallions, sliced
2 cloves of fresh garlic, finely chopped
1 tablespoon of fresh lemon juice
2 tablespoons of Nova Scotia dulse

Sauté onions in 1/8 inch (3 mm) of water in a frying pan for three minutes. Add celery, carrots, shiitake mushrooms, fresh ginger, garlic, peas, kidney beans, tofu and lemon juice, and sauté for two more minutes.
Put 4 cups of water in a large pot, bring to a boil.

Add miso paste to warm water only (1 cup), and mash with a fork until smooth. Take boiling water off the heat and add sautéed vegetables. Once cooled to eating temperature, add miso broth. Stir once before serving in soup bowls. Garnish with scallion slices, sesame seeds, grated carrot and diced red pepper.

ZESTY COTTAGE CHEESE SALAD FOR TWO

Large bowl of mesclun greens (combination of baby lettuce)
2 yellow tomatoes, sliced
2 orange tomatoes, sliced
1/2 avocado, chopped
1 orange pepper, chopped
8 stems parsley, chopped
8 stems watercress, chopped
8 stems fresh dill, chopped
1 tablespoon ginger, peeled and chopped
2 cloves garlic, peeled and chopped
1 large carrot, diced
2 stems of celery, chopped
6-inch-long cucumber piece, sliced into rounds
4 red radishes, thinly sliced
3-inch (7.5 cm) piece daikon (Chinese radish), peeled and finely grated
1 small red beet, washed, peeled and finely grated
2 tablespoons pan-roasted sunflower seeds
1 cup dry curd, fat-free cottage cheese

Mix all ingredients in a large glass, clear bowl with the olive oil dressing, except the chopped orange pepper, diced carrot and grated red beet, which are added on top of the mixed salad for visual appeal. Add 1 cup of dry curd, fat-free cottage cheese to the top and middle of each salad. Sprinkle with pan-roasted sunflower seeds. To pan-roast the sunflower seeds, simply put them in a dry frying pan with no oil, at medium heat for five minutes, while you constantly stir. They will lightly brown as they roast.

CURRIED TEMPEH, TOFU AND VEGETABLES FOR TWO

1 1/2 teaspoons canola oil
2 tablespoons curry powder
2 cups water
1/2 cup of tomato purée
1/2 teaspoon saffron
2 cloves garlic, chopped
1 tablespoon fresh grated ginger
1 medium red onion, chopped

10 yellow beans

10 green beans

11/2 cups cauliflower, cut into small pieces

1 cup broccoli, cut into small pieces

3 oz (85 g) of extra-firm herbal tofu

3 oz (85 g) of tempeh

2 tablespoons of Nova Scotia dulse, crumbled

Heat oil on low in large frying pan and whisk in curry. Roast curry for ten to 12 seconds and remove from heat. In a small saucepan add water, tomato purée, saffron, garlic, dulse, ginger and bring to a boil. Add onions, beans, broccoli, cauliflower, tofu and tempeh and simmer for 15 minutes to desired tenderness. Add roasted curry and stir. Add water to make more soupy if necessary.

NEW MEXICO BLACK BEAN ROLLUPS FOR TWO

1 16-oz (455 g) can of black beans, drained and rinsed

6 tablespoons of salsa

1 4-oz (115 g) can of peeled, chopped green chilies

6 tablespoons of fat-free sour cream or mashed soft silken tofu

6 tablespoons fresh cilantro, chopped

2 scallions, finely chopped

1 medium green pepper, finely chopped

1 medium carrot, finely grated

1 small beet, finely grated

6 sprouted, whole wheat tortillas, 10-inch (25 cm)

In a medium bowl combine beans, chilies, salsa, cilantro and sour cream (or mashed soft silken tofu). Evenly divide the mixture and spread over each tortilla within one inch (2.5 cm) of edges. Sprinkle on top of each one the green peppers, carrots, beets and scallions. Tuck in one end and tightly roll each tortilla.

TARRAGON-LEMON CHICKEN BREAST FOR TWO

2 tablespoons canola oil

1 lemon, thinly sliced

1/4 cup fresh tarragon, chopped

2 tablespoons of peeled and finely grated ginger

8 oz (230 g) boneless skinless chicken, all visible fat removed

3 garlic cloves, minced

1/3 cup of water

Mix all ingredients except for the tarragon and chicken. Rub this mixture onto the chicken and let it marinate, covered well, for ten minutes while the oven heats to 400°F (200°C). Bake the chicken in a pan with 1/4 inch (6 mm) of water for 20 minutes. Add tarragon on top of chicken and cook for another ten minutes.

LENTILS WITH KALE

    1 red pepper, chopped
    1 large onion, chopped
    2 teaspoons chili powder
    1 teaspoon Celtic sea salt mixed with 1/2 teaspoon salt-free Spike
    1 teaspoon fresh, dried cumin
    3 cloves of garlic, chopped
    1 can of peeled, plum tomatoes
    4 cups water
    1 cup dried lentils, sorted and rinsed
    1 can chopped green chilies (4 oz /115 g)
    2 small carrots, thinly sliced
    2 stalks of celery, thinly sliced
    1 small yam or sweet potato, diced small
    2 small zucchini, diced
    10 large leaves of kale, washed and hand-torn
    10 stalks of parsley, chopped
    2 cups sunflower or broccoli sprouts, or a combination
    4 tablespoons of dry, pan-roasted sunflower seeds

In a medium saucepan, heat onion, sea salt mixture, cumin, garlic, chili powder and plum tomatoes, to boiling; reduce heat. Cover and simmer for three minutes. Stir in water, lentils and chilies. Heat to boiling, reduce heat, cover and simmer for 40 minutes. Stir in carrots, zucchini, yam, celery and kale and simmer for five minutes maximum or until lentils are tender but not mushy. Put into attractive soup bowls and top with red peppers, parsley, roasted sunflower seeds and either sunflower or broccoli sprouts or both.

MEDLEY OF STEAMED VEGETABLES WITH MISO-TAHINI SAUCE FOR TWO

    2 small Chinese eggplants
    2 cups of finely chopped red cabbage
    1 small sweet potato, chopped
    1 6-inch square of butternut squash, chopped
    12 stems of asparagus
    6 okra
    2 small turnips, chopped
    1 small leek, diced
    2 large stems of Swiss chard, hand broken
    10 stems of cilantro, diced
    10 stems of watercress, diced
    1/2 red pepper, diced
    1/2 green pepper, diced

Wash and cut all vegetables into irregular bite-sized pieces. Bring 1/2 inch of water in a pot to a boil. In a steaming tray above the water, add the red cabbage, sweet potato, okra, turnips and the squash. Turn heat to medium and steam only five minutes. Add eggplant, asparagus, leeks, Swiss chard and steam for only another five minutes until "crunchy tender." Put into serving bowls and top with cilantro, watercress, red and green diced peppers.

In a 1-quart saucepan mix 2 tablespoons of tahini into 6 tablespoons of boiling water. Remove from heat, add 2 tablespoons of any miso paste. Mash until smooth and drizzle over vegetables.

Yummy Peaches-n-Cream Power Yogurt Sundae

    3 cups plain fat-free yogurt
    2 scoops of whey protein isolate powder
    1 tablespoon raw, unpasteurized honey OR organic unsulphured molasses
    4 tablespoons organic flax seeds
    2 tablespoons sunflower seeds
    2 tablespoons pumpkin seeds
    10 whole almonds
    8 walnut halves
    2 tablespoons of pine nuts
    4 heaping tablespoons of peeled and chopped ginger
    4 fresh peaches skinned or 1 bag of frozen peaches, quartered
    2 tablespoons cornstarch

Put fresh or frozen peaches in a 3-quart pot with 1 cup of water and add the ginger. In a small bowl mix 2 tablespoons of cornstarch in 1/4 cup of water. Bring peaches and ginger to a boil and immediately reduce heat to low. Slowly add the cornstarch liquid while stirring the peaches. Stir the cornstarch, peaches and ginger for three more minutes, adding 1 tablespoon of honey (or molasses); then promptly remove from heat and let cool.

Put the flax seeds, sunflower seeds and pumpkin seeds in a coffee grinder and grind to a powder for five seconds.

Mix the yogurt and whey protein isolate powder together. Put the ground seed powder on top. Add the peach-ginger sauce on top and finally decorate with almonds, walnut halves and pine nuts.

Eggplant-Walnut Baked Tofu

    1/4 cup water
    1 pound (455 g) eggplant, unpeeled and diced
    2 tablespoons extra-virgin olive oil
    1 medium onion, chopped
    2 garlic cloves, minced
    1 stalk celery, finely chopped

1 cup yellow squash, thinly sliced
1 cup red pepper, seeded and chopped
8 black olives, pitted and cut in half
1 teaspoon Italian herb seasoning, pepper to taste
8 oz (230 g) Italian-style peeled tomatoes, drained and chopped
2 tablespoons capers, drained
8 oz (230 g) of extra-firm herbal tofu cut into 4 slices
16 walnut halves
2 tablespoons of Nova Scotia dulse

Preheat oven to 375°F (190°C). On stovetop pour water into a stainless-steel skillet. Combine eggplant, onion, garlic, celery, yellow squash and Italian tomatoes. Cook five minutes, stirring often, until onions are translucent.

Remove from heat. Combine Italian seasoning, capers, dulse and olive oil, and pour into skillet ingredients. Put tofu slices in an oven-proof casserole, dust with fresh black pepper and spread the eggplant caponata mixture evenly over the tofu slices. Bake ten minutes uncovered.

Sprinkle chopped red pepper, black olives and walnuts on top of the eggplant caponata sauce and serve.

GREEN BEANS, ALMONDS AND RED PEPPERS

1 pound fresh young green beans, washed and stem ends removed
1 cup red pepper, seeded and chopped
1 tablespoon organic flax seed oil
2 teaspoons apple cider or balsamic vinegar
1/2 teaspoon dried dill
Nova Scotia dulse and pepper to taste
10 whole almonds

Steam the green beans in a steamer basket for five minutes or until "crunchy-tender." Add water if necessary to prevent pan from boiling dry. Transfer beans to a serving bowl; pour flax seed oil, apple cider or balsamic vinegar, dried dill, dulse and pepper on beans and toss. Garnish with whole almonds and red peppers.

HERBAL BAKED LEMON-GINGER SALMON

1 pound salmon fillet, 1 inch (2.5 cm) thick
2 teaspoons paprika
2 tablespoons of fresh dill
2 tablespoons of fresh tarragon
4 tablespoons minced fresh ginger
4 tablespoons fresh parsley, chopped
2 large lemons, 1 juiced, 1 cut into thin slices
1 cup carrots, diced large

    1 1/2 cups cauliflower flowerets

    1 1/2 cups broccoli flowerets

    1 tablespoon extra-virgin olive oil

    Black pepper and Celtic sea salt to taste

Preheat broiler at 350°F (175°C). Steam cauliflower and broccoli flowerets for four minutes; add carrots and steam for one more minute. Remove from heat and keep warm. Mix fresh lemon juice, dill, tarragon, ginger and olive oil together with pepper and Celtic sea salt to taste. Brush both sides of salmon with herbal mixture. Broil until opaque in center (approximately five minutes per side), basting occasionally with remaining herbal mixture.

During last minute, spread lemon slices over the salmon. Transfer salmon to a long platter and sprinkle paprika and parsley on top of the salmon. Decorate edges of salmon with cauliflower and broccoli flowerets and carrots.

GRATED ROOT SALAD FOR TWO

    1 cup sunflower sprouts

    1 tablespoon chopped fresh mint

    1 teaspoon chopped fresh basil

    1/2 teaspoon dried oregano

    1/2 lemon, juiced

    2 tablespoons of Eden seaweed gomasio

    1 cup chopped tomatoes

    1/2 cup sliced celery

    1/2 cup sliced radishes

    1 cup grated squash

    1 small sweet potato, grated

    2 medium-sized parsnips, grated

    1 medium-sized rutabaga or turnip, grated

    1 medium-sized beet, grated

    6 stems of cilantro, finely chopped

    4 tablespoons of dry, pan-roasted sunflower seeds

Mix mint, basil, oregano, lemon juice, olive oil and seaweed gomasio dressing in a small bowl. Mix all chopped, sliced and grated vegetables in a bowl except cilantro, sunflower sprouts and carrots. Mix dressing into raw vegetables. Serve in high mounds, sprinkled with grated carrots, sunflower sprouts, chopped cilantro and sunflower seeds.

TOFU VEGETABLE KEBOBS ON SPICY GARLIC SPINACH

    6 wooden skewers, soaked in water overnight

    8 oz (230 g) extra-firm tofu, patted dry, cut into 1-inch (2.5 cm) cubes

    1 large red pepper, seeded and cut into large squares

    1 large green pepper, seeded and cut into large squares

2 red onions, cut into large pieces
2 medium zucchini, cut into 1-inch (2.5 cm) pieces
2 medium summer squash, cut into 1-inch (2.5 cm) pieces
1 tablespoon extra-virgin olive oil
4 tablespoons dried thyme
2 tablespoons garlic powder
1 teaspoon freshly ground black pepper
4 tablespoons dried oregano
1 teaspoon dried rosemary, crumbled
2 portobello mushrooms cut into 1-inch (2.5 cm) slices
2 cups steamed spinach
1/2 teaspoon of cayenne pepper
1 cup watercress, stemmed and chopped
2 tablespoons of kombu, crumbled

Put tofu and vegetables on wooden skewers, being gentle with tofu so it doesn't break. Lay vegetable kebobs at bottom of shallow pan or bowl. In a small bowl mix olive oil, kombu, thyme, garlic, black pepper, oregano, rosemary and cayenne pepper. Pour mixture over kebobs and let marinate, refrigerated, for two hours. Preheat broiler or grill to 300°F (150°C). Place kebobs in shallow pan and turn frequently. Watch carefully so vegetables don't burn. Cook until vegetables are tender. Serve warm on steamed spinach. Top with chopped watercress.

MARINARA SAUCE ON KAMUT LINGUINI WITH TUNA OR SOY BEANS

2/3 cup canned water chestnuts, drained
2 teaspoons fresh lemon juice
16 vine-ripened cherry tomatoes, cut in half
3 large garlic cloves, minced
1 small jar capers, drained
1/4 cup extra-virgin olive oil
2 tablespoons fresh basil, chopped
1 leek, thinly sliced
4 tablespoons fresh parsley, chopped
1 teaspoon fresh oregano or 1/2 teaspoon dried
1/2 teaspoon fresh thyme or 1/4 teaspoon dried
3 tablespoons sapsago cheese or soy cheese, grated
12 oz kamut linguine pasta (preferably fresh)
Nova Scotia dulse flakes and pepper to taste
12 black Italian spicy olives, pitted and cut in half
1 small fennel bulb, sliced very thin
1 can (7.5 oz / 213 mL) of water-packed, low-sodium, solid, albacore tuna
or

1 can of low-sodium soybeans, drained and rinsed   or

1 cup of edamame soy beans

In a large bowl, combine all the ingredients except linguini, cheese, parsley, tuna or soy beans and olives. Mix well. Cook kamut linguini as directed on package, al dente (don't overcook). While kamut linguini pasta is cooking, pour mixed ingredients into a large skillet and heat over medium heat for two or three minutes. Drain pasta and place in a large pasta bowl or dish. Pour hot vegetable mixture on top and toss. Sprinkle with parsley, olives, sapsago cheese or soy cheese, and tuna or soybeans.

OPEN-FACE SAVORY WEST COAST VEGGIE BURGER

4 tempeh or veggie burger patties

2 large red tomatoes, thickly sliced

1 medium sweet onion, thickly sliced

4 red lettuce leaves, washed and patted dry

2 large carrots, grated

1 medium red beet, grated

Mustard to taste

4 teaspoons extra-virgin olive oil

2 tablespoons of pickled ginger slices (available in Asian markets)

4 fistfuls of fresh sunflower sprouts

4 scallions, chopped

2 tablespoons fresh cilantro, chopped

4 thick slices of organic sourdough bread made with spelt, rice or rye, but not wheat

Put 1/8 inch (3 mm) of water in a skillet and cook burgers for three minutes on each side. Remove from skillet. Spread olive oil and mustard on bread slices. Next add lettuce, burger, onion slices, tomato slices, ginger, grated carrots and beets, cilantro, scallions and top with sunflower sprouts.

ROAST TURKEY WITH HERB RUB, WILD RICE, ROASTED VEGETABLES

Wild Rice:

1 cup wild rice

1 can water chestnuts, drained and sliced

1/2 cup minced onion

1/2 cup sliced almonds

3 cups water or vegetable broth

Rinse wild rice well under running water using a strainer. Combine all ingredients in 3-quart saucepan, bring to a boil, reduce heat and let simmer for 60 minutes.

Roasted Vegetables:
2 tablespoons extra-virgin olive oil
1 medium yam, cubed
1 medium sweet potato, cubed
1 large parsnip, cubed
1 large yellow pepper, cut into 1-inch (2.5 cm) squares
1 large orange pepper, cut into 1-inch (2.5 cm) squares
1 small turnip, cubed
2 small carrots, sliced large

Put all vegetables in a shallow pan with 1/4 inch of water. Bake for 15 minutes covered. Remove cover and bake for five minutes. Rub olive oil on vegetables and broil for three minutes.

Ingredients for Roast Turkey:
3 tablespoons fresh rosemary, chopped
3 tablespoons fresh thyme, chopped
3 tablespoons fresh tarragon, chopped
1 tablespoon fresh ground black pepper
1 1/2 teaspoons Celtic sea salt
18-pound (8 kg), free-range, organic turkey
2 tablespoons canola oil
2 cups canned, low-salt chicken broth
4 parsley, fresh herb sprigs
4 watercress, fresh herb sprigs
4 cilantro, fresh herb sprigs
6 cloves of garlic, quartered

Mix herbs (but not fresh herb sprigs), pepper, garlic and salt in a small bowl. Place turkey on a rack and set in a large roasting pan. Add canola oil to herb mix and rub all over turkey. Preheat oven to 425°F (220°C). Pour 2 cups of broth into pan. Place turkey in lowest third of oven. Roast turkey 45 minutes, then remove turkey from oven and cover with pan top. Reduce oven temperature to 350°F (175°C). Return turkey to oven and baste with pan juices every hour until done. Total cooking time will be approximately four hours for non-stuffed turkey.

Transfer turkey to platter. Tent with foil and let stand for 30 minutes. Carve and serve with fresh herbal sprigs on top. Serves 16.

NEW MEXICO CHILI
2 large carrots, grated
2 tablespoons whey protein isolate powder
1 1/2 teaspoons extra-virgin olive oil
1/2 medium red onion, chopped
1/2 medium green pepper, seeded and chopped

1/2 medium red pepper, seeded and chopped

1 teaspoon New Mexico (preferably from Hatch) chili powder

1/2 teaspoon ground cumin

1/4 teaspoon Celtic sea salt

2 cloves garlic, chopped

6 oz of tempeh, crumbled

1/2 cup water

1 1/4 cups canned, crushed tomatoes

1 cup fresh diced tomatoes

1/2 cup canned red kidney beans, drained and rinsed

1/2 cup canned pinto beans, drained and rinsed

2 oz (55 g) of soy cheese

4 tablespoons roasted hemp seeds

2 tablespoons roasted pine nuts

2 cups cilantro, washed and chopped

1 cup broccoli pieces, chopped small

In a large non-stick sauté pan with cover, sauté the broccoli, onions, peppers and garlic in water for five minutes. Add chili powder, cumin, salt, crushed tomatoes, fresh tomatoes, tempeh, red kidney beans and pinto beans. Cook another two minutes. Add olive oil, cover and simmer for two minutes to blend flavours. Remove from heat; add 2 tablespoons whey protein isolate powder. Serve in a bowl and sprinkle with cilantro, hemp seeds, pine nuts, grated carrots and soy cheese.

Variation:

You can use low-fat Monterey cheese instead of soy cheese. Organic, sprouted whole-wheat 10-inch (25 cm) tortillas can be eaten with this chili.

My Favorite Vegetable Juice Recipe

2 medium-sized carrots (no more than 2 because of their high sugar content)

1/2 –1 medium red beet

Large piece of fresh ginger chopped (equivalent to 1 heaping tablespoon)

1 stalk of celery with leaves

6 stems of watercress

6 stems of parsley

1/2 yellow or orange pepper

1 red tomato

1 level tablespoon of a high-quality "green drink" powder

Optional:

1/2–1 tablespoon of lemon juice

Dash of just one of cayenne pepper, curry or turmeric

1 teaspoon of salt-free Spike or any salt-free, non-irradiated herbal seasoning

THE SEVEN GATES OF STABILITY

The "Seven Gates of Stability" is a rather ancient system of life management I was made aware of, quite by accident, while in South Korea in the 1980s. It is a balanced, steady, conscious effort to control the most fundamental aspects of your body chemistry.

Follow these easy steps and you will increase your anabolic capacity and maintain your anabolic drive so your body can quickly self-diagnose and self-heal on a daily basis.

These seven steps or "gates" allow you to live, sleep and eat in harmony with your longstanding genetic predisposition to food and the circadian rhythms of nature: your bones will become stronger; your energy will increase and be steady; your mental acuity will be heightened; wrinkles may well disappear; body fat will dissolve layer after layer; your rejuvenated heart will beat strongly and regularly; every cell in your body will be protected from chemical intruders, inhaled toxins and carcinogens; you will look revitalized and feel better than ever before; you will be grounded and balanced; you will maintain your anabolic drive as well as your anabolic capacity; and once and for all you can successfully balance your hormone production so you feel strong, vital and clear—physically, emotionally, mentally and spiritually.

THE SEVEN GATES OF STABILITY

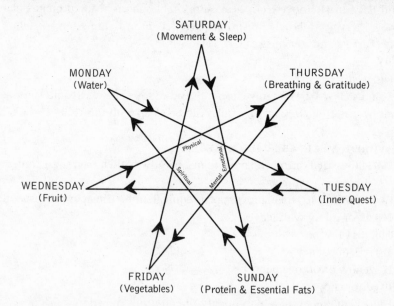

SATURDAY
(Movement & Sleep)

MONDAY
(Water)

THURSDAY
(Breathing & Gratitude)

Physical   Emotional
Spiritual   Mental

WEDNESDAY
(Fruit)

TUESDAY
(Inner Quest)

FRIDAY
(Vegetables)

SUNDAY
(Protein & Essential Fats)

The Seven Gates of Stability allow you to focus on **just one** aspect of good mental and physical health, one conscious day at a time. It is as easy as focusing on the one main theme for that day and controlling your fundamental body chemistry for clean blood and a strong immune system.

Soon, one day's theme will be effortlessly incorporated into the other days of the week. For instance, although Monday's main theme may be water, after a while it will extend to all days.

We are all creatures of habit and we must replace destructive habits with new lifestyle habits that I call a "progressive dietary strategy."

Your Dietary Strategy: Bioenergetic Fuel

On the Seven Gates of Stability diagram, each day of the week is independent, but if you carefully follow each line, each day is really interdependent. Your health is won or lost at the cellular level, on a daily basis, depending on the dietary strategy of all seven days. The constructive (anabolic) or destructive (catabolic) effort of each day is cumulative. We call this the regenerative anabolic capacity if your food choices are health-supportive or a declining catabolic capacity if your food choices are health-destructive. Lin, in the Introduction to this book, was consuming an anabolic supportive dietary strategy, while Lynn was consuming a steadily declining catabolic dietary strategy.

A health-supporting dietary strategy is not a "hit or miss" approach but an enlightened awareness of how you are fueling your 100 trillion molecular motors, your cells. Fuel them wisely with bioenergetic foods. Your body and mind will respond with peak performance in every facet of your life. It is your call! You can immediately modulate your hormonal imbalances, return to homeostasis and stop being fat, hungry, impotent, hypertensive and cancerous with a weak heart.

Monday: Pay strict attention to how much water you drink on this particular day. Your goal is to drink six to eight 8-oz glasses of water a day for sedentary lifestyles; eight to ten 8-oz glasses of water for an active lifestyle or if your work causes you to perspire; ten to twelve 8-oz glasses of water for those on a rigorous exercise or training routine. You can include 1 to 2 cups of herbal tea daily to replace one of those glasses of water.

Increase your water intake gradually to allow your kidneys, which are like a sponge, to properly adjust to the additional water.

Drink all your water through a straw. Weight Watchers or sports shops sell convenient containers that have a firm plastic straw that can be removed daily for washing. These containers also have the added benefit of indicating how much water they hold, 8 oz (1 cup), 16 oz, 24 oz or 32 oz. You can successfully monitor your water intake. Do not wait to drink your daily water quota all at one time. Hydrate by drinking small amounts continually.

The most critical time to drink water is as soon as you wake up in the morning. Your body, organs, tissues and cells were detoxifying and "cleaning house" while you were sleeping. Room-temperature water will help you flush out all the cellular waste and debris your body cleansed, so your cells will be capable of another day of peak performance.

Results: You will have a wonderful skin tone, less desire to overeat, mental clarity, enhanced bowel movements, more abundant energy.

Tip: Add 1 teaspoon of fresh lemon or lime juice to every 32 oz (four glasses) of water you drink.

Tuesday: This is a day dedicated to your inner quest. It is a day you consciously become aware of "being and becoming." You acknowledge who you are (being) and make a concerted effort to develop (becoming) the type of thinking, talking, acting, dreaming personality that will make you a better human being.

Begin by spending one-half hour upon rising and one-half hour before retiring for the night, in meditation, prayer, pondering or self-analysis. Be gentle and kind to yourself.

Forgive all those who have transgressed against you and ask for forgiveness of all those you have transgressed against, in one way or another.

Eventually dedicate a lovely spot in your dwelling for the exclusive use of meditation, prayer, pondering or self-analysis. When you enter this area, be sure to turn off all radios, telephones, televisions, CD units, computers, pagers and cell phones, and be daring enough to put a "Please do not disturb" sign on your door.

Go to a quality bookstore and check out the various books on meditation, prayer and self-analysis.

Consider writing a poem or short story or keeping a simple journal of your inspired thoughts.

Consider, if you can, using part or all of this day for a quiet spiritual day of retreat in nature. You may also go to an organized meditation group, church service, self-help group or choir. Watch the moon and stars—be a stargazer at night!

Results: You will become more focused, grounded, loving, compassionate and kind. You will touch a deep part of yourself that is far beyond the physical limitations of the mind and body.

Tip: Consider keeping a daily journal or diary of just these times; carry a small book of wise sayings, short inspiring life stories, poetry or prayers that you refer to several times a day.

Wednesday: Go out of your way to eat two pieces or servings of whole, ripe, in-season, organic colorful berries, a slice of melon or fresh fruit. Blueberries or any strongly colored berries such as blackberries or raspberries are at the top of the scale for containing enormous amounts of phytonutrients and antioxidants.

Organic citrus such as oranges, tangerines and pink grapefruit are jam-packed with many unique phytonutrients that keep your anabolic drive and health at optimum. Try to eat a little of the white pulp and skin where some of the unique and powerful phytonutrients are found.

Your third choice could be an apple, a pear, some black cherries, a slice of watermelon, some pineapple, a peach, a plum or a few prunes.

Results: The colorful flavonoids and carotenoids will actually add some color to your complexion; they also act as an internal "suntan lotion," protecting and quenching the reactive free radical singlet-oxygen, when you get a little necessary early-morning or late-afternoon sun on your skin. They are potent "network" antioxidants that protect you from degenerative and oxidative diseases such as arthritis or cancer.

Tip: Purchase fruits a few days before you plan to use them so you always have a steady supply of fresh, ripe fruit handy.

Thursday: This is the day to both become more conscious of how deeply we are breathing or not breathing, and to give gratitude.

Most of us breathe shallowly and never get all the stale carbon dioxide out of our lungs or a full capacity of empowering oxygen into our lungs. Most of us are simply oxygen deprived! Sit outside or at a semi-open window, carefully looking at and admiring nature. Take ten minutes twice a day to breathe in deeply and breathe out deeply with a rhythmic concentration, neither favoring the inhalation or exhalation, but feeling the chest cavity expand and contract.

Results: You will immediately experience clearer thinking, more vibrant energy, better and deeper sleep patterns. Stopping to deep-breathe also naturally calms us down quickly, without the use of drugs. It is a superior lifestyle component. I wish we could all experience this kind of medicine daily. Just stopping to slow down is significant.

Tip: Give thanks before eating or sharing food. Food and nourishment combines art, science and spirituality; it merges technology and philosophy. Have great gratitude for the blessing of food and consume your food with a spirit of gratitude, not mindlessness.

Friday: We want to consume a wide variety of colors in our salad and vegetable choices. Vary your vegetable and salad choices by color, texture, shape, growing style and season:

- *By color*: Choose vegetables of every color: green, red, yellow, orange, white, purple, brown.
- By *flavor*: Try bland in lettuce, pungent in garlic, sweet in beets, or sharp in cilantro.
- *By texture*: Incorporate tender sunflower sprouts, hearty squashes, irregular roots like sweet potatoes, and various leaves like arugula.
- *By growing style*: Consider vegetables that are upward growing (broccoli, dandelions, cauliflower); downward growing (carrots, yams, parsnips,

turnips, red or purple potatoes); and hanging ones (yellow summer squash, zucchini, eggplant, pole beans).

- *By season*:
  - *Fall:* Nova Scotia dulse, fall squashes, grapes, apples, pears, yams, parsnips, potatoes, kale, Swiss chard, spinach, carrots, beets, thyme, basil, parsley, cilantro, onions, garlic.
  - *Winter:* Spirulina, chlorella, celery, carrots, beets, turnips, fresh sunflower or broccoli sprouts, apples, pears, chard, kale, mint, spearmint, garlic, horseradish, Nova Scotia dulse.
  - *Spring:* Fresh pears, asparagus, dill, strawberries, blueberries, blackberries, mints, parsley, chives, avocados, spirulina, chlorella.
  - *Summer:* Peaches, plums, grapes, tomatoes, lettuces, melons, green onions, shallots, cucumbers, radishes, carrots.

Results: You will consume lots of soluble and insoluble fiber that will thoroughly clean out the gastrointestinal tract. You will also benefit from huge varieties of phytonutrients, antioxidants, vitamins, minerals, trace minerals and cell salts.

You may never have eaten sea vegetables (sea weeds) but I highly recommend them both as a gourmet food and as a terrific source of the rare, micronutrient organic sodium.

Tip: Use a "green drink" daily as nutritional insurance, mixed in water, unsweetened fruit juice or fresh vegetable juice to ensure you have all your basic plant-based nutrients and to make your body more alkaline by reducing corrosive acids that build up in your cells.

Saturday: This is the day to pay attention to your exercise routine and your sleep patterns. Your exercise program should include:

- Aerobic exercise: walking, swimming, bicycling, Feldenkrais, Tai Chi, hatha yoga, running, spinning, rowing, stair master, etc.
- Anaerobic exercise: weight-resistance training at a gym with a qualified instructor or in your own home.

Make a concerted effort to do one hour of a combination of aerobic and anaerobic exercise at least four to five days a week. Start with a ten minute warm-up, then do 30 minutes of anaerobic exercise, and finish with 20 minutes of aerobic exercise.

Results: You will gain more abundant energy, your blood will flow more freely, your internal organs will be massaged and exercised indirectly, your heart will become stronger, your blood purer, and you will eliminate toxins and toxic debris from your cells more readily.

Tip: Take some class action. Join a YMCA, YWCA, community center or fitness club, and join organized classes in some form of aerobic and anaerobic exercise to increase strength, flexibility, sensitivity and awareness.

Saturday is also a critical time to consider your sleep patterns. You may be sleep-deprived in a society that prides itself on being "up and ready" 24 hours a day, seven days a week, 365 days a year. We may be able to live to 80 with surgery and antibiotics, but think how long we could live if we had sufficient sleep. If you don't get enough sleep, you are headed for extinction because you are out of circadian rhythm and evolution, plain and simple.

Try to get 8.25 to 8.5 hours of sleep each night. Sleep is the only way to reduce cortisol, our means of dealing with episodic stress, which, when continually elevated, is highly corrosive to our lean muscle mass and brain cells.

Tip: Sleep ultimately controls homeostasis, the state where all your hormones are fully balanced, engaged and in harmony. Research clearly demonstrates that you must take care to prevent light leaks in your sleeping area during the dark phase of a day—the night cycle. Use heavy shades on windows, have no electronic equipment with blinking lights. Sleep in an absolutely dark room.

Sunday: This is the day to focus on essential fats and the protein that is responsible for cellular building and repair. Your body needs protein on a daily basis. One-fifth of your total body weight is protein. Protein is second only to water as the most plentiful substance in the body. Skin, hair, nails, eyes, muscles, hormones, enzymes and nerve-transmission chemicals are mostly protein. Eat some protein at each of your three daily meals (women should consume about 27 grams of protein and men about 35 grams of protein on average per meal) each day. (See Chapter 12, "Protein: The Building Blocks of Life.")

Vegetarian protein sources can be chosen from a variety of legumes, beans, peas, seeds, nuts, sea vegetables, soy protein powders, yogurt, free-range organic eggs, fresh sprouts and nutritional yeast.

If you get your protein from animal sources, cook your meat with all visible fat and skin removed. Eat primarily free-range, organic eggs; ocean fish (such as salmon); chicken; turkey and lamb. Limit or eliminate your red meat intake and do consider one meal a day of plant-based protein, especially a power protein shake at breakfast.

Results: Your energy will be stabilized and consistent. Protein helps you to moderate your appetite and enhance your performance and anabolic drive. Your hormones will be better balanced, allowing you to feel emotionally centered.

Tip: For one of your meals try a lactose-reduced, undenatured, whey protein isolate, or non-GMO, water-extracted soy protein isolate powder daily in a protein shake. It is best to equally combine the two.

We all have a love of fat that we inherited from our hunter-gatherer ancestors. Today, fat is not the problem per se, but rather the kinds of fat that have become dominant in our diets. We do need some fat on a daily basis and those fats must supply, or be able to be converted to, eicosapentaenoic acid (EPA) and docosa-hexaenoic acid (DHA), both longer-chain essential fatty acids (EFAs) in the Omega-3 series. The best sources are fatty fish such as mackerel, sardines, cod, krill, anchovies, albacore tuna, salmon and herring, or other dark fresh fish, fish oils, egg yolks and sea algae. (See Chapter 13, "Fats: Not All Bad.")

Many people use flax seeds, flax seed oil, hemp seeds, hemp seed oil, pumpkin seeds, pumpkin seed oil, or walnuts to derive their Omega-3 EFAs. The trouble is it requires nine very intricate, biochemical transactions to convert these vegetable oils to EPA and DHA. Even if you are in extraordinary health, you would only convert about 10 percent of these oils to the necessary EPA and DHA. Be prudent and use fish oil capsules, cod liver oil or algae-derived EPA and DHA daily for stable moods and superior mental acuity. If you use flax or hemp seeds or their oils daily for your Omega-3 EFAs, use 1 to 2 tablespoons of ground seeds or 1 tablespoon of their oils.

If you consume fish, you may eat salmon, tuna or sardines, broiled, three times a week to ensure you have sufficient EPA and DHA. It is the fat you want, so as you broil these fish, baste them several times with their own juices.

Also there needs to be a balance of consumption of one part Omega-3 to two parts Omega-6 EFAs. Omega-6 EFAs are in a disproportionately high intake in Western countries and our average consumption is 20 parts Omega-6 EFAs to one part Omega-3 EFAs. It is certain that the Western diet is seriously deficient in Omega-3 EFAs. Dark leafy greens also supply small amounts of Omega-3 EFAs.

Omega-6 EFAs are also necessary in your diet and you must have them regularly to live and be healthy. Omega-6 EFAs come from both animal and vegetable oils, and from the bakery items that use these oils as an ingredient. Omega-6 EFA oils are from meat, poultry, sunflower, soybean, sesame, safflower oil, peanut, grape-seed, cottonseed, corn, borage, black currant and evening primrose.

Extra-virgin, cold-pressed olive oil is an Omega-9 EFA and is best consumed on salads, averaging about 1 to 2 tablespoons a day. Olive oil is hormonally neutral.

It is interesting to note that even if you have enough of the right starting material from flax or hemp seeds, from walnuts, from ocean algae such as spirulina or chlorella, or from grasses such as alfalfa grass or wheatgrass, your body cannot make EPA if there are too many Omega-6 fatty acids in the diet.

Results: If you reduce your intake of saturated fat from red meat, full-fat dairy and Omega-6 EFAs from vegetable oils, except for borage oil—and increase your Omega-3 EFAs—you will notice more mental acuity and more stable, uplifting moods. Inflammation such as in arthritis is reduced dramatically when you do this.

Too many Omega-6 EFAs in a ratio of 20 to one to Omega-3 EFAs, standard in North America, make defective hormones. Don't pay that price.

Tip: Use two capsules daily of sardine, anchovy, mackerel, salmon or cod liver oil, molecularly distilled, rich in Omega-3 EFAs or 1 tablespoon of cod liver oil. Also use 1/2 teaspoon of Omega-6, GLA rich borage oil daily.

Vegetarians and vegans are encouraged to use 2 tablespoons of organic flax seeds or hemp seeds ground in a coffee grinder, or 1 tablespoon of their oils daily; dark leafy vegetables (especially purslane, a common weed in most vegetable gardens); grasses such as alfalfa, barley and wheatgrass; ocean algae such as spirulina, chlorella and Nova Scotia dulse; and supplement with algae oil capsules. This will give you at least 120 grams of DHA, the key to brain functions, and 180 grams of EPA, the key to optimal immunological and cardiovascular function.

WE ARE BUILT FOR WELLNESS—NOT ILLNESS

In the Divine Blueprint, you have been given everyday foods to keep the activities of your cellular, sub-cellular, molecular and even atomic levels running with accuracy and precision. Where are they? My goodness, right in your garden, your whole food store, farmers' market or produce section of your favorite grocery store as fruits, vegetables, herbs, and sea vegetables. You can also find them in nutritional food stores in bins of grains, legumes, nuts, seeds, beans and peas. Right now, as you read these very words, they are probably right in your refrigerator, vegetable garden or cupboard.

Look for them vigilantly and use them wisely because, if you haven't noticed, you're running out of time!

18

CHOCOLATE AND COFFEE REVISITED: NOT SO BAD AFTER ALL

CHOCOLATE REVISITED

Our Favorite Flavor

Our obsession with chocolate could be partially cultural. Men may receive a pen set as a gift and women receive chocolates. Chocolate is associated with pleasure and indulgence. February 14th, Valentine's Day, has become a tribute to chocolate for many people.

Chocolate has the perfect mix of fat and sugar to turn on almost every appetite-triggering neurotransmitter. The sugar in chocolate sparks serotonin release and soothes NPY levels and ignites endorphins, and this combination gives you a deep sense of well-being. Chocolate also contains caffeine and theobromine, compounds that give you a mental lift. Chocolate also contains another unique compound called phenylethylamine (PEA). It increases the heart rate and blood pressure and stimulates the nervous system. PEA and endorphins combine to give a genuine pleasure response.

Chocolate has a melt-in-your-mouth texture, a remarkable aroma and comes with various names such as "wickedly rich." Cocoa contains over 400 distinct flavor compounds. This is 200 percent more than any other food. Perhaps there are many unexplored compounds in chocolate that trigger euphoria and cravings.

The ancient Olmec, Mayan and Aztec Indians, who gave cocoa its name, worshipped it as "food for the gods," the literal meaning of its Latin name, *Theobroma cacao*. Chocolate was introduced to Europe by the mid-1500s and spread throughout the world, leading to cocoa plantations in the Caribbean, the

Philippines and western Africa. Chocolate is still used by traditional healers in Oaxaca, Mexico, for conditions ranging from bronchitis to scorpion and bee stings.

Chocolate Can Be Good For You

What could be better than hearing that chocolate is truly good for you? Chocolate contains powerful disease-fighting phytonutrients, as found in grapes and green tea, that protect you from heart disease and cancer.

Dark bitter-sweet chocolate that is a minimum of 70 percent cocoa contains less sugar and more phytonutrients than regular milk chocolate because of its higher cocoa content.

Lindt is a Swiss brand that makes a Lindt Excellence dark semi-sweet chocolate made with 70 percent cocoa butter, lecithin and sugar. The only chocolate I recommend must be 70 percent or more of cocoa butter, as it has the least sugar and the greatest phytonutrient profile.

The major fatty acid in cocoa butter—stearic acid—is converted to oleic acid, a monounsaturated fatty acid, the same fat as olive oil, which does not raise blood cholesterol levels as do saturated fats. The low-calorie amount of 1/2 oz (14 g) of dark semi-sweet chocolate averages only 30 calories. If eaten in mid-afternoon, it can raise endorphin and serotonin levels to give you a genuine pleasure response.

Recent studies have dispelled the claim that chocolate aggravates acne. Chocolate is a good source of magnesium and copper. Chocolate does not promote dental cavities, primarily because the fat helps protect the teeth from acids otherwise formed from sugar. Chocolate appears to fight plaque formation and contains an antibacterial agent.

A 5-oz (155 mL) glass of dry red wine contains about 150 milligrams of a protective antioxidant called phenols. Dark, semi-sweet chocolate that is a minimum 70 percent cocoa butter contains the most phenols of any chocolate or red wine, about 160 milligrams per ounce.

In a study conducted at the University of Pennsylvania, researchers found that chocolate is liked by everyone, but women more than men crave chocolate, especially when they are premenstrual. Most chocolate is eaten as an afternoon or evening snack.

Final Thoughts on Chocolate

If you use the right chocolate, at the right time, it can have very healthful properties. A 1/2 oz (14 g) serving of milk chocolate has 75 calories and 8 milligrams of caffeine. Dark semi-sweet chocolate has only 30 calories and 8 milligrams of caffeine in a 1/2 oz. Dark semi-sweet chocolate contains cocoa butter, which is like olive oil. Cocoa butter does not raise cholesterol and has a beneficial effect on blood lipid profile. Milk chocolate contains butter fat, which raises cholesterol levels. Cheaper milk chocolate products replace cocoa butter with unhealthy, undesirable fats like palm oil, which is highly saturated, or even with partially hydrogenated oils full of dangerous trans-fatty acids. Read the labels carefully!

Good-quality, dark semi-sweet chocolate from Switzerland, France and Belgium is particularly good. It is not unhealthy and makes a pleasant treat or dessert, if eaten once or twice a week in moderation. As long as you do not exceed 1 1/2 oz (42 g) per serving, you can enjoy the rich taste of this unique food.

Dark, semi-sweet chocolate contains more protective phytonutrients with antioxidant activity. Read and compare labels of milk chocolate and dark semi-sweet chocolate. Sugar makes up 75 percent of milk chocolate and is the first ingredient. Dark semi-sweet chocolate that is 70 to 75 percent cocoa butter has cocoa as the first ingredient and is only 20 to 25 percent sugar. It also contains no allergy-causing dairy products but does contain soy lecithin, a food I highly recommend (see the section "Soy Lecithin Granules" in Chapter 14 for more details). The lecithin emulsifies the cocoa butter, giving a rich, smooth, creamy melt to the chocolate in your mouth.

On an island off the British Columbia coast, close to an island I live on, is the Denman Island Chocolate Company, which uses both Belgian dark chocolate and sugar certified organically grown, with non-genetically modified (non-GMO) lecithin. You can get in touch with them at www.denmanislandchocolate.com.

There is no denying that worldwide, people find chocolate a remarkable food. Chocolate contains phenylethylamine, a mood enhancer, and theobromine, which has stimulating, caffeine-like effects and triggers the release of endorphins. But make sure that you're not using chocolate as an emotional crutch for coping with day-to-day stresses.

And a Bonus

Dark, semi-sweet chocolate that is 70 to 75 percent cocoa is very rich in the amino acid tyrosine. Tyrosine, as I mentioned in Chapter 2, is the building block for the hormone dopamine. Dopamine levels rise once the first rays of light appear in the morning and decline toward sundown. Dopamine makes you alert, motivated, decisive and clear. It gives you the edge to survive.

If you do consume chocolate, only consume dark, semi-sweet chocolate that is 70 to 75 percent cocoa butter or cocoa mass. Do consume small amounts of it at about 3:00 p.m. to raise your dopamine levels, improve your mood and give yourself an afternoon boost in alertness. The small sugar content will immediately trigger the release of endorphins, which make you feel euphoric, followed by a steady supply of a glucose fuel mix to your brain. This still maintains your homeostasis. In 60 to 90 minutes, tyrosine produces the hormone dopamine and you continue to maintain a sense of wellness.

The ultimate dietary strategy, if you do consume chocolate, would be to consume 7 grams of protein from a whey or soy protein isolate powder (half of an enclosed scoop) in 4 oz (125 mL) of water, unsweetened almond milk or rice milk—then sit back and savor your dark, semi-sweet chocolate. The whey or soy protein isolate powder supplies 7 grams of biologically complete protein plus 350 milligrams of additional tyrosine. In addition, the protein from the whey or soy protein isolate powder acts as a "braking mechanism" on the sugar in the chocolate, slowing the rise in blood glucose levels and spacing the release of insulin.

If you do it right, you can enjoy, in moderation, the exotic taste of dark, semi-sweet chocolate and regulate hormone fidelity by increasing both dopamine and serotonin levels for heightened alertness and calmness—while avoiding the mood-altering roller-coaster ride produced from high-density processed carbohydrates that raise blood glucose levels and cause devastating insulin spikes as a detrimental consequence.

People who attempt to quit smoking report that they have increased appetite and mood changes. Nicotine—the addictive drug in tobacco—stimulates serotonin release. "When people quit smoking, they turn to sweets to get the same serotonin effect. In essence, the sweet cravings of ex-smokers are an attempt to self-medicate and improve mood, diminishing the uncomfortable nicotine withdrawal symptoms they are experiencing," writes Elizabeth Somer in *Food and Mood*. Many ex-smokers tell me they binge on inexpensive milk chocolate to relieve the nicotine withdrawal pain. It works, but two hours later they have negative mood swings and crave sugar. The chocolate protein recipe above—plus consuming complex, low-density carbohydrates like whole grain pasta and bread, ripe fruit, vegetables and legumes like lentils—boost moods and help to curb carbohydrate cravings because they increase serotonin levels. Combine this with protein meals high in the amino acid tyrosine and we can help people "kick" destructive addictions to nicotine and alcohol. There is always hope if people get the right information.

COFFEE REVISITED

Caffeine is what makes coffee the morning cup of "get up and go." Coffee's aroma and promise of instant energy have made it the number-one mind-altering drug and the second most popular drink, after soft drinks, in North America. As of 2000, we consume half of the world's coffee, averaging about 1,000 cups a year per person.

Virtually all of the caffeine in coffee is absorbed, and within half an hour of consuming it, caffeine's stimulating effects leave you more alert, less tired and faster to react. The initial high from coffee can be followed by a mild symptom of fatigue. You can get caught in a vicious cycle if you drink more coffee to prevent the inevitable letdown. People's tolerance to coffee varies widely. Caffeine also lingers in the body for hours. It acts as a diuretic, contributing to dehydration, itself a cause of fatigue. For every cup of coffee you drink, consume two 8-oz (250 mL) glasses of water.

North Americans spend US$2.3 billion on coffee, specialty blends and flavored beans annually. A cup of coffee is one of the few pleasures that remains calorie-free, as long as it is ordered black. If coffee overstimulates you or gives you the "jitters," don't drink it—you are caffeine-sensitive. Those who are pregnant or breast-feeding should not consume caffeinated beverages.

The Caffeine Buzz

Studies indicate that up to 300 milligrams of caffeine a day, equal to the caffeine in about 2 cups of freshly brewed coffee, is safe. (On a typical day, 49 percent of North American adults drink an average of 3.3 cups of coffee.) The caffeine in coffee can actually assist in the stimulation of some cognitive abilities. Computer programmers, mechanics, think-tankers, seminar participants, travelers and students have used coffee to give them that slight mental alertness advantage. But the downside is that caffeine in more than moderate doses has other bad effects, including accentuating gastric acid secretion and ulcers, and can lead to blood sugar, cortisol and insulin imbalances.

As nerve cells in the brain ignite, they use energy and produce adenosine in the process. Adenosine is related to the energy molecule adenosine triphosphate (ATP). As adenosine builds up on neurons, it operates as a natural brake to keep neurons from overfiring.

Caffeine has a similar structure to adenosine and easily fits into adenosine receptor sites, but the fit is not perfect and caffeine does not have the sedating effect of adenosine. It therefore blocks the nerve-soothing job of adenosine. The nervous system stays revved, you think more clearly, are more alert, have a faster reaction time and can concentrate better.

Just because some caffeine boosts thought processes does not mean drinking more of it makes you smarter. The stimulating effects of caffeine linger in your system for up to six hours. A cup of coffee or a mid-afternoon cola could disrupt your sleep at 10:30 p.m., resulting in mental fatigue and poor judgment the next day. Caffeine is effective only up to your "jitter threshold"; add more caffeine after this and you're too buzzed to think clearly. Recent research also suggests that caffeine and its related methylxanthines may encourage the release of two amino acids, glutamate and aspartate, which are the main excitatory neurotransmitters in the brain.

Caffeine and Athletic Performance

At the cellular level, caffeine enhances neuromuscular transmission and improves muscle contraction. Athletes have used coffee to aid performance in high-intensity exercise. Most athletes consume the equivalent of 2 to 4 cups of regular coffee without harsh side effects.

CAFFEINE CONTENT	
Beverage-Food-Medication	Milligrams of Caffeine
Coffee (5 oz / 155 mL)	
brewed, drip method	115–180
Instant	65–120
Decaffeinated	2–5
Café latte, café mocha	55–57
Cappuccino (8 oz / 250 mL)	110–130
Green tea (organic, 5 oz / 155 mL cup)	60–70
Tea (5 oz / 155 mL)	
Brewed	60–110
Instant	30–50
Iced	70–75
Cocoa beverage (5 oz / 155 mL)	2–20
Chocolate milk (8 oz / 250 mL)	2–7
Dark chocolate, semi-sweet (1 oz/ 28 g)	15–35
Mountain Dew (8 oz / 250 mL)	55.0
Coca Cola (8 oz / 250 mL)	45.6
Diet Cola (8 oz / 250 mL)	45.6
Pepsi Cola (8 oz / 250 mL)	37.2
Diet Pepsi (8 oz / 250 mL)	35.4
Canada Dry Cola (8 oz / 250 mL)	30.0
Canada Dry Diet Cola (8 oz / 250 mL)	1.2
Cadbury milk chocolate bar (1 oz / 28 g)	15
Excedrin (2)	65
Anacin, Midol, Vanquish, Dristan (2)	30–33
Cafergot (prescription for migraine headaches) (2)	100
Darvon (prescription pain medication) (2)	30–32

Caffeine does increase the level of fatty acids in the blood, and research has shown it can boost the oxidation of these fats to be burned as fuel. It is for this reason that endurance athletes have used caffeine for years to promote the burning of fat and the spacing of muscle glycogen.

To ignite the fat-burning, you must consume 2 cups of black, preferably organic, freshly brewed coffee a full two hours before a major event or a hard, all-out training session. It takes this much time for caffeine to work in your metabolic pathways to burn fat, even though you feel the buzz earlier.

Coffee and caffeine work only if you do not use them daily as your body will compensate for their daily use. Use coffee only once a week if you use it for athletic or training reasons. Pre-race caffeine can stave off feelings of fatigue and definitely boost alertness if it is not used daily, but saved for once a week hard training or competition events. The conversion of fat to energy is about 35 percent more efficient when caffeine is consumed prior to exercise. When your body burns fat, it reduces its reliance on glycogen, glucose and amino acids, so your bloodstream glucose fuel mix levels remain higher for longer.

> The International Olympic Committee sets a limit on caffeine levels acceptable in urine tests corresponding to about 5 cups of coffee drunk in 30 minutes. It allows an upper limit of 12 mcg/mL of urine tested. Over a two to three hour period, 1 cup of coffee with 150 milligrams of caffeine results in a urine concentration of about 2.0 mcg/mL.

Many athletes and weight lifters use dopamine-like stimulants, such as caffeine, Ma-Huang herb, guarana herb and ephedrine, to get a more powerful workout from increased motivation and drive. You can quickly overstimulate your system with these stimulants, speeding up the aging auto-oxidation and degeneration of the sensitive dopamine-producing brain cells.

Take It Easy

The optimum amount of coffee is 2 cups a day. That's enough caffeine to combine with the entire day's fat and sugar intake to balance mood swings, sleep problems and fatigue. The phytonutrients in coffee may also exert a protective effect against colon cancer. Top any coffee with whipped cream and you add 110 calories of fat. Keep coffee black, if you can, and request that your coffeehouse have at least one organic coffee available.

You might experience caffeine withdrawal within hours of your last cup, which leaves you mentally sluggish and a little grumpy. Coffee contains compounds called tannins, which reduce other brain-boosting nutrients, such as magnesium, by 75 percent. If you consume more than 2 cups a day, gradually cut back to 2 cups of black, organic coffee daily. Black, organic coffee is alkaline-forming, but once you add a sweetener and/or dairy or rice milk, the coffee is acidic to your system.

You are most likely to feel tired or experience other symptoms of coffee withdrawal, such as headaches, if coffee intake is reduced too quickly. As you cut back, try a decaffeinated coffee for any coffee you drink after noon. Try a grain-based drink such as Cafix, Postum or Krakus, which taste and smell somewhat like coffee but only average 12 calories a cup and have no caffeine.

As you reduce your daily coffee intake, try switching to green tea, which has 60 to 70 mg of caffeine per cup, about one half that of freshly brewed coffee.

The pharmacological effects of caffeine are transient, usually only lasting a few hours. Caffeine does not accumulate in the body. Any discomfort caused by abruptly reducing caffeine consumption can be avoided by progressively decreasing intake over a few days.

People who are caffeine-sensitive (experience headaches, anxiety, "jitters," irritability) may feel as though they've overdosed on just half a cup of regular brewed coffee. Virtually all of the caffeine in coffee is absorbed and distributed throughout your body in one half hour. Caffeine's stimulating effects can last for up to six hours. Caffeine can behave as an appetite suppressant if you do not add sugar or a sweetener to your coffee or consume a sugary donut or muffin. Caffeine in coffee revs up your metabolic rate and releases stored fat to be burned as energy, although it is debatable as to whether it truly makes a difference during a diet.

Caffeine does cause you to lose some calcium so take a calcium-magnesium supplement that gives you 100 mg of elemental calcium and 100 mg of elemental magnesium and 100 IU of vitamin D3 per capsule. Use three capsules before you go to sleep along with your garlic, flax or hemp seed oil, and several tablespoons of organic, unsweetened, plain yogurt or quark cheese. The calcium and magnesium should be in a citrate or bis-glycinate form.

Studies of long-time caffeine intake show that people develop a tolerance to the blood pressure-raising effects of caffeine over time. If you have high blood pressure or are elderly, the acute effects of caffeine can be extremely significant, so avoid or limit your daily consumption to half a cup a day, mixed with half a cup of hot water. You may try to incorporate a healthy, non-caffeinated herbal tea into your day.

Caffeine-sensitive people, who get a severe buzz on half a cup of coffee, may experience a transient rise in blood pressure, usually lasting for two to three hours. It also appears unfiltered coffee has natural constituents that are responsible for raising cholesterol. A 1989 report from the Framingham Heart Study, which is still ongoing, examined all potential links between caffeine intake and cardiovascular disease, and found no harmful effects from drinking coffee in moderate amounts.

Natural Stimulant Substitutes for Coffee

Guarana is an herb from the Amazon jungle. The active ingredient in guarana is called guaranine, very similar to caffeine. Some retailers sell it as an aphrodisiac, but there is absolutely no evidence to support such claims.

Guarana is showing up daily in sports and "smart" drinks for those who want extra neurological energy and mental focus. "Smart" drinks or energy drinks use guarana that has been standardized for its "caffeine" content, to allow them to use a measured dose. A measured dose is equal to about 100 to 150 mg of caffeine, or 1 cup of brewed coffee. I am opposed to using guarana.

Another Peruvian rainforest herb is maca, or lepidium meyenii. Native Peruvians have used maca since before the time of the Incas for both its nutritional and adaptogenic properties. The plant grows at an altitude of approximately 4,000 meters. There is no caffeine in maca and its use gives strength, vitality, mental clarity and a sense of well-being.

A great coffee substitute is to use a "green drink" supplemented with 400 IU of mixed tocopheryl (or tocopherol) vitamin E; 500 mg of vitamin C as calcium, magnesium and potassium ascorbate; and 1,000 mg of maca. The finest maca should bear a seal of approval from Dr. Ramon Ferreya, Ph.D., of the National University of San Marcos, Lima, Peru, and president of the Peruvian Botanical Society.

Another herbal coffee substitute is organic yerba maté, ecologically harvested in cooperation with indigenous communities from the Paraguay and Argentina rainforests in South America. Yerba maté contains a compound called mateine, a natural energizer without the jittery side effects of caffeine.

I personally have 1 cup of organic yerba maté once a week, on hard training days, and the herb maca with a "green drink" every two weeks to support an intense training session. Guarana and the herbs cola nut and Ma-Huang (ephedra) overstimulate dopamine production and can cause the dopamine neurons to become depleted and die prematurely. I do not recommend their use.

Final Thoughts on Caffeine

Caffeine can cause excessive body odors in some individuals. Caffeinated soft drinks are to be avoided as the additional phosphoric acid they contain leeches excessive calcium from your bones. Caffeine can overwhelm the adrenal glands, which produce the hormone cortisol, causing short-term stress.

If you do use caffeinated coffee, green tea or soft drinks, I highly recommend you daily use two capsules of adrena+, a very potent herbal combination that reduces the sheer stress in, and supports the proper metabolic functions of, your two adrenal glands, located one on top of each kidney.

19

ANSWERS TO FREQUENTLY ASKED QUESTIONS ABOUT FOOD AND NUTRITION

Weren't we designed to be vegetarian?

In the very beginning of human history, humans' primary source of protein came from scavenging dead animals. Humans could not compete with many of the large predators. Approximately 100,000 years ago, Dr. Boyd Eaton of Emory University writes, modern humans (Homo sapiens) appeared and intelligence levels increased quickly as humans learned to use their five-finger dexterity and make hunting tools as well as fire and protective shelters. Humans now became the main predator, hunter and gatherer. The first tools were rocks used to open the skulls of dead animals, to make available their brains for consumption— which were exceedingly high in the long-chain Omega-3 fatty acids DHA and EPA. Humans also began to catch fish and eat shellfish, which furthered their cognitive and neurological processes by supplying a steady supply of DHA and EPA, which now make up 50 percent of the structure of our brains and central nervous systems. Once humans became proficient hunters, they consumed from 100 to 200 grams of lean animal protein per day. Overhunting forced some people to develop agriculture just 10,000 years ago. Grains and starches now became the staple and provided a much lower protein, but far greater carbohydrate intake, than they had ever consumed in the 90,000 years as hunters and gatherers, whose main diet was fruit, vegetables, herbs and lean animal protein. Anthropologists, such as Hugh Brody in his recent book *The Other Side of Eden*, have found that the skeletal remains of hunter-gatherers show fewer signs of degenerative disease than the remains of early farmers or even modern people.

Depending on your genetic inheritance, 90 percent of us are either blood type O (and should utilize 10 to 40 percent lean animal protein sources, since you are still somewhat of a "hunter-gatherer" and 60 to 90 percent plant-based protein sources) or blood type A (and are a descendant of the agriculturist and should consume 100 percent plant-based protein sources). I am blood type O and eat only six organic, free-range eggs a week plus fat-free organic yogurt to fulfill my type. The rest of my protein sources are whey protein isolates and plant-based proteins.

I want to eat more fruits, vegetables and herbs. Do I have to worry about pesticides on them?

Yes you do! You can wash all commercial produce for ten seconds in warm water and biodegradable dish detergent or purchase a premade fruit and vegetable liquid cleanser. Scrub sturdier fruit and vegetables. Peel waxed cucumbers and apples. This will remove 85 percent of all pesticides. I highly recommend that you purchase organically grown, chemical-free fruit and vegetables whenever possible.

Why balance protein, carbohydrates and fats at all three meals?

I advocate that you plan to eat three meals a day and two snacks. This will allow food to constantly be digested, broken down to glucose, and enter your bloodstream as your ideal fuel-mix. You want a continuous balance of glucose bloodstream fuel, which can only be achieved by consuming bioenergetic whole foods every three to four hours.

A small amount of fat makes foods smell good, taste good and builds your brain and central nervous system. The right amount of low-density carbohydrates helps synthesize the hormone serotonin, which makes you feel good and keeps insulin levels steady. The right amount of protein also balances insulin levels and hormonal glucagon levels for four hours between meals. If you eat too much protein and too few carbohydrates, your insulin levels will be very depressed and you will feel exhausted. Eat too many carbohydrates and not enough protein, and your insulin levels will rise too high and cause hormonal imbalances. The body wants homeostasis or supersymmetry from meal-to-snack-to-meal and a balanced glucagon/insulin hormone axis.

Why all this talk about excess insulin being harmful?

The number one cause of accelerated aging for anyone is chronically elevated insulin levels. Insulin drives nutrients and bloodstream glucose fuel into your cells, so too little of it and your 100 trillion cells die of starvation. Too much insulin, a response to eating high-density, processed carbohydrates day after day, stores extra glucose in "long-term" storage tanks as fat, your portable energy reserve. Excess insulin levels raise levels of your stress hormone cortisol and their elevated combinations cause obesity, decreased mental focus, decreased robust energy, diminishing strength, sagging skin, poor hair texture and chronic disease.

What is the nutritional difference between raw food versus cooked food?

Supporters of raw food diets have long felt that cooking foods destroys all enzymes contained in raw foods, which makes it more difficult to digest food. The basic theory is that cooking destroys nutrients. In reality, the opposite may be more true. Cooking breaks down indigestible cell walls so your body's digestive enzymes can better digest the nutrients and successfully absorb them. Of particular note, the phytonutrient lycopene, a major health-supportive ingredient in tomatoes, is made more available and is more concentrated in tomato juice or tomato sauce than in raw tomatoes. It is also absorbed better if it is accompanied by a fat, such as olive oil, than if you eat the tomato raw by itself.

Obviously, overcooking does destroy vitamins and enzymes and you lose many of the minerals. I recommend that vegetables be cooked "crunchy-tender"; fruits, salad, herbs, sprouts, nuts, seeds and spices be eaten raw for the most part; and that legumes, peas and grains be presoaked or sprouted and thoroughly cooked to be digested properly. My dietary strategy would be that you do have some raw food at each meal and a colorful glass of fresh vegetable juice daily. Lean meats and eggs should be thoroughly cooked.

Always use a stainless steel food grater and grate a huge variety of raw, colorful vegetable specks over your entrées, salads, soups, stews, casseroles, stir-fries and in your sandwiches.

Does eating more fruits, vegetables, salads and herbs prevent cancer and heart disease?

Yes, yes, yes! As a matter of fact, 75 percent of North Americans will die from diseases of the heart, arteries or veins and cancer. Truly, 85 percent of these diseases are caused by diet and lifestyle and 15 percent by genetics. Those eating the most fruits, vegetables, lean protein, salads, herbs and "green drinks" experience 70 to 90 percent less of these two main chronic ailments. Therefore, you can live a longer, healthier life, disease free.

What is the difference between eating ripe fruits and drinking fruit juices?

Fruit juices are concentrated high-density carbohydrates, which are sugar-intense, without any fiber to slow their entry into your bloodstream. I suggest you eat one serving of fresh berries, fruit or melon at a time. An 8 oz (250 mL) glass of juice can be equivalent to six to eight pieces of the fruit. This huge amount of unopposed carbohydrate, as sugar, causes a "giant hit" of insulin that initiates hormonal malfunction and imbalances. Your body does not know if this huge burst of sugar came from candy or fruit juice. The more often your cells experience "giant hits" of insulin, the less responsive your cells become to insulin.

What are the differences between low-density complex carbohydrates and high-density simple carbohydrates?

Low-density complex carbohydrates are fruits, legumes, peas, seeds, nuts and whole grains. They are made up of simple carbohydrates complexed with a lot of fiber in a natural state. Vegetables are very-low-density complex carbohydrates.

High-density simple carbohydrates have a lot of carbohydrates with very little fiber. They break down to bloodstream glucose faster than table sugar and cause a "giant hit" of insulin to forcefully drive the excessive blood glucose levels down. They are found mostly in refined grain products and processed "food."

Are grains essential for optimal health?

No! Remember, 10,000 years ago there were no grains. Just 100 years ago there were no processed "foods" with refined wheat as the base. Your longstanding genetic predisposition is to low-density carbohydrate consumption—from fruits, vegetables, salads, herbs and sea vegetables. Try to eliminate wheat in favor of other sourdough or sprouted grain products made from spelt, rye, amaranth, kamut and millet, but only use them sparingly. Use organic grains whenever possible, but use them sparingly. Pasta and bread do not occur in nature. There are no pasta trees or bread plants.

I have no energy. Could my diet be the problem?

Low energy levels are caused by poor nutrition, skipping meals, too much protein, too much fat, too many processed "foods," lack of quality sleep that causes hormones to be "out-of-whack," not exercising and stimulating your blood movement, dependence on caffeine, depression and paralyzing stress.

Are artificial sweeteners safe?

No—I repeat, No! I refuse to consume them. Don't let your body be a toxic chemical dump! The down side to all artificial sweeteners is that none of these sweeteners help curb carbohydrate cravings, boost moods or help to manage weight.

Should I eat eggs?

Yes! Eat three to nine organic, free-range eggs a week—poached, soft-boiled or hard-boiled. Eat the yolks unless you have inflammation or high cholesterol. If you do have inflammation or high cholesterol, eat two eggs at a time, discarding one yolk; if you eat three at a time, discard two yolks. Eggs have sulfur-bearing amino acids your immune system needs. Yolks of chickens fed organic flax seeds are high in the necessary long-chain Omega-3 fatty acid DHA that you daily need for superior neurological and central nervous system functioning. Yolks are a potent source of choline, vitamin B12 and the powerful antioxidants superoxide dismutase (SOD) and catalase. If you fry or scramble eggs, the exposed DHA and pre-formed cholesterol in the yolk, upon contact with the heat, oxidizes and forms a number of cell-damaging, toxic byproducts called free radicals.

Chocolate tastes great. Is it bad for me?

Good quality, semi-sweet, 70 percent or more cocoa, dark Belgian, Swiss or French chocolate is not unhealthy and can make a wonderful treat. It actually contains large amounts of protective phytonutrients and antioxidants. Use this chocolate in moderation at about 3:00 to 4:00 p.m. for a genuine pick-me-up caused by elevated endorphins and an increase in stabilizing serotonin levels as well as a decrease in the stress hormone cortisol. Simply limit your intake.

I eat well. Do I need vitamins?

Humanity has never lived with as high an amount of non-stop stress, environmental toxins, agrichemicals, suspect water supplies, TV and newspapers reporting constant high-level drama, financial crises, relationship crises, family crises and personal crises as we do today. Yes definitely, you require vitamin supplements, antioxidant supplements, mineral supplements and medicinal herbal supplements to help your body and mind withstand the extreme stress and pressure of a faster-is-better, 24-7-365 society.

Remember, always let food be your first remedy, your first line of defense. You were created that way. Food is the strongest modulator of hormone biosynthesis, hormone fidelity and hormone receptivity. Time-honored herbal formulas are a powerful and dramatically effective means of helping you reach greater hormonal harmony—which eventually means physical, emotional, psychological and spiritual balance. You only need to include them in your daily eating routine. Natural, bioenergetic whole foods are your foundation to living a longer, healthier life and preserving the Earth's future. Do use supplements in small quantities three or four times a day to maintain bloodstream homeostasis of each nutrient, rather than a mega-dose all at once.

Why should I take a "green drink"?

Green is the color of chlorophyll, the most phytonutrient-rich color of all. "Green drinks" are pure cellular health insurance. They contain huge varieties of alkaline-forming, bioenergetic, colorful, organically grown grasses, sea vegetables, unique water-extracted herbal extracts and the most nutrient-dense hormone-supporting vegetables. They are extremely low in calories, contain virtually no fats and are jammed with fiber, phytonutrients, antioxidants, vitamins, minerals and the glutathione-flavonoid sub-network of herbal extracts that make glutathione.

As a nutrient-rich, low-calorie, virtually no-sugar-content food, a high-quality "green drink" is the perfect example of the calorie-restricted foods proven to reverse the aging process, and they approach an ideal food. Take a "green drink" once before breakfast and a second time at about 3:00 p.m. to prevent the afternoon doldrums.

"Green drinks" are the most nutrient-rich foods you can consume.

What should I look for in a good antioxidant formula?

You want a convenient, cost-effective, high-quality, synergistic blend of antioxidants for full free radical protection. This is critical in modern society. I recommend capsules or softgels, never tablets that contain binders, fillers, excipients (materials used to make tablet ingredients flow easily through mechanical, high-pressure tablet machines), glaze agents and so on. This is true for vitamins, herbs, minerals and antioxidants. Antioxidants must be "networked" and combined together.

The basic, full-spectrum, ideal network blend would include, in two capsules:

- Carotenoid complex (alpha and beta carotene)   5,000 to 7,000 IU
- Vitamin C as an ascorbate complex   250 to 350 mg
- Vitamin E as a succinate with
  beta, delta, gamma fractions   200 to 270 IU
- Selenium   20 to 40 mcg
- N-Acetyl Cysteine (NAC)   65 to 70 mg
- Full-spectrum grape extract
  with resveratrol and ellagic acid   30 to 40 mg
- Alpha lipoic acid   30 to 40 mg
- Citrus bioflavonoids   30 to 40 mg
- Coenzyme Q10 (CoQ10)   10 to 20 mg
- Lycopene   10 mg
- European bilberry   5 to 10 mg

I would use four single capsules: one at each meal and one before going to sleep. This combination will synthesize your cells' most important endogenous antioxidant enzyme, glutathione peroxidase, and protect your mitochrondria.

How do you feel about genetically modified foods?

I am utterly suspicious that they have been brought into the food chain far too quickly. While the jury is still out, I strictly avoid them in grains, corn, potatoes and tomatoes. As of 2001, global acreage of genetically modified crops is 109.2 million acres—twice the size of England.

What critical hormone ratio should we all try to balance?

DHEA hormones are the most abundant steroids in the human body. Low levels of DHEA are associated with most disease states, such as heart disease, osteoporosis, immune dysfunction and a greater risk of certain cancers. The dramatic aging-related drop in DHEA levels is accompanied by an equally dramatic rise in cardiovascular disease—our number one killer. DHEA is incorporated into both high and low-density cholesterol, protecting it from oxidation. After age 30, cholesterol-bound DHEA steadily declines and cholesterol oxidizes more readily. DHEA also increases the activity of superoxide dismutase (SOD), one of your most important antioxidant enzymes in the cell.

Meditation has long been known to increase DHEA and reduce corrosive cortisol hormone levels. This is a critical ratio to watch after age 30. High insulin, high cortisol and low DHEA are the cornerstone of accelerated aging for all. Stress reduction causes a shift in adrenal cortex steroidogenesis from cortisor to DHEA.

DHEA and its metabolite 7 alpha-hydroxy-DHEA protect the thymus gland and brain against progressive atrophy induced by excessive cortisol stress hormones (glucocorticoids). Thymus atrophy triggers immunosenescence and is the most destructive mechanism that accelerates aging. We need some stress so we can learn to be adaptable. Too little stress (cortisol) and the adrenal glands would atrophy. Too much stress (cortisol) reduces protective DHEA levels and quickly accelerates biological aging in a declining catabolic drive.

Who Lives the Longest –What Do They Eat?

The 1997 American Heart Association's *Statistical Supplement* compiled mortality rates for both women and men from countries with very distinct dietary habits. In particular, they looked at the death rates in the 35 to 74 age group, where a death could be considered to be premature.

MORTALITY RATES (PER 100,000) OF ADULTS (AGES 35 TO 74)

Country	Male Death Rate	Female Death Rate
Rural China	1,433	914
United States	1,209	688
Canada	1,150	599
France	1,065	438
Japan	814	380

As you can see, Americans fared only slightly better than the rural Chinese who eat mostly a rice-based diet with some protein. Americans spend a far greater amount of money on health care, especially heroic life-saving attempts, than the rural Chinese do. It may be this huge expenditure (plus the additional protein in the American diet) that gives them a very slight edge in living longer than rural Chinese do. Canadians, on average, outlive Americans.

The Japanese are the healthiest and longest lived of any people; they eat less processed food, more fruit, more vegetables, more fish and more quality soy protein than any other population in the world. Their diet is more protein-rich than the Chinese diet, with more fish, as well as more vegetables and more fruit. Also, since the end of World War II, along with more protein, the Japanese have consumed much less rice.

The longest to live of the Japanese people live on the island of Okinawa, a part of Japan, but close to 400 miles from Japan, southeast in the Pacific Ocean. Compared to mainland Japanese, the Okinawan population has close to 40 percent lower death rates in every age range from heart disease, stroke and both breast and prostate cancer. Okinawans have nearly five times the percentage of people living healthfully over 100 compared to their Japanese counterparts, who themselves are long lived and healthy compared to the rest of the world's population. Okinawans have the largest percentage of healthy 100-year-olds of any region in the world.

Okinawans eat 40 percent more protein, especially soy protein and twice as much fish abundant in long chain Omega-3 fatty acids (rich in heart-healthy EPA and brain-healthy DHA), many more vegetables and fruits, and 20 to 40 percent fewer calories from rice and processed carbohydrates than the mainland Japanese do. They are the healthiest, longest living population.

What dietary strategy will allow me to live the longest, healthiest life?

This is the single most important question that I am constantly asked. There are really two critical questions being asked. The unspoken one is, "How should I die?"

The January 1996 edition of *Scientific American* magazine published the results of many years of research on reduced-calorie diets by Roy Walford, M.D., of UCLA Medical School; Dr. George S. Roth of the National Institute on Aging; and a brilliant researcher, Richard Weindrich, Ph.D., of the University of Wisconsin.

Since 1900, advances in health practices have greatly increased the average lifespan of North Americans, mainly by improving prevention and treatment of diseases that end life prematurely. But those interventions have not substantially affected the maximum lifespan. As of 2001, to favorably round it off, the average North American lives to be 80 years of age. Researchers feel that the human body is designed to function well to age 100 or 120, with the longest living of our species reaching 150.

The only clinically proven way to markedly increase the maximum as well as the average lifespan has been the research of Walford, Roth and Weindrich. Simply put, a reduced-calorie diet not only prolongs the life of rodents and other animals, it also enables animals to remain youthful longer with few chronic diseases.

Voluntary calorie-restriction, eating bioenergetic whole foods to modulate hormones, avoiding salty/sugary/fatty processed "foods," stress reduction, drinking plenty of water, getting 8.5 hours of sleep a night, and eating a huge variety of organic, colorful fruits, vegetables, herbs and sea vegetables—these add up to the simple formula for optimum health and longevity.

Even more exciting, beyond extending survival, calorie-restricted (or low-calorie) diets in rodents have postponed most major diseases that are common late in life, including cancers of the breast, prostate and colon. Moreover, with respect to the 300 or so measures of aging that have been studied, some 90 percent stay "younger" (and disease-free) longer in calorie-restricted rodents than in well-fed ones. Restriction of fat, protein or carbohydrate without overall calorie restriction does not increase the maximum lifespan of animals.

The actual research results are based on taking four groups of mice, each group having an unrestricted, natural living habitat. They all received the same water and the same food. The only difference is that the four groups received different amounts of the same food:

- Group A could eat all the food they wanted, called an unrestricted caloric diet. They ate when they wanted, how much they wanted.
- Group B got 80 calories a week.
- Group C got 60 calories a week.
- Group D got 40 calories a week.

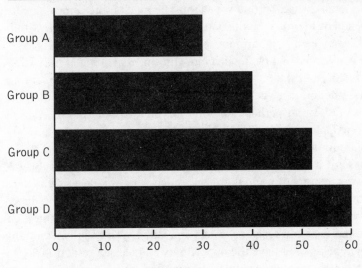

TEST RESULTS OF CALORIE-RESTRICTED DIETS IN MICE

How many months they lived

Remember, the mice on the calorie-restricted diets not only lived longer, they remained youthful longer and had very few chronic diseases. The mice who ate an unrestricted diet lived, on average, for 36 months and were very ill for one month before they died. Their fur got gray, dry and lifeless. The majority of mice put weight on and, to some degree, experienced diabetes, high blood pressure, mental confusion and cancer.

The mice who ate 40 calories of the very same food per week, lived to be 62 months of age, on average, and were not sick for a month. They ran around doing all the things mice do and one day they just fell over dead. They expired without the excessive weight gain, diabetes or cancer. They wore out. Their fur and skin still had color, sheen and a relatively healthy appearance. They did not languish in painful illness like group A mice.

For humans to practice voluntary calorie-restriction, it is not fasting or starvation. It is about consciously eating a wide variety of nutrient-rich, low-calorie, fresh, bioenergetic whole foods. Please refer to page 142 in Chapter 10 to understand the basis of "The World's Best Diet" that will help you get to age 110, 120 or 150 with complete mental clarity, robust energy and optimum vitality. The average North American eats the opposite—a high-calorie, low-nutrient diet with far too many sugary, salty, fatty, refined grains and processed "foods" that look good, smell good and taste good, but destroy your beautifully crafted mind and body by rusting them out far too soon. You're causing yourself to languish in what Karlis Ullis, M.D., calls the four Ds—discomfort, doctors, disease and drugs—that you can avoid.

How should we pass on then?

It is my own personal conviction that we all must be much more compassionate with ourselves, and be in sync with the natural, intrinsic healing rhythms within our elegant bodies by eating in harmony with our longstanding genetic predisposition to the bioenergetic whole food chain. Our understanding of life extension, already enhanced in the last five to ten years, is about to take a quantum leap forward. Decades of never-before-experienced vigor and vitality in our 80s, 90s, 100s, 110s, 120s—and perhaps for some beyond—should be the natural experience for the majority of human beings. It is not a promise just to prolong life; it is a promise to make the quality of life much better.

The only reason I want you to experience more vigor, vitality and a disease-free life is that we are humanity and there is so much work we have to do. There are too many hungry, lonely, heart-broken, sad, forgotten, angry, violent, directionless, frightened, dysfunctional, naked, homeless children, women and men of all countries, nationalities, religions, colors and faiths. As a healthy, emotionally stable human being, you have the opportunity and blessed responsibility to help through—thought, word, deed, action or prayer—to heal, help and uplift humanity and support the evolution of our species. Make the goal of your life a blessed endeavor.

Today we have sophisticated medical imaging tools and ultrasound scanners; we have the ability to assess genetic information screened from an egg or sperm; we have satellites and wireless telecommunications; we can manipulate defective genes, turn a gene called p53 "off" from spreading cancer, and use nanotechnology to build computer-controlled molecular tools, much smaller than a human cell, with programmable intelligence that can enter the bloodstream to kill cancer cells or take over the function of sub-cellular organelles; we have cryonics; we have cloning, with the debut of Dolly in Scotland; and we have germ-line engineering that can insert "better" artificial chromosomes and other genetic material at the egg stage of human development rather than correct a difficult defect after birth.

Maybe we are ultimately looking for help in all the wrong places.

I don't pretend to know the answers to the ethical questions about lifespan extension and genetic selection using these increasingly advanced and soon-available genetic interventions. I do know that both you and I can grow into more loving, kind, considerate, wholesome, compassionate, consciously conscientious human beings. I do know that we can truly help ourselves, our partners, our families, our friends, our community, our country, our Earth—one person at a time. Create your own clear vision!

20

TEN TIPS FOR LIVING LONGER AND HEALTHIER—NOW

1. Maintain an Anabolic Survival Advantage

You have a natural cellular repair system called an anabolic drive, which continuously regenerates healthy cellular structures and tissues if all the parts of the bioenergetic whole food are eaten.

Anabolic Capacity
(eating bioenergetic whole foods)
+
Anabolic Regulatory Hormones
(insulin, testosterone, estrogen
growth hormone, thyroid)

=

Anabolic Drive
(cellular regeneration,
restoration and revitalization)

If your body spends less time in an anabolic state and moves toward entropy, a state of cellular hormonal dysfunction and metabolic disrepair that leads to rapid accelerated aging, it moves into a catabolic drive. Your goal is to remain primarily in an anabolic drive and build up an anabolic reserve by "eating smart" and promoting anabolic hormonal fidelity and balance.

The downward spiraling decline from a vital anabolic drive to a catabolic drive begins at age 25 and is at only 15–20 percent by the time we are 70.

You must conscientiously remove both the internal and external catabolic (accelerated aging) factors from your life and environment.

2. Timing Is Everything

Anabolic capacity and anabolic drive are both at their maximum levels when all your body's hormones are in supersymmetry (balance) and at their peak levels.

Most people do not realize how immediate the food–mood connection is! What you ate at your last meal or snack, prior to reading these words, is having a profound hormonal effect directly upon your present mood, energy, clarity of thinking and emotional stability.

Big "hits" of insulin from eating refined or processed foods full of fat, salt, sugar or an artificial sweetener throw your balanced hormonal state out of whack. When you eat excess simple or refined carbohydrates, such as chips, pop, bread, muffins, pies, cakes, cookies, candies, beer, alcohol, chocolate bars, gum, etc., you trigger excess insulin production that shuts down growth hormone (GH) and you go through mood swings. Meanwhile, cortisol levels (stress hormone) increase as insulin increases and your internal biochemistry ages quickly with these elevated hormones.

I highly recommend that you eat three well-planned meals and two snacks each and every day, never going more than 3 1/2 hours between eating. Balance your carbohydrate intake by eating more lean protein at each of your meals as this will regulate your insulin swings—modifying your internal stress by reducing cortisol levels and keeping your serotonin (feel good) hormones balanced and your dopamine (full alert) hormones balanced. A smart breakfast should be a power protein shake using the most bioavailable advanced protein—99 percent undenatured whey protein isolate powder.

You must get a minimum of 8.25 hours of sleep in a dark environment each night, going to sleep as soon as possible after the sun sets to produce growth hormone (GH), which revitalizes, repairs or renews each of your cells in a deep sleep state.

Never eat food, especially "sweet treat" carbohydrates, after 7:30 p.m., as you will increase insulin and cortisol levels (accelerate aging) and not produce sufficient growth hormone, whose job it is to slow down premature aging and keep you in a revitalizing anabolic drive.

The Food Connection is not a diet—it is a life-long hormonal control program.

3. Eat Bioenergetic Whole Foods

The earth naturally produces all sorts of healing bioenergetic foods. Bioenergetic foods are plant-based foods grown under the direct energy pathway of the sun and equally infused with the energies of the soil and rain. They convert their energy (energetic) to the efficient and effective biological (bio) rejuvenation and revitalization of every cell in your body. They promote "high-fidelity" hormone communication in supersymmetry, so they can instantaneously turn any chemical relay system "on" or "off." Hormones left to run at random create senseless chemical reactions that put your symmetry dangerously "out of order."

Bioenergetic whole foods are natural, unrefined foods, such as colourful vegetables, herbs, ripe fruits, berries, whole grains, beans, nuts, seeds, pollen, sea vegetables, and alfalfa, barley and wheat grasses. You may also consume them indirectly by eating the fish, chickens, animals or wild game that initially ate these bioenergetic whole foods.

Our "hunter-gatherer" ancestors developed sophisticated hormonal systems to send messages to instantaneously turn "on" or "off" any message relay system between the brain and the many various biochemical interactions in their bodies. Hormones such as testosterone, estrogen, DHEA, melatonin, cortisol, growth hormone (GH), dopamine and phosphatidyl choline developed and were based on the natural bioenergetic food chain. Today, these hormones are directly regulated by your diet and have the greatest effect on your healthy survival if you can optimize their performance with bioenergetic whole foods.

4. Protect Yourself From Premature Aging

Researchers worldwide have recently discovered that all bioenergetic fruits, vegetables, whole grains, herbs, nuts, seeds and sea vegetables contain unique groups of health-promoting nutrients called phytonutrients. We estimate that there are 30,000 to 50,000 bio-dynamic phytonutrients in plants, though only 1,000 of these have been isolated so far, and only about 100 of these disease-preventing plant compounds have been analyzed.

Phytonutrients may prevent elusive, age-related illnesses, such as heart disease and cancer. Phytonutrients have two cancer-preventing mechanisms. The first is that they block the **initiation** of the cancer process and the second is that they suppress the **promotion** of cells already initiated into the cancer growth process. Phytonutrients, with rigorous precision, help to keep you disease and stress free, abundantly adding to your anabolic capacity.

Phytonutrients are powerful enough to:
- seek out,
- confront,
- destroy and
- eliminate

  yeast, bacteria, viruses, fungi, parasites and carcinogens from each of your 100 trillion cells. They are toxic garbage cops guaranteed to keep you healthier and younger—longer.

Remember, phytonutrients come from the variety of colors found in fruits, vegetables, herbs and sea vegetables. Go out of your way to add color and flair to each meal. Eat a wide variety (up to 18 various colors each day) in your fruit and vegetable selections. "Color your plate" for great eye appeal and make your meals outrageously delicious. Pause before you eat, and be grateful for your food.

5. Adaptability

There is no need to flip-flop from diet to diet to diet. You must simply eat in harmony with your long-standing genetic predisposition to bioenergetic whole foods grown in Nature, and eaten in sync with your daily and seasonal circadian rhythms.

You need to have great adaptability to survive successfully and do what no generation before you has done—live longer and healthier.

6. Rejuvenate and Revitalize With Deep Sleep

We are the "great unslept." Loss of sleep has been shown in recent research to have a cumulative negative effect on the overall outcome of your vital hormones, critical neurotransmitters, functional energy, sharp mental acuity and an efficient, responsive immune surveillance.

Please note, it is only—I want to repeat it—it is only in the dark cycle (night) of the daily circadian rhythm that you replenish your energy reserves, renew and repair muscle tissue, cleanse the brain of accumulated cellular debris and revitalize your immune system. Keep your immune system revitalized and it will reward you by keeping you alive!

Your nightly sleep quota as an adult is between 8.25 and nine hours each and every night. Your children require nine to ten hours a night. Sleep is not a waste of time. For deep, rejuvenating sleep you must sleep in as complete darkness as possible, with no light contamination from lighted alarm clocks, night lights, blinking lights on TVs or VCRs or light coming through the windows.

Try to go to bed and rise at the same time each night and day. Take all stress out of the bedroom. In the summer try to go to sleep by 10:30 p.m. and in the winter by 9:30 p.m., whenever possible.

Do not eat, especially high-density carbohydrate foods, after 7:30 p.m., as these foods raise your insulin levels for four full hours and prevent the critical synthesis of the hormone melatonin, which is needed for deep sleep, as well as being a cancer protector, and is secreted about 1 1/2 hours after you go to sleep. It also reduces the production of growth hormone (secreted two hours after initial melatonin secretion and vital, as your "youth hormone," for burning fat and building lean muscle mass, as well as rejuvenating all your 100 trillion cells).

An accumulated loss of sleep is the number one factor in your premature aging and is also implicated in all degenerative diseases, such as cancer. Lose sleep and you fall out of rhythm with nature, which causes an early extinction event, even if it is by your very own hands.

7. The Most Powerful Drink for a More Vital You

After oxygen, water is the second most important nutrient in your body. Women's bodies are composed of about 63 to 65 percent water and men's bodies about 68 percent. Water is critical to maintaining an anabolic drive and for your optimal survival advantage.

You may often misinterpret thirst signals as hunger signs and eat when you really should be drinking the powerful revitalizer, pure H_2O.

The average body contains 95 to 96 pints of water, 65 pints inside your cells and the remainder outside your cells. Your body's critical water supply is the only fluid responsible for and involved in regulating every biological process, especially synthesizing hormones, neurotransmitters and maintaining ultimate mental acuity, body balance and supersymmetry—homeostatis.

You require six to 12 8-oz glasses of water a day. Do not wait to drink your water quota for the day all at once. Prehydrate by drinking water every one or two hours. Your skin is 80 percent water. The most important cosmetic help you can give yourself to successfully promote a clear, smooth, soft, radiant complexion is to drink, throughout the day, clean, pure water. To know if you are drinking enough water, simply monitor the color of your urine. If your urine is pale yellow to clear throughout the day you are consuming enough water to satisfy your body's requirements.

Drink your water from a closed container and through a straw to avoid excess air and prevent bloating.

8. Fats for a Sharp Brain and a Strong Heart

Consume your necessary fats on a daily basis, especially the Omega-3 essential fatty acid derivatives DHA/EPA and the Omega-6 essential fatty acid derivative gamma linolenic acid (GLA). The three best sources of GLA are borage seed oil (23 percent), followed by black currant seed oil (15-18 percent) and evening primrose seed oil (8-12 percent). I recommend that you use 1/2 teaspoon of borage oil daily.

You want to consume 1,000 mg of EPA and 650 mg of DHA daily. Good sources are high DHA/EPA cod liver oil, two to four fish oil capsules or four to nine algae oil capsules. Cold-water fish, such as herring, mackerel, anchovies, salmon, sardines, trout and albacore tuna, are the richest sources of DHA/EPA. All sea algae such as chlorella, Nova Scotia dulse and spirulina are also excellent sources. You need to eat the algae daily or eat at least three servings of one of the above fish weekly, preferably broiled, since you want to eat these necessary and good fats.

In addition, I highly recommend that you consume 1 tablespoon of one of: flax seed, hemp seed or perilla seed oil, or grind 2 tablespoons of their fresh seeds in a coffee grinder and add to your power protein shake each morning. Furthermore, add 1 tablespoon of extra virgin olive oil to your salad each day for its oleic acid content. Olive oil is a hormonally neutral Omega-9 fat.

Omega-3 EFAs and Omega-6 EFAs are absolutely necessary for superior neurological processes, intelligence, memory, hormone synthesis, central nervous system coordination, cell wall development and cardiovascular health.

9. For Optimum Vim and Vigor, Exercise Regularly

As you age, beginning at about age 30, you lose lean body mass and gain fat in its place. Proper exercise can actually reverse all the biomarkers of aging.

Aerobic activity, such as walking, bicycling, rowing, treadmill, swimming, dancing, Tai Chi, hatha yoga, stairmaster, etc., allows you to burn calories very efficiently and expel carbon dioxide from your lungs and breathe in fresh oxygen supplies to the deep (generally unused) recesses of your lungs. Aerobic (using oxygen) activity stimulates vital blood flow to all of your 100 trillion cells, promoting nutrient delivery and efficient waste removal.

Anaerobic (without oxygen) activity, such as weight training, causes you to gain lean muscle mass and is one of your most critical tools in achieving and maintaining a young biological age, much younger than your chronological age.

Proper daily activity is necessary to allow for your maximum anti-aging hormonal release. You need to be involved in daily activity for a minimum of 30 minutes or more to burn 300 calories, which will extend your healthy life. Quadralateral movement, such as brisk walking, is a biological miracle for stimulating your internal organs and glands, as well as for promoting efficient, regular bowel movements. I recommend 45 to 60 minutes of exercise four times a week. In a 45-minute session, do 15 minutes of aerobics, 25 minutes of weight training and five minutes of stretching. In a 60-minute session, do 15 minutes of aerobics, 25 minutes of weight training, 15 minutes of aerobics and five minutes of stretching.

Ideally, you should do your preferred activity in the morning, which raises your resting metabolism rate (RMR) so you burn extra calories for a full 12 hours after your activity. In order to keep yourself strong, flexible, agile and independent well into your 90s, 100s, 110s or beyond, keep your body well toned and in a constant anabolic environment.

In his book *The Antioxidant Revolution*, Kenneth Cooper, the promoter of aerobic activity, comes to a startling conclusion: "No pain, no gain" is not true, but "steady low-threshold activity can produce enormous longevity gains." Be moderate, but consistent.

10. Smart Network Supplementation—Your Life Insurance Policy

You originated from a single cell, which combined the unique genetic message from your mother's ovum and your father's sperm. These genes have been passed down from your hunter-gatherer ancestors.

Your genetic inheritance, your gene pool, is called your "genome." Your genetic inheritance, plus your lifestyle and diet, is called your "phenotype."

We now know that about 15 percent of any premature aging or age-related disease is related to a weakness in your "genome." That means that 85 percent of all biological aging or disease states can be brought on or eliminated by your choice of lifestyle and diet by giving you a stronger, or weaker, "phenotype."

You can modify your genes for better energy, clearer skin, better metabolic function and a vigorous immune system by "eating smart" and supplementing your diet with phytonutrients, antioxidants, medicinal herbs, vitamins and minerals.

In our busier-is-better lifestyle of this modern era—where we push our bodies to a new 24-7-365 pace—proper supplementation is absolutely necessary to function mentally, physically and emotionally at optimum levels.

Lester Packer, Ph.D., and co-author Carol Colman, in their ground-breaking book *The Antioxidant Miracle*, state that it is not a single antioxidant, phytonutrient or vitamin, but the entire "network" that produces the manifold effects of preventing or reversing disease. The "network" of nutrients reverses your declining catabolic drive and reinstates your regenerative anabolic drive. As a "network," each nutrient actually significantly boosts and regenerates the level of effectiveness of every other nutrient.

I highly recommend that you supplement daily with the following smart "network" nutrients:

- A high-quality "green drink" containing the six glutathione-boosting sub-network of antioxidants and phytonutrients from the water-extracted herbs: full-spectrum grape, European bilberry, Japanese green tea, Siberian ginseng, milk thistle extract and ginkgo biloba extract.
- A vitamin C complex of calcium ascorbate with bioflavonoids (500 mg to 5 g daily).
- A vitamin A complex of alpha-carotene, beta-carotene, lycopene, crytoxanthin, zeaxanthin and luten (two softgels daily).
- A vitamin B complex with 50 mg of each B vitamin, 1 mg of folic acid and 60 mcg of biotin (one capsule with breakfast, one with lunch).
- A vitamin E (400–1,200 IU daily) of the easy-to-absorb form d-alpha tocopheryl succinate and also a capsule of the other vitamin E subfractions, beta, delta and gamma tocopheryls or tocopherols. Use 400 IU at each meal.
- Vitamin D3 (1,000 IU) in the months when you do not get sunlight on your skin. Sunlight increases the production of l-alpha 25-hydroxyvitamin D3 in the colon, which, along with the enzyme l-alpha-hydroxylase, prevents cancer cell initiation or promotion in your colon. Sunscreens prevent sunburn, but also prevent vitamin D3 formation by sunlight.
- Full-spectrum grape extract with 95 percent procyanidolic value, 463 ppm resveratrol and 200 ppm ellagic acid (two a day: one at breakfast and one at lunch).
- After 40 years of age, use two broad-range, plant-based digestive enzymes at the beginning of each meal.
- Use three capsules of A•G•E inhibitors™ daily to prevent advanced glycated end products from damaging your brain, heart, cell walls and mitochondria.
- Use four capsules of protect+, the most advanced "network" of synergistic antioxidants, phytonutrients, standardized herbs, vitamins and amino acids. Take one with each meal and one before sleep.
- Use 50 to 300 mg of CoEnzyme Q10 (CoQ10) each day when you take your oil, as it is fat soluble.

- Take two capsules a day of L. acidophilus and B. bifidum and other "friendly bacteria" in a base of 200 mg of FOS. You may choose to use an enteric-coated capsule for better delivery to the small intestine or one container of BioK+ with the CL1285 strain of acidophilus.
- Use three capsules of the potent immune builder, Moducare, at about 8:00 p.m.
- Use 2 scoops (30 grams of protein) of Alphapure™ whey protein isolate powder (as found in transform+ and proteins+) in your protein power shake each morning for the highest biological value protein in the world that contains powerful subfractions, such as lactoferrin, immunoglobulins and alpha-lactalbumin, to fully energize your immune system.
- Use a high-quality multimineral supplement plus silica, half with supper and half before sleep.

NOTE: Take a high-quality "green drink," such as greens+, before breakfast and again at about 3:00 p.m. to prevent the afternoon doldrums, to maintain robust energy, and to boost your mental acuity, attention span and good mood.

Many supplements, such as vitamins B, C and alpha lipoic acid, are water soluble and stay active in the bloodstream for only three to four hours. Vitamins A, E and CoQ10 are fat soluble and must be taken at a meal that contains fats such as flax or hemp oil, extra virgin olive oil, nuts, seeds, animal-based protein or fish oil supplements. Alpha lipoic acid is both fat and water soluble.

Vitamins are enzymatic initiators and must be taken with breakfast and lunch. Antioxidants should be taken with each meal and before sleep. Minerals are constructive and need to be taken half at supper and half before sleep.

Do not take your supplement quota all at one time each day. For a steady supply of nutrients to your 100 trillion cells and for homeostasis (biochemical balance), I highly recommend that you take your supplement quota spread out between your three meals and before sleep. This is "smart" supplementing.

Powerful herbal supplements or teas should be taken before breakfast, between meals, before sleep or when you awake after several hours of sleep to go to the washroom.

EPILOGUE

THE POWER OF CHANGE

I would like to briefly share a story about my father's passing on to illustrate how I would hope we should all pass on.

Before the age of 85, my father, whom his family and many friends affectionately called "Papa Joe," surpassed his total load capacity of cumulative toxic damage and became critically ill. He had 22 inches of his descending colon removed from cancer, had arthritis in his knees, and was hard of hearing and had advanced cataracts. Up to this point he had felt invincible. Papa Joe, at 84, made drastic changes in his lifestyle and diet. He full-heartedly lived and ate by the recommendations in this book. These changes were so powerful and decisive that he fully revived his health. His hair grew in thicker, 60 percent of the black color returned, the cancer was neutralized and the arthritis subsided.

Papa Joe's facial skin became taut, clear and radiant. He began to sing and dance because he had such robust energy and deep unassisted sleep. From 85 to 94, Papa Joe had brilliant health, the best decade of his life. He became a crusader to enlighten seniors about the possibility and the power of change. Papa Joe began at 85 with serious ailments, and look at his results. Imagine if you *really* begin before this. At 94, the cancer in his liver was bringing the vibrant chapter of his life to an end.

Surrounded by his loving children, grandchildren and great grandchildren, as well as wonderful neighbours and friends, he spent his last month of life at home. He was not feeling well for a month, was ill for a week and very ill for one day. He was alert, conscious, loving, accepting and totally present. I am so very blessed to have spent 24 hours a day with him for that month.

As Papa Joe passed on, he gently placed my hand on his heart, raised his arms and shouted, "I am ready to go home, I want to go now, I took good care of Grace, (my mother), I love all my children equally, I want to go home now, take me home Mother." He pulled me to his chest, we embraced in great celebration, he called out again, "I Love You God, I Love You God, I Love You God," and he exquisitely expired, so calmly and joyously—elegantly passing beyond the shores of life.

Papa Joe provides an example of a diet combined with a low-caloric, but bioenergetic nutrient-rich dietary strategy. I stand by the conviction that his passing on was in rhythm with his faith, lifestyle and diet. Perhaps for the majority of people this model of being not well for a month, ill for a week and very ill for one day should be the norm. The majority of you should not languish in seniors' homes with an ever-increasing litany of ailments that continue to escalate—alone and isolated.

Papa Joe began in earnest, he got in hormonal sync, with two strikes against him at 84 years of age. Imagine if you started earlier. What then would be your rewards and results? *The Food Connection* is not a diet—it is a lifelong hormonal control program. The time is now to stand up and be counted. A good start would be to incorporate, slowly or quickly, the recommendations in this book into your daily lifestyle and dietary strategy with balance and moderation. Either you are a "tip-toer" or "plunger."

You're saying, "Yeah, but this will upset my habits, lifestyle and social life." True—but cancer, strokes and heart attacks will probably upset them a heck of lot more! Remember, the addition or omission of a single nutrient in your diet can make or break your immune response, attention span, learning capability, mental acuity, deep sleep and vibrant energy.

All of us must be continually adaptable to ignite a longer, more fruitful life where optimum mental, emotional, physical and spiritual health exists. It has always been about adaptability; it is about adaptability and will always be about adaptability.

Today, genetics and lifestyle are colliding. Can you be creatively adaptable? If you can, your immune system will thank you by keeping you alive. You need to have great adaptability to survive successfully and do what no generation before you has done—live longer and healthier. Remember that the environment—through food, water, light, oxygen and stress—flips switches "on" or "off" to produce hormones, which in turn flip other switches for growth, repair or death. You are one with the dynamics of the ecosystem, an integral part of it.

We now have to adapt to our new potentiality and knowledge. We may, indeed, be on the verge of creating a new type of human being—hopefully, a better type. We are creatively adaptable beings who can create by adapting ourselves anew, under novel conditions. We will do it—and if our enquiring minds earnestly seek the Truth from the illuminating light of wider vistas, then, who knows, perhaps the Truth will set us all free.

The words of J.W. Goethe echo in my ears:

> *What you can do, or*
> *Dream you can do, begin it.*
> *Boldness has genius, power and magic in it.*
> *Only engage, and then*
> *The mind grows heartened.*
> *Begin it, and the work will be completed.*

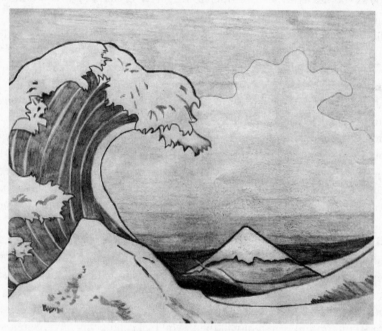

(Illus. by Karen Corley)

APPENDIX A

ONE IMMUNE ORGAN TO KEEP PRISTINE

---

1. Your blood absorbs vitamins, minerals, antioxidants, phytonutrients, fat, protein, carbohydrates and water through a network of blood vessels that wrap around the stomach, small intestine and colon. These very sensitive blood vessels absorb dissolved nutrients out of the intestines. They are transported to the liver, via the portal vein ("door to the liver").

2. The portal vein carries nutrients (from the Latin *nutrire*, meaning "to keep alive" or "to feed well") to the liver where they are further broken down, recombined and given an electrical charge to promote cellular recognition and absorption.

3. Your heart pumps these nutrients from the liver to your 100 trillion cells.

4. Your bloodstream delivers nutrients, mostly carried on the albumin-transporting molecule, to each cell, and after unloading nutrients the bloodstream loads up cellular waste from the byproduct of cellular metabolism and safely delivers wastes to the elimination stations of the colon, kidney, lungs or skin where they are excreted.

5. It is fiber that literally soaks up the waste, binds it and eliminates it safely from the small intestine or colon. For superior inner hygiene, keep your intestinal tract clean with many sources of soluble and insoluble fiber.

6. Clean water and 40 grams of fiber a day from bioenergetic whole foods gently sweep out your intestinal "garbage disposal" system daily to:
   a) eliminate waste quickly before it can putrefy, harden and block the "portals of entry" to the nutrient-absorbing blood vessels; and
   b) promote proper bowel transit times (BTT); waste products that are not eliminated quickly will literally begin putrefying—giving off toxins and polluting the colon—while they remain stagnant in the intestinal tract.

These toxins, such as mucus or fecal matter, reabsorb into the body causing toxic overload, accelerated aging and chronic disease.

7. A healthy intestinal tract is critical for it is also an immune system organ, the site of 70 percent of all your body's immune defense system. Gut-associated lymphoid tissue (GALT) is a specialized tissue surrounding the intestinal lining.

   GALT tissues produce antibody proteins that roam your bloodstream to destroy infections, bacteria, viruses, parasites, fungi and carcinogens. The GALT secretions destroy toxins in your stomach and intestines that enter your body daily through your food, beverage and water intake.

8. The small intestine and the large intestine (colon) are the home to many "friendly bacteria" that help to thoroughly digest the food you consume and, in concert with GALT, destroy invading toxins and pathogens. These friendly bacteria are called Lactobacilli casei, plantarum, rhamnosus, acidophilus, bifidobacteria bifidum, breve and longum.

   They adhere to the mucosal lining in the small intestine and on the colonocytes—special cells in the large intestine designed for the purpose of clearing body waste and preventing autointoxication of stagnant fecal matter or toxins.

HEALTHY INNER ECOLOGY

Smart Support for Your Gastrointestinal Tract (GIT)

- Exercise three to four times a week in a gym doing both aerobic and anaerobic movements. Try to walk briskly, daily for 30 minutes. Both of these strategies massage and promote a flexible GIT to keep it healthy and clean.
- Use a high-quality "green drink" once or twice a day to receive billions of non-dairy probiotic (meaning "in favor of life") bacterial cultures in a base of special food they consume called FOS (fructo-oligo-saccharides). "Green drinks" set the proper pH in the intestinal tract and supply deodorizing chlorophyll. Chlorophyll, formed by sunlight in the process of photosynthesis, is the green pigment in vegetation that destroys viruses, bacteria and fungi in the GIT. Chlorophyll is antiseptic. "Green drinks" should also contain a non-GMO, organic phosphatidyl complex of phosphatidyl choline (PC) and phosphatidyl serine (PS) that ignites the process of peristalsis (the rhythm of contraction and expansion of the muscle lining around the intestines that quickly and safely moves waste products out of the body). Both PC and PS are fundamentally needed to make the neurotransmitters critical for good memory and abstract thinking.
- Use a non-dairy encapsulated supplement of L. acidophilus and B. bifidum and other "friendly bacteria" in a base of 200 mg of FOS in your power protein shake to keep the 350 to 400 strains of gastrointestinal flora living in your GIT repopulated. L. acidophilus is the primary beneficial bacteria in the small intestine, while B. bifidum is the major bacteria of the large intestine. You may choose to use an enteric-coated capsule that passes undigested through the acids in the stomach and may help "friendly bacteria" to be

absorbed better in the small intestine. A fiber called arabinogalactan, which naturally occurs in fruits and vegetables such as carrots and tomatoes, is called a probiotic, as beneficial bacteria appear to preferentially feed off of arabinogalactans.

- Consume 1 cup of fat-free, organic plain yogurt daily or 3.5 oz (100 g) of the potent Bio-K+ with the CL1285 strain of acidophilus.
- Consume 40 grams of soluble and insoluble fiber daily from a large variety of colourful bioenergetic whole foods to scrub clean your "garbage disposal" system.
- Use two cloves of garlic finely chopped, or four capsules of a garlic supplement, with fat-free organic yogurt or Bio-K+, with 1/2 tablespoon of high-lignan, organic flax seed or hemp seed oil before going to sleep to kill pathogens in your GIT.
- Sublingually take between 5 to 10 grams of the tasteless and easily dissolved amino acid glutamine before you go to sleep. Glutamine provides energy for the intestines where it also helps to control fluid loss and strengthens the mucosal lining. It also fuels the activity of the colonocyte cells in the large intestine that clear body waste out of the large intestine (colon).
- In your vegetable selection, choose bitter vegetables such as kale, Swiss chard, mustard greens, arugula, watercress, red beets, escarole, endive, commercial dandelions, beet tops and parsley, which promote the growth of probiotic "friendly bacteria."
- The photoelectric cryptochrome cells on your skin, which monitor the circadian rhythm and the amounts of photons of direct light you are exposed to, are in direct communication with the bacteria in your gastrointestinal tract. Every hormone has its origin here and is eventually synthesized in the "control center" in the hypothalamus-pituitary axis of the brain.

It is in deep sleep when your core temperature drops and your body is in an anabolic restorative state that the GIT cleanses, heals, rejuvenates and replenishes itself. For this critical restorative process to happen, you must get 8.25 to 8.5 hours of sleep each and every night. Be sure your deep sleep is in utter darkness with no light contamination.

Furthermore, it is only in the anabolic early phases of deep sleep (stages 3 and 4), just before REM sleep (rapid eye movement) when you dream, that the "youth hormone," growth hormone (GH), is synthesized and secreted from the pituitary gland in spurts.

- Drink your water quota of six to 12 glasses of clean water a day. Drink more if you exercise or work in an environment where you perspire. The water washes toxins and cellular debris out of the intestinal tract and keeps the delicate mucosal lining moist, as well as flexible.
- Once or twice a week drink 2 tablespoons of aloe vera gel in 4 oz (125 mL) of water to reduce any inflammation in the GIT. Ginger (the oils called

gingerols) is also very anti-inflammatory, so use it liberally in cooking. Additionally, ginger tones the circulatory system and has anti-cancer effects, blocking the ability of some carcinogens to cause mutations in the DNA.

- The liver is the largest internal organ in our body. It is the primary pathway for removing metabolic wastes and toxins. To keep your liver functioning smoothly, I recommend detoxifying it every six months with a liver and gallbladder flush. This will help the intestinal tract to function at full capacity.

  Dr. Robert Atkins' book *Dr. Atkins' Age-Defying Diet* and Dr. Hulda Clarke's book *The Cure for All Diseases* both explain a liver and gallbladder cleanse step-by-step.

- Once a year, consider doing a "spring cleaning" of the colon and receive a professional colonic; or do a similar colon cleanse at home on your own.

  During the course of a lifetime, you consume—and the gastrointestinal tract processes—more than 25 tons of food. In a compromised gastrointestinal environment, with impaired digestion or increased intestinal permeability, significantly more problems with "leaky gut" syndrome or problems with indigestion and severe food allergens will be aggravated.

APPENDIX B

MITOCHONDRIA AND PROTEIN INTEGRITY HOLD THE KEY TO CELLULAR LIFE AND DEATH

Australian scientist Anthony Linnane, Ph.D., began observing that mutations accumulate in mitochondrial DNA as humans age. A decline in the capacity of a cell to generate energy and respond to stress leads to disease and biological degeneration.

Mitochondria are the power plants of the cell. They transform oxygen and nutrients into energy and water through a process called cellular respiration. There are hundreds of mitochondria in a typical cell. Each contains a unique form of DNA inherited from the mother alone. However, recent research points to the mitochondria as the crucial targets of oxidative stress (excess free radicals) and as regulators of cell death.

According to Linnane's theory, as defects accumulate in mitochondrial DNA, cellular energy goes into a rapidly declining catabolic deterioration.

In the 1990s, Linnane discovered a way to restore cellular vitality by improving energy production and resistance to stress in cells without intact mitochondrial DNA.

Each species of mammal has a known Maximum Lifespan Potential (MLSP). Anthony Linnane's theory suggests that the MLSP of each species corresponds to the level of a free radical called **superoxide**. Superoxide is a free radical formed from oxygen, especially when electrons leak out of mitochondria in the cellular respiration chain, when energy is being produced. The lower the mitochondrial superoxide level in a given species, the longer the species lives. While this does

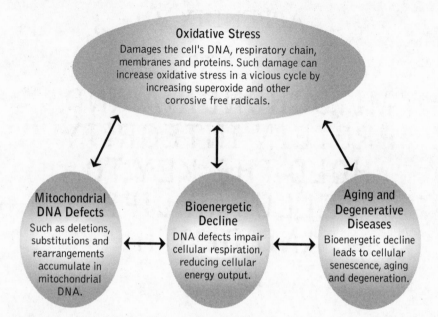

Adapted from the work of Anthony Linnane, Ph.D., and *Life Extension Magazine*, February, 2001.

not necessarily mean that superoxide is a direct cause of aging, it does open up some fascinating lines of inquiry.

In mammals, CoQ10 exists alongside the related form CoQ9. The proportions of CoQ10 and CoQ9 vary greatly among species. For example, mice and rats have mostly CoQ9, while humans have mostly CoQ10 in heart cell mitochondria.

Antioxidant researchers Rajindar Sohal, Ph.D., Achim Lass, Ph.D., and their colleagues discovered that the higher the proportion of CoQ9 in a species, the more superoxide is generated in its heart mitochondria. As Sohal and Lass wrote in 1997, this finding is "consistent with the speculative notion that longevity co-evolved with a relative increase in the amounts of CoQ10." In other words, the evolution of longer lifespan in mammals such as humans is connected with the evolution of higher proportions of CoQ10. This is a thought-provoking hypothesis. You make endogenous CoQ10 in your cells but from the age of 35 onward, your production of CoQ10 declines yearly and the spiralling decline mirrors the catabolic aging cycle.

Finally, Anthony W. Linnane and fellow researchers wrote in 1998:

Dietary supplementation with coenzyme Q10 is thus indicated as a treatment to improve the quality of life of aging individuals and to provide protection against age-related conditions such as heart failure and neurodegenerative diseases.

He writes that CoQ10 operates at three levels to slow down the bioenergetic decline:

CoQ10 protects mitochondria DNA and the cellular respiratory chain from oxidative damage from superoxide and other free radicals.

CoQ10 enhances cellular respiration, drawing maximum performance from aging mitochondria.

CoQ10 fuels an alternative energy source in the cell called glycolysis. Glycolysis produces energy directly from glucose which helps compensate for declining cellular respiration.

PROGRAMMED CELL DEATH

When cellular energy production declines in a mild, gradual way, cells adapt to produce energy through compensatory systems such as glycolysis. However, when cellular energy levels drop more sharply, cells activate a process called "programmed cell death," also called apoptosis. Programmed cell death dismantles the cell in an orderly way, with minimal damage to surrounding tissues.

Linnane proposed that programmed cell death by energy-starved cells figures prominently in the pathology of age-associated disorders such as heart disease, cancer and neurodegeneration. It is now established that mitochondria regulate the process of programmed cell death. The mitochondrial "decision to die" appears to spring largely from bioenergetic energy failure and oxidative stress that opens the mitochondrial "mega-channel" (also called the permeability transition pore, or PTP) that sets in motion the self-destruction of the cell. Anthony Linnane, Ph.D., and F. Rosenfeldt, Ph.D., demonstrated that supplemental CoQ10 restores vitality, energy and stress recovery in aged heart tissue to youthful levels. Mitochondrial aging depletes vitality—but mitochondrial rejuvenation with a synergistic antioxidant formula and CoQ10 may help to restore it.

WHEN CELLULAR ENERGY DECLINES

When the mega-channel or the PTP opens, the mitochondrial membrane becomes highly permeable and loses its electrical charge. According to the research of Dr. Seamus J. Martin (a professor of medical genetics at Smurfit Institute, Trinity College, in Dublin, Ireland), Cytochrome c, a cell death-promoting factor from the mitochondria inner membrane space, is released into the cytoplasm where it is bound to a caspase-activating protein, Apaf-1, which triggers a self-destructive cascade. When this happens in large enough proportions of the cell's mitochondria, the cell cannot survive. This process can lead to either programmed cell death, or to the more destructive cell death pathway called necrosis. What determines whether the mega-channel opens and which path the dying cell takes?

We now know that programmed cell death is controlled by the mitochondria. It is believed that when a sudden bioenergetic catastrophe opens the mega-channel before the cell can adapt, the cell undergoes explosive necrotic death. On the other hand, when the mega-channel opens gradually over a sufficient period of time, an orderly programmed cellular entropy process unfolds instead.

A binding site for the CoQ10 family of compounds has been shown to regulate the opening of the mega-channel in rat liver and muscle cells. Moreover, ground-breaking new laboratory research shows that supplemental CoQ10 directly inhibits the opening of the mega-channel.

I firmly believe that a dietary strategy based on bioenergetic whole foods; clean water; stress management and reduction; exercise; avoiding processed "foods" and smoking; minimizing alcohol; as well as the proactive approach of using antioxidants, especially Coenzyme Q10, prevents degradation of cellular respiration and allows the cell to function and live longer at optimal well-being. It also prevents age-involution and promotes immunological responsiveness.

CELLULAR SELF-DESTRUCTION

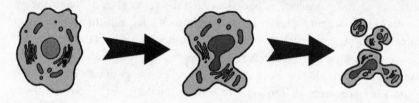

Programmed cell death is a well-orchestrated process of cellular self-destruction. As the cell shrinks and then fragments, its organelles remain relatively intact and enclosed by membranes. Neighboring cells or macrophages safely digest the fragments.

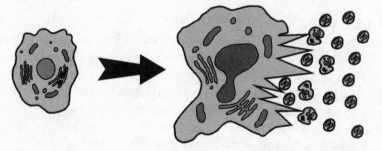

In necrotic cell death, the mitochondria swells to form a "mega-mitochondria" and the permeability transition pore (PTP), referred to as the megachannel, bursts open violently, ruptures, spewing cellular debris and causing the organelles to disintegrate.

Source: Adapted from Adachi, K. et al., 1995 and *Life Extension Magazine* February 2001.

CELLULAR PROTEIN INTEGRITY

Every one of your cells contains carnosine, a multifunctional dipeptide protein made up of a chemical combination of the amino acids beta-alanine and l-histidine. Long-lived cells such as nerve cells (neurons) and muscle cells (myocytes) contain high levels of carnosine.

Laboratory research on cellular senescence (the end of the life cycle of dividing cells) demonstrates that carnosine has the remarkable ability to rejuvenate cells approaching senescence, restoring normal appearance and extending cellular lifespan.

The body is made up largely of proteins. Unfortunately, proteins tend to undergo destructive changes as we age, due largely to oxidation and interactions with sugars and aldehydes. These interrelated protein modifications include oxidation, glycation, cross-linking, carbonylation, and advanced glycation end product (AGE) formation. They figure prominently not only in the process of aging but also by accumulation in proteins, causing the familiar signs such as skin aging, wrinkling, sagging skin and loss of elasticity, brown spots on skin, cataracts and neurodegeneration. Studies show that carnosine is effective against all these forms of protein modification. In fact, carnosine is the only antioxidant to significantly protect chromosomes from oxidative damage due to 90 percent oxygen exposure.

In a remarkable series of experiments, the Australian researchers Dr. G. McFarland and Dr. R. Holliday have shown that carnosine rejuvenates cells as they approach senescence. These scientists cultured human fibroblasts (connective tissue cells) from the lung and the foreskin. Fibroblasts that went through many rounds of division, known as late-passage cells, displayed a disorganized, irregular appearance before ceasing to divide. Fibroblasts cultured with carnosine lived longer and retained youthful appearance and growth patterns.

What is most exciting is the ability of carnosine to reverse the signs of aging in cells approaching senescence. When scientists transferred late-passage fibroblasts to a culture medium containing carnosine, the fibroblasts exhibited a rejuvenated appearance and often an enhanced capacity to divide, thus preventing programmed cell death (by keeping the mega-channel closed) and necrotic cell death (by protecting the cell's DNA and chromosomes). The carnosine medium also increased lifespan, even for old cells. The number of population doublings (PDs) provides a convenient measure of cell division.

When late-passage lung fibroblasts at 55 PDs were transferred to the carnosine medium, they lived to 69 to 70 PDs, compared to 57 to 61 PDs for the fibroblasts that were not transferred. Moreover, the fibroblasts transferred to the carnosine medium attained an average lifespan of 413 days, compared to 126 to 139 days for the control fibroblasts.

Modified proteins accumulate as we age, while carnosine levels decline. Once a protein is modified, it has lost its ability to function normally, and when a significant portion of the body's protein has reached this point, the body becomes prone to age-related degenerative diseases, CoQ10 levels decline—and the mega-channels open.

The tell-tale sign of destructive protein modification is the protein carbonyl group. Accumulation of proteins with carbonyl groups is a molecular indicator of cell aging. In humans, approximately 30 to 40 percent of all proteins become carbonylated in the age range from 50 to 75 years of age. Antioxidants do not slow down carbonyl groups, but the pluripotent carnosine does.

Brain aging and degeneration are marked by protein carbonylation, a major source of oxidative damage and cellular dysfunction with the oxidation of polyunsaturated lipids in the membranes of brain cells and their extensions such as axons. This chain reaction spreads oxidative damage and generates highly neurotoxic byproducts such as aldehydes, which are neutralized or "quenched" by carnosine.

Glycation and AGE Formation

One of the processes that carbonylates proteins, glycation is itself recognized as a major cause of aging and degenerative disease. Glycation occurs when proteins react with sugars. Then, through a series of reactions including oxidation, advanced glycated end products (aptly called AGEs) form.

AGEs accelerate the aging process and turn proteins brown, making them "sticky-gooey." This physically impairs the function of proteins, DNA and lipids, which can lead to blindness, cardiovascular disease, stroke and cancer. When AGEs attach to their cellular binding sites, they interfere with hormone fidelity, changing the cellular signals, triggering a cascade of destructive events that open the mega-channel. Carnosine is a natural anti-glycating agent. Studies in a wide variety of experimental models demonstrate that carnosine inhibits protein glycation and AGE formation, both of which grind your cell cycle to a halt. Carnosine is not presently available in Canada.

Another powerful, safe, synergistic and natural anti-glycating agent I highly recommend you use daily is the product, A•G•E inhibitors™. This is a remarkable formula, which in three capsules contains reduced glutathione, N-Acetyl-Cysteine, alpha lipoic acid, Alphapure™, lactoferrin, full-spectrum grape extract, thyme extract, turmeric extract, inositol, quercitin, aqueous extract of stinging nettle, ginger extract and the amino acid taurine.

Your main food source of carnosine is red meat and whey protein isolate powders. Since I recommend that you minimize or eliminate red meat, I strongly suggest that you use whey protein isolate powder daily in your power protein shake, and after the age of 40, supplement daily with three capsules of A•G•E inhibitors™ or 1,000 mg of carnosine. Your body produces an enzyme

that limits carnosine production called carnosinase enzyme. To derive carnosine's multiple benefits, you must take 1,000 mg to saturate carnosinase enzyme,
so as to make enough free carnosine available to the rest of your body to give
you a broad spectrum shield against protein degradation.

Once advanced glycation endproducts (AGEs) are formed by glucose-amino
acid complexes, they interact with neighboring proteins to permanently produce
pathological crosslinks that inhibit protein physiological function and restrict
protein's flexibility. The formation of AGE-crosslinks are non-enzymatic processes
and cannot be reversed by enzymes that disrupt protein bonds.

The rate of AGEs accumulation and the degree of stiffness they produce are
proportional to blood glucose levels and the length of time these levels persist.
It is therefore critical that you reduce or eliminate as many sugars, sweeteners
and artificial sweeteners from your dietary strategy as possible. Be vigilant!

It is interesting to note that the research company Alteon has developed a
new class of pharmaceutical compound called ALT-711 that inserts itself into
AGE crosslinks, separates and cleaves the linked molecules and releases the
proteins. ALT-711 reverses AGEs. ALT-711 has not yet been approved and is in
final clinical trials.

In conclusion, CoQ10 and carnosine production dramatically decline each
year after the age of 25. They are both implicated in cellular protein integrity
and in optimum mitochondrial well-being. CoQ10 and A•G•E inhibitors™ or
carnosine should be natural supplements after the age of 40. I would suggest
that you take three capsules of A•G•E inhibitors™ daily or 1,000 mg of carnosine with your power protein shake daily and age-relate your CoQ10 use. From
age 40 to 50 use 100 mg of CoQ10 daily, from 50 to 55 use 200 mg daily, and
from 55 onward use 300 mg of CoQ10 daily, especially when it is combined
with the vitamin-E-like subfractions from red palm oil—tocotrienols. For every
100 mg of pharmaceutical-grade Coenzyme Q10, make sure your supplement
contains 20 or more milligrams of tocotrienols from red palm oil. Red palm oil
is rich in carotenoids and tocotrienols and should not be confused with palm
kernel oil, which has a notably different profile and which I do not recommend
you ever use.

BIOENERGETIC FOODS FOR RADIANT SKIN AND HAIR

BIOENERGETIC FOODS FOR RADIANT SKIN

Thanks to recent breakthroughs in skin-care technology, you can restore a youthful tone and quality to your skin. The best part is that it won't take you more than a few minutes a day.

Skin Composition

Skin is very amazing. It's actually the body's largest organ, weighing 4 to 6 pounds (2 to 3 kg) and, if laid out flat, measures to an average of 20 square feet (1.8 square meters). A single square inch of skin contains about 19 feet of blood vessels, 19 million cells, 65 hairs, 620 sweat glands and about 90 oil glands, so there's a lot going on in your skin. Skin makes up 15 percent of the total dry weight of the body. More importantly, it is the first line of defense between you and an otherwise hostile environment full of bacteria, yeast, fungi, viruses and toxins. Unlike most organs, skin cells (fibroblasts) are constantly growing, being made to renew the outer layers of the skin, which are constantly lost to the environment. By the age of 30, the rate of new skin cell synthesis declines and by the age of 60 can drop by nearly 50 percent.

The skin is made up of two basic layers: the epidermis and the dermis. The epidermis is the thin outer layer that we can see and feel, and consists mostly of dead skin cells that have pushed their way to the surface. The epidermis is composed primarily of an upper layer, the stratum corneum, whose dead cells have a lipid composition. The stratum corneum is a hydrophobic barrier to the outside environment. These dead skin cells are constantly shed to reveal new skin underneath. They are surrounded by a structural protein called keratin, which prevents the dead cells from flaking off. The entire process from the actual synthesis of a new skin cell to it becoming an integral part of the stratum corneum takes anywhere from 15 to 30 days.

The epidermis also contains cells called melanocytes that release melanin, the compound responsible for tanning and protecting the skin from UV radiation. As the melanocytes decrease with age, your protection against UV radiation also decreases. This leads to brown spots ("age spots") on the skin, which are an accumulation of cross-linked proteins and oxidized fats (lipids) catalyzed by UV radiation in the absence of sufficient melanin. Likewise, a decrease in the number of melanocytes within hair follicles causes hair to go gray. The number of melanocytes is controlled by melanocyte-stimulating hormone (MSH). MSH is secreted from the kidney-bean-sized pituitary gland in the brain but requires a second messenger, cyclic AMP, to do so. Age spots and graying hair are visible indications that cyclic AMP levels may be low in the pituitary gland and could also indicate that other pituitary hormones (the pituitary secretes ten hormones) such as vital growth hormone (GH) may also be running low.

The dermis is the thick underlying layer that delivers nourishment and removes metabolic waste from newly developed skin cells. The dermis also helps regulate collagen and elastin, protein fibers that keep skin soft and also help it to adjust its size to accommodate your growing body—and provide the scaffolding that supports the outer layer of cells, the epidermis.

Skin aging involves structural protein changes in the collagen and elastin that maintain skin's elasticity and flexibility. Wrinkled skin is mostly a combination of reduced collagen synthesis combined with the free radical-induced cross-linking of collagen fibers.

Some of you may feel we should simply accept wrinkled, sagging skin gracefully because it is an inevitable part of growing older. Actually, the condition of your skin is a good barometer of what is going on inside your body.

Skin is not a decorative container. Healthy skin is a hard-working organ, instrumental in the production and storage of vitamin D, which is essential for the absorption of calcium. Skin is vital for maintaining critical body temperature and enables you to retain essential fluids such as blood and water. It plays an important role in the operation of the endocrine system, which is responsible for producing the hormones that govern all bodily functions. The skin contains the cytochrome cells that are constantly monitoring the light (day) and the dark (night) circadian rhythms each day to keep you in supersymmetry with the ecosystem and cosmos.

How Skin Ages

The Scaffolding Collapses: The actual structure of the skin is maintained by elastin and collagen, the scaffolding in the dermis. With age, both of these structural proteins decrease. Another structural protein, keratin (the protein component of the hair and fingernails), which is the protein component of the stratum corneum necessary to maintain the integrity of this barrier to the outside environment, decreases.

You Lose Water: Healthy vibrant skin is plump and filled with 80 percent water. After the age of 30, each year we lose cells that retain moisture and as a result skin becomes drier. By age 50, skin loses about 30 percent of its water. Even though the stratum corneum is composed of dead cells, their ability to form a tight junction is critical for keeping the skin from losing water.

You Lose Lipid Composition: When people go on a no-fat diet, within a very short period of time, significant deterioration of the skin takes place, almost as if the skin were undergoing accelerated aging. Unknowingly, they are depriving themselves of both Omega-3 and Omega-6 essential fatty acids (EFAs). Incidentally, when you regularly add olive oil and cod liver oil to your dog's food, its coat becomes shiny and vibrant. The first sign of an essential fatty acid deficiency is a breakdown in the lipid structure of the dead cells in the stratum corneum, so their tight junction is broken, resulting in dry, flaking skin. Omega-6 EFAs are responsible for this structural function and Omega-3 EFAs are responsible for stimulating the synthesis of keratin, the structural protein in the stratum corneum.

It is easy to visually determine if keratin is being synthesized or not. Fingernails and hair are mostly composed of keratin. Once you begin to eat a balanced bioenergetic, whole-food diet sufficient in lean protein, low-density, unrefined carbohydrates, and essential fats, you quickly observe significant increases in hair and fingernail growth.

The functioning of sweat and oil glands begins to decline at about age 35 and further contributes to moisture loss in older skin.

You Lose Blood Flow: The dermis is extremely rich in capillaries that bring in fresh nutrients and oxygen for the continued manufacture of new skin cells. Once the capillaries "download" the oxygen and nutrients to a cell, they collect and remove the metabolic waste from each cell.

With age, the number of these capillaries decrease, giving rise to the appearance of paler skin. Fewer capillaries mean less oxygen and nutrients "in," as well as less waste "out."

Sun Damage: The vast majority of skin problems are due to what dermatologists call "photo-aging," or excessive damage caused by ultraviolet (UV) rays of the sun. Damage from UV light is cumulative and can take years before it is apparent. There are two types of ultraviolet rays: UVA and UVB. Both types stimulate the formation of free radicals in the skin. UVB rays, commonly referred to as the burning rays, cause immediate damage on the epidermis. UVA rays do not cause a reddening of the skin, but cause injury to the cells of the dermis and the subcutaneous layer of fat that is underneath the outer layer. This damage can show up years later as lines and wrinkles.

The March 2001 edition of the *Journal of the American Academy of Dermatology* presents research showing that green tea extract is remarkably effective at protecting your skin from sunburning. A 2.5 percent solution of extract gave excellent protection, and a 10 percent solution gave complete protection from sunburn. Look for it in topical sun-protective products.

Restoring the Micro-Environment of the Skin

We know that melanocyte-stimulating hormone (MSH) controls the number of melanocytes. The release of MSH from the pituitary gland requires cyclic AMP as a second messenger. Therefore you need to avoid excess saturated fat but consume the Omega-3 EFAs from eating salmon, mackerel, tuna, sardines, trout, cod liver oil, fish oil supplements or algae oil supplements, soybeans, green leafy vegetables, walnuts, flax seeds, hemp seeds, perilla oil and high-DHA eggs from chickens fed organic flax seeds. Also consume a moderate amount of Omega-6 EFAs from legumes, nuts, seeds, organic free-range egg yolks, organic cold-pressed sesame oil (rich in sesamin, sesamol and sesaminol, which are potent antioxidants and act as anti-inflammatory agents), hemp seeds, meat, poultry, evening primrose oil and organic vegetable oils (which must be kept to a minimum). The balance of Omega-6 EFAs to Omega-3 EFAs in your diet should be in an approximate 2:1 ratio. For most people living on modern-day diets, initially consuming more Omega-3 EFAs may be necessary to restore a balance offset by far too many Omega-6 EFAs. The Omega-3 EFAs must supply 1,000 mg of EPA and 650 mg of DHA daily to restore cyclic AMP second messenger levels. Also consume 1/2 teaspoon of Omega-6, GLA-rich borage oil daily.

Both elastin and collagen in the dermis and keratin (all three are structural proteins) in the stratum corneum are restored to optimum levels if you consume sufficient, high-biological-value proteins daily at each of your three meals. Sufficient lean protein consumption stimulates the microproduction of collagen that fills in wrinkles. The drug Retin-A removes wrinkles in this way—but you can do it by "eating smart." As of this writing, a weaker cousin of retinoic acid, retinal, is being used in over-the-counter skin-care products. Retinal can help reduce fine lines and wrinkles, and reduce age-associated skin discolorations, causing the skin to redden and peel as did Retin-A or retinoic acid. Also, the "friendly" prostaglandins, PGE1 and PGE2, formed from eating the proper amounts and ratios of Omega-3 and Omega-6 EFAs, restimulate the synthesis of elastin, collagen and keratin so you re-establish tight, taut, radiant skin. These essential fatty acids improve the tight junction between the dead cells in the stratum corneum so you keep water in the skin cells for a full, vibrant look.

Exercising with a combination of aerobic and anaerobic exercise at least four times a week stimulates blood flow through the capillaries, so the delivery of nutrients and removal of waste debris is encouraged. Exercise also increases the flexibility of capillaries.

Network Antioxidants: The oral supplements of network antioxidants, such as alpha lipoic acid, Co-enzyme Q10, vitamin C-complex, vitamin E-complex with gamma tocopherol, selenium, N-Acetyl Cysteine, lycopene, European bilberry, a carotenoid complex with alpha- and beta-carotene, citrus bioflavonoids and full-spectrum grape extract, keep the capillaries elastic, flexible and healthy. These antioxidants prevent UVA and UVB sun damage and can also rejuvenate collagen, elastin and keratin. They are available in one convenient formula.

The vitamin E-like tocotrienols derived from red palm oil tend to concentrate in the skin and, like the essential fatty acids, maintain youthful skin. The Malaysians, famous for their lovely complexions, liberally use red palm oil, the richest natural source of tocotrienols, in cooking. Antioxidant creams are the ideal way of transdermally bringing antioxidant protection into your skin. The ideal cream, not yet on the market, would contain:
- tocotrienols from red palm oil,
- CoQ10,
- alpha lipoic acid,
- fat-soluble vitamin C as ascorbyl palmitate,
- vitamin A-complex,
- RNA and DNA for cellular regeneration,
- vitamin E-complex, and
- MSM (methyl sulfany methane).

There is at present little doubt that skin stays less wrinkled and more youthful when supplied with antioxidants both from the inside (supplements and a bioenergetic diet) and from the outside (antioxidant creams). High levels of antioxidants, taken orally and topically, slow down the aging of skin cells. Ideally, DHEA and melatonin, both hormones, could be added to a night-time facial cream in a liposome delivery form.

Rehydrate: Since your skin is 80 percent water, ensure that you drink your daily water quota of at least six to 12 full 8 oz glasses of clean water spread throughout the day.

Cleanse Naturally as an Alchemist: Be an alchemist in your washroom and easily create the finest cleansing solution. Grind organic oatmeal in a coffee grinder and put the powdered oatmeal in a jar next to your sink. Morning and night, use this powder to wash your face and neck. Put 2 tablespoons of powdered rolled oats onto the palm of your hand and sprinkle water into it until a thick, but not runny, composition is produced. First, wet your face with warm water, then wash with the "muddy" oatmeal. Wash for one minute, then leave the oatmeal on for three minutes. The oatmeal cleanses your skin of dead cells and old oils. It also is a humectant and adds moisture to your skin. Wash off with cold water and pat dry.

Rejuvenate Your Face with Fruit: You can teach your older skin new tricks by encouraging it to shed old cells and replace them with new ones. Over the last 15 years, dermatologists have developed a system of using chemical peels to exfoliate dead skin cells and reveal glowing new skin. The chemicals used in this process are typically Retin-A or tretinoin, but these agents, while effective, can lead to burning, irritation and elevated sensitivity to the sun in many people.

There is a natural and more gentle way to renew a lifeless complexion—fruit-derived alpha-hydroxy acids (AHAs) and beta-hydroxy acids (BHAs). Glycolic acid is the best-known member of the alpha-hydroxy family and is useful in treating age spots, acne, fine lines and shallow wrinkles. There are many commercial products available, but for best results a product should have a concentration of 4 to 8 percent glycolic acid and a pH between 3.0 and 4.0. Papaya and pineapple are two popular fruits used in natural peels because they are both rich in AHAs. Both fruits contain a protein-dissolving enzyme that sloughs off dead cells and stimulates collagen production. In papaya this enzyme is papain, and in pineapple it is bromelain. You can mix lemon or grapefruit with these fruits as they are also high in AHAs.

Since free radical damage plays a role in photo-aging of the skin, the addition of certain antioxidants to AHA products is essential. Look for products with L-ascorbic acid, ascorbyl palmitate (synthetic, fat-soluble vitamin C), vitamin E, CoQ10 and alpha lipoic acid. These antioxidants have a synergistic effect on reversing the evidence of sun-damaged skin. They further protect the skin from the sun's UVA and UVB rays, as well as stimulate the synthesis of pro-collagen genes.

Face peels should be applied to skin that has been cleansed. Dry skin responds to peels containing either glycolic acid or lactic acid, or both. Both acids are water-binding and act as humectants. Those with blemish-prone skin, should use a BHA peel that includes salicylic acid derived from willow bark. Salicylic acid breaks up and clears away excess oil without drying the skin. Normal or oily skin responds well to either AHA or BHA peels, or a combination of both. Before sleep, spread peels on your face, leave on for five to ten minutes and wash off with cold water. Follow this with a moisturizer rich in CoQ10.

Make Your Own Peel—in the Evening: Once a week, be an alchemist and take 1 teaspoon of fresh, organic lemon juice, and mash it up with 2 tablespoons of either ripe papaya or pineapple. Add this to your ground oatmeal and add a little water to make a fluid paste. To this, add 1/2 teaspoon of a "green drink," and then add 1 teaspoon of aloe vera gel and 1/2 teaspoon of witch hazel. Apply to your clean face and neck. Gently scrub for two to three minutes. Leave on for one-half hour to one hour. The oatmeal draws out toxins and waxes. The "green drink" adds colored pigments to your skin and acts as a toner; the BHAs and AHAs from the fruits slough off dead skin from a deep level; the witch hazel tighten pores; and the aloe vera gel soothes irritated skin.

Wash this mixture off with cold water and pat your face dry. Use a moisturizing cream rich in CoQ10 or break open a softgel containing 100 mg of CoQ10. Spread the contents of the softgel over your face, concentrating on wrinkles, age spots and troubled skin. On top of this, gently pat in a moisturizing cream rich in CoQ10, or a serum or cream rich in CoQ10 and designed as a wrinkle-defense system. Do this on a weekend or evening so you can take time and relax afterwards or go to sleep.

The Evening Herbal Face Sauna: Boil 1 quart of pure water. My favorite herbs to mix in the water are 2 tablespoons of lavender essential oils and 1 tablespoon each of the powdered herbs: orange blossoms, peppermint, chamomile and fennel seeds.

Mix herbs in the boiling water, turn off the heat, remove the pot from the burner, cover the pot and let stand for two minutes. Make a tent-like cover out of a towel and cover your head and the pot as you lean over the hot pot. Close your eyes and take a few deep relaxing breaths. Steam your face for ten minutes. Splash cool water on your face and apply your CoQ10 moisturizing serum, cream or gel. Your skin will be ultra-clean and radiant.

Vitamin C Serum or Cream—in the Morning: Gently massage a small amount of a commercial vitamin C washing solution into your face and neck, using upward circular motions. Let set for two minutes and rinse well with warm water. Follow with a little vitamin C serum, cream or lotion. A little vitamin C goes a long way, and too much can be irritating. Wait five minutes for the vitamin C to be fully absorbed and then apply your favorite moisturizer. Vitamin C stimulates collagen production. It stimulates the microproduction of collagen that fills in wrinkles.

The old saying that beauty is skin deep is correct. You can successfully control the appearance of your skin by altering the hormonal micro-environment with bioenergetic whole foods. Bioenergetic foods are your "smart drugs" for radiant and clear skin.

BIOENERGETIC FOODS FOR RADIANT HAIR

The Biochemical Background

For most people the shock sets in when they find their shower drain clogged with hair or their pillow covered with loose hair. If your once-thick hair is falling out in small clumps, or you've got bald patches appearing, you're not alone. Although there are many types of hair loss, the most common type—androgenetic alopecia (AGA)—affects up to 60 percent of men and 25 percent of women, beginning at about the age of 35 to 40.

AGA in both sexes is caused by a combination of heredity and hormonal forces. Women with AGA generally have diffuse hair-thinning all over the scalp, most noticeably over the top of the scalp. Men with AGA typically get receding hairlines and large patches of hair loss fringed by a horseshoe-shaped tuft of hair. Most people have referred to male hair loss as "male pattern baldness." In genetically susceptible hair follicles of the scalp, an enzyme known as 5-alpha-reductase enzyme converts the hormone testosterone into another metabolite hormone called dihydrotestosterone (DHT). In a process called miniaturization, DHT shrinks hair follicles and causes them to lose function and deteriorate over time. Scalp hair becomes thinner and starts to fall out. DHT also stimulates prostate growth, leading to enlargement of the prostate gland called benign prostatic hyperplasia (BPH). The prostate swells and squeezes the urethra partially or completely closed.

Increased levels of sebum, the oily substance that can clog pores, is also thought to contribute to hair loss by holding DHT inside hair follicles. Poor scalp circulation is attributable to a combination of a fatty buildup in the blood vessels from excess saturated fat from meat and dairy; plus excess arachidonic acid (AA) primarily from meat, egg yolks, full-fat dairy; excess Omega-6 fats from vegetable oils; unfriendly trans-fatty acids in processed foods; and not enough long-chain Omega-3 essential fatty acids rich in DHA and EPA. Furthermore, inadequate vitamin C, vitamin E and antioxidants (such as zinc, selenium, alpha lipoic acid, full-spectrum grape seed and skin extract and CoQ10 with tocotrienols) adds to the problem.

As people age (beginning at 25 but becoming pronounced by 40), testosterone in men and women becomes bound to sex hormone-binding globulin (SHBG), the component in blood that renders free testosterone inactive.

In young males, low amounts of estrogen are used to "turn off" the powerful cell-stimulating effects of testosterone. As estrogen (specifically estradiol) levels increase in men, beginning at about 35, testosterone cell stimulation may be locked in the "off" position. As more and more testosterone is converted to estrogen (estradiol), the estradiol is taken up by testosterone receptor sites in cells. When an estradiol molecule occupies a testosterone receptor site on a cell membrane, it blocks the ability of serum testosterone to induce a healthy hormonal signal. It does not matter how much free testosterone is available if excess estrogen (estradiol) is competing for the same cellular receptor sites. For testosterone to function as a support for hair growth, it must be "freely" available to cell receptor sites in hair follicles and not be "bound" in the bloodstream by SHBG or competing with excess estradiol. To complicate matters even more, the large volume of estradiol tricks the brain into thinking that enough testosterone is being produced, thereby slowing the natural production of testosterone.

For men, it is desirable to suppress excess levels of both sex hormone-binding globulin (SHBG) and estrogen (estradiol), while boosting free testosterone levels. The safest and easiest way to increase free testosterone is to prevent it from being converted (aromatized) into excess estradiol. If blood test results show your estradiol levels are greater than 30 pg/mL, men should consider using an aromatase-inhibiting agent. Certain herbs and plant medicines, such as saw palmetto, pygeum, stinging nettle root, corn silk, chrysin (a bioflavonoid) and diindolylmethane (DIM), are natural aromatase inhibitors.

Research indicates that chrysin is not absorbed well on its own, but the addition of a black pepper extract ingredient called piperine significantly enhances the bioavailability of chrysin, so it can act as a potent aromatase-inhibiting agent preventing the conversion of testosterone to dihydrotestosterone (DHT).

Testosterone is the substrate to make estrogens. The more insulin you produce, the greater the accumulation of body fat. It is that stored body fat that contains the enzyme that converts testosterone to estradiol. The only way to reduce estrogen (estradiol) formation is to reduce excess body fat. That can only be done by lowering insulin levels. Lowered insulin levels can quickly be achieved by removing from your diet processed, sweet foods and eating more bioenergetic whole foods such as fruit, lean protein, vegetables, whole grains, herbs, legumes, salads and sea vegetables. Finally, to increase testosterone levels, you must reduce cortisol levels by reducing your overall stress. As cortisol levels rise, testosterone levels drop.

Counteracting Hair Loss

There are four distinct remedial steps that you can take to naturally keep your hair growing radiant and reasonably thick.

Step 1—Reduce Estradiol: Do not put weight on, and systematically eliminate any excess fat you are carrying, especially abdominal fat. It is in this fat pad that the enzyme is synthesized and converts testosterone to estradiol (estrogen). Lose the excess body fat and this enzyme's activity declines dramatically. Elk velvet antler extracts, stinging nettle root, wild oats, ashwagandha (an Indian herb) and yohimbine (derivative of yohimbe tree bark) all raise free testosterone.

Step 2—Support Free Testosterone: Generally, physicians prescribe the drug Proscar (finasteride) or Propecia (finasteride) at 1 mg daily to inhibit the action of 5-alpha-reductase enzyme and prevent the conversion of testosterone to dihydrotestosterone (DHT).

In Europe, in 90 percent of the cases, physicians use a combination of four powerful herbal extracts to successfully block the conversion of testosterone to dihydrotestosterone (DHT). These potent plant medicines have documented remarkable blocker therapeutic effects, working just as well as Proscar or Propecia. The herbal extracts are saw palmetto (450 mg a day), pygeum (125 mg of a 30:1 extract daily), stinging nettle root (30 mg of a 10:1 extract daily) and corn silk (120 mg of a 4:1 extract). In addition, the plant medicine from licorice root (at least 200 mg daily) aids as an herbal transporter to ensure these four herbs are absorbed and delivered. These herbal extracts, aided by licorice, also have prostate-specific anti-inflammatory effects and should be used twice daily by all men 35 years of age and older. Use two capsules of this formula in the morning, between meals, and two capsules in the afternoon. These herbs prevent free testosterone from binding to sex hormone-binding globulin (SHBG), which renders free testosterone inactive.

Step 3—Aromatize: Inhibiting the conversion of valuable free testosterone into estradiol (estrogen) is a process called aromatization. It is not uncommon for a 65-year-old male to have higher estradiol levels in his body than a woman of the same age.

Stinging nettle root extract is a medicinal herb that prevents this unfortunate conversion from taking place, as does diindolylmethane (DIM).

Another aromatizing agent is the bioflavonoid extracted from plants called chrysin. To be absorbed it must be in combination with an extract from black pepper called piperine. From the time you notice your hair thinning, use an encapsulated supplement containing 1,000 mg of chrysin and 10 mg of piperine.

There is a Chinese herb called He Shou Wu that has been used for centuries as an effective aromatizing agent. In the extract of He Shou Wu, researchers isolate the active ingredient, chrysophanics, a metabolite of chrysin. He Shou Wu can be taken by supplement—generally I recommend three capsules daily containing at least 1,500 mg of a 12:1 standardized extract of He Shou Wu. It is also available in topical solutions that you rub on your scalp before going to sleep.

In India the aryuvedic herb ashwagandha has been used as an herbal arom-atizing agent for centuries.

Plant phytosteroids have testosterone-enhancing effects that activate and accelerate the body's anabolic rate. A remarkable new product called enact+ combines a proprietary Suma extract (Ekdisten) and Sambaia—two plants very high in natural ecdysterones—with an aqueous extract of stinging nettle root that supports testosterone functions in the body.

Step 4—Feeding Hair from Within: No matter which hair-loss treatment you choose, it is important to follow a balanced diet of bioenergetic foods. Men in particular should follow a low-cholesterol diet, since research has found a link between AGA and high-cholesterol diets. Because protein is a chief constituent of hair, both men and women should eat an adequate amount of high-biological-value protein foods each day.

Minerals

Iron, zinc, copper and silica are the minerals most closely associated with healthy hair. In lab experiments, zinc inhibits 5-alpha-reductase activity. The effect was strengthened when vitamin B6 was added.

Found in all body tissue, copper is involved in normal hair growth. It also inhibits the activity of 5-alpha-reductase enzyme. A number of topical hair-growth lotions contain copper peptides (a copper/protein combination) and have shown good results in preventing hair loss. Remember, zinc prevents excess copper activity. If you use any copper peptide solutions on your hair, ensure that you supplement them with at least 30 mg of zinc daily, and have your physician test your blood for copper and zinc levels.

Silica is a mineral involved in the formation of collagen and is essential for healthy hair. The herb horsetail is rich in silica. You can supplement before sleep, with one cup of horsetail tea or two capsules totaling 1,000 mg of atomized aqueous extract of spring horsetail (equisetum arvense), supplying about 20 mg of pure organic silica. Or, you can use ten to 20 drops of a liquid containing 2 percent elemental silicon as stabilized orthosilic acid. Each drop has 1 mg of silica and is extremely bioavailable.

Twenty men with AGA were given two capsules daily of a supplement containing silica and a fish oil extract daily for six months. As a control, 20 other men took only two capsules of fish oil daily. The group with the silica-fish oil combination grew 38 percent more hair, compared to just 2 percent in the other group. Massaging essential oils into the scalp for just two minutes a day with a combination of rosemary, thyme, lavender and cedarwood, blended with jojoba oil and grape seed oil, is gaining a dedicated following.

Conclusion

Every hair on your head adheres to a genetically programmed schedule that includes growth, resting and shedding. About 90 percent of the hair on your head grows approximately 1/2 inch (12 mm) per month and continues for two to six years. There are three hair growth cycles:

1. Anagen Phase: the active cycle of hair growth and may last for several years. At any given time, 90 percent of hair is in this phase.
2. Catagen Phase: a cycle of several months in which the hair follicle regresses and begins to shrink.
3. Telogen Phase: the cycle at the end of the Catagen Phase when hair is released from the shriveled follicles and the Anagen Phase begins again.

When the growth phase ends, usually the hair shaft begins a rest period and then sheds. Only 10 percent of your hair is resting at any one time. On the average, 50 to 150 hairs are lost each day, but most hair regrows because the follicle (root) remains. Considering the typical adult head has about 100,000 shafts of hair, 50 to 150 hairs is not a lot of loss. Eventually, a new hair shaft begins to grow from the root embedded inside the hair follicle, pushing out the old shaft as it grows. When shedding significantly exceeds growth, excessive thinning occurs.

Wash your hair daily with a high-quality antioxidant shampoo to clear away excess sebum and feed the scalp with antioxidant nutrients. Use thorough brushing, scalp massage and even inverted yoga poses to improve scalp circulation. Avoid the excessive use of electric hair dryers, which dry your hair out too much. Vitamins and herbs can reverse or stabilize the miniaturization process. Vitamin B6 and biotin inhibit the action of 5-alpha-reductase enzyme from converting testosterone into follicle-killing DHT. Research indicates that you may require 50 mg of vitamin B6 three times a day, and 100 mcg of biotin three times a day to help in this process.

A bioenergetic, anabolic, whole-foods dietary strategy can make your existing hair healthier and more radiant than ever.

APPENDIX D

RESOURCES

Please note that I have thoroughly researched each of the following companies and their products. In the case of greens+ I developed the product myself after years of research. Each company has superior products and continually is committed to maintaining their superior quality. I highly recommend each and every one of these companies because I also personally use these products, publications or online services. Each company offers 100 percent guarantee to protect you, the consumer.

LONG-CHAIN OMEGA-3 FATTY ACIDS, FISH OILS, DHA AND EPA

In Canada
Ocean Nutrition Canada Ltd.
Bedford, Nova Scotia
Toll-free: (800) 980-8889
Web site: www.ocean-nutrition.com

In the United States
Roche Vitamins
Parsippany, New Jersey
Toll-free: (800) 526-8413

Quest Vitamins
Triple Fish Oil
(Anchovy, mackerel, sardine)
Vancouver, British Columbia
Toll-free: (888) 683-4653
Web site: www.questvitamins.com

Martek Biosciences Corp.
Columbia, Maryland
Tel: (410) 740-0081
producer of algae oils
rich in DHA and EPA

GOOD ESSENTIAL FATTY ACID (EFA) MANUFACTURERS

Udo's Choice Oil and Flax Oil

In Canada
Flora Distributors Ltd.
Burnaby, British Columbia
Toll-free: (800) 663-0617
Web site: www.florahealth.com

In the United States
Flora Distributors Ltd.
Lynden, Washington
Toll-free: (800) 446-2110
Web site: www.florahealth.com

Omega Balance Oil and Flax Oil

In Canada
Omega Nutrition Canada Inc.
Vancouver, British Columbia
Toll-free: (800) 661-3529
Web site: www.omegaflo.com

In the United States
Omega Nutrition U.S.A. Inc.
Bellingham, Washington
Toll-free: (800) 661-3529
Web site: www.omegaflo.com

Hemp Oil and Bioriginal Oil

In Canada
Bioriginal Food and Science Corp.
Saskatoon, Saskatchewan
Tel: (306) 975-9268
Fax: (306) 242-3829
Web site:
   intro@freshhempfoods.com

In Canada and the United States:
Manitoba Harvest
Fresh Hemp Foods (oil and seeds)
Winnipeg, Manitoba
Toll-free: (800) 665-4367
(I have personally followed
the growth and development of
this young company and
their exceptional quality.)

CONCENTRATED GREEN FOODS

Not all concentrated "green drinks" are of the same quality. **greens+** is the only multi-award-winning formula in Canada and the United States. It has won a gold prize as "Product of the Year" in both countries on several occasions. greens+ contains the green drink formula noted in Chapters 8 and 15.

In Canada
ehn inc. (greens+ Canada)
Toronto, Ontario
Toll-free: (877) 500-7888
Web site: www.greenspluscanada.com

In the United States
Orange Peel Enterprises Inc.
Vero Beach, Florida
Toll-free: (800) 643-1210
Web site: www.greensplus.com

HERBAL PRODUCTS AND PREPARATIONS RECOMMENDED

In Canada and the United States
ehn inc. (greens+ Canada)
Toronto, Ontario
Toll-free: (877) 500-7888
Web site: www.greenspluscanada.com

VITAMINS, MINERALS, ANTIOXIDANTS AND FLAVONOIDS

Look for formulas that contain as close a mix to the network I recommend in this book. There are many various qualities on the market, so choose wisely. For instance, full-spectrum grape seed extract formulas should contain 95 percent procyanidolic values with resveratrol and ellagic acid. A superior brand is called **grapes+**, which contains all the values mentioned in Chapter 20, page 324.

IN CANADA AND THE U.S.

grapes+ (formula listed in Chapter 20, page 324), **protect+** (formula listed in Chapter 8, page 113 and Chapter 19, page 312), **A·G·E inhibitors** (formula listed in Appendix B, page 338) and **diindolylmethane** (DIM) (formula listed in Chapter 4, page 58) are distributed by:
ehn inc. (greens+ Canada)
Toronto, Ontario
Toll-free: (877) 500-7888
Web site: www.greenspluscanada.com

Each of the following Canadian companies produce a large array of superior supplements that I highly recommend:
Flora
Burnaby, British Columbia
Toll-free: (888) 436-6697 or
(800) 663-0617
Web site: www.florahealth.com

Natural Factors
Burnaby, British Columbia
Toll-free: (800) 669-4241
Web site: www.naturalfactors.com

Quest Vitamins
Boehringer Ingelheim
Vancouver, British Columbia
Toll-free: (888) 683-4653
Web site: www.questvitamins.com

SISU Enterprises Co. Inc.
Burnaby, British Columbia
Toll-free: (800) 663-4163
Web site: www.sisuhealth.com

IN THE UNITED STATES

Dr. Julian Whitaker's Healthy Directions, Inc. produces superior supplements targeted for specific needs. I highly recommend:
Heart Essentials; Joint Essentials; Memory Essentials; Osteo Essentials; Pain Essentials; Vision Essentials

These superior lines are distributed by:
Healthy Directions, Inc.
Potomac, Maryland
Toll-free: (800) 722-8008
Web site: www.drwhitaker.com

Another superior line of supplements is distributed by:
Life Extension Foundation
Hollywood, Florida
Toll-free: (800) 544-4440
Web site: www.LifeExtension.com

I highly recommend:
Life Extension Mix
(multivitamin-mineral-herbal-amino
  acid formula)
Super CoQ10 with Tocotrineols
Herbal Mix
Vitamin K
Super Carnosine Capsules
Gamma E Tocopherol
Vitamin B12 (methyl cobalamin)

Prairie Naturals
Essential Phytosterinolins Inc.
Port Coquitlam, British Columbia
Toll-free: (800) 931-4247
Web site: www.prairienaturalsi.com

Purity Life
Acton, Ontario
Toll-free: (877) 297-7332
Web site: www.moducare.com
This company distributes the award-winning
product Moducare, which has been clinically tested
to balance the immune system.

WHEY PROTEIN ISOLATE (POWDERS proteins+ [Alphapure™],
formula listed in Chapter 14, pages 206–208; **transform+**, formula listed in
Chapter 14, page 208)
Alphapure™ is a patented isolation process for whey protein isolate, creating the
highest biological value of any protein on the market today. In the U.S.A. another
excellent whey protein isolate is Enhanced Life Extension Protein (ELEP).

In Canada	**In the United States**
Alphapure™ is distributed	Life Extension Foundation
exclusively	Hollywood, Florida
in Canada by ehn inc.	Toll-free: (800) 544-4440
ehn inc. (greens+ Canada)	Web site: www.LifeExtension.com
Toronto, Ontario	
Toll-free: (877) 500-7888	
Web site: www.greenspluscanada.com	

BOVINE COLOSTRUM
A superior bovine colostrum in liquid or powder is **Symbiotics Colostrum™**,
distributed by:

In Canada	**In the United States**
Smarte Brand Laboratories, Ltd.	Symbiotics, Inc.
Calgary, Alberta	Sedona, Arizona
Tel: (403) 252-7150	Toll-free: (800) 784-4355
E-mail: smarte@smarte.ab.ca	Web site: www.symbiotics.com

SOY PROTEIN ISOLATE
The Supro® non-GMO brand of soy protein isolate contains the highest quality
water-extracted soy protein on the market today. Soy protein is a very good
source of the amino acid tryptophan, as well as the muscle-building branched-
chain amino acids (BCAAs).

In Canada and in the United States
Supro®
Protein Technologies International
St. Louis, Missouri
Toll-free: (877) 769-4432 or (800) 325-7108

WHEY PROTEIN ISOLATE AND SOY PROTEIN ISOLATE

The award winning product, **transform+**, is a unique combination of **greens+**, Alphapure™ whey protein isolates, Supro® soy protein isolates and all the necessary plant-based digestive enzymes.

In Canada
ehn inc. (GREENS+ Canada)
Toronto, Ontario
Toll-free: (877) 500-7888
Web site: www.greenspluscanada.com

In the United States
sorry, not available

SPECIAL FORMULATIONS

For Weight Loss

For maximum fat burning, you can find the most effective and safest combination available as **lean+**.

lean+ contains:

Cayenne
Citrus aurantium
Coleus forskohlii
Grapefruit juice powder

Green tea extract
Guggulipids (plant compounds)
Hydroxycitric acid (HCA)
    from Garcinia Cambogia

For Muscle Growth and Anabolic Acceleration

Various plant phytosteroids are effective in increasing the anabolic rate and reducing the declining catabolic rate of metabolism. All these natural phyto-steroids can now be found in one product that also incorporates the testos-terone-enhancing effects of stinging nettle root extracts. The product is called **enact+** and it makes use of safe natural phytosteroids found in plants to activate and accelerate the body's anabolic rate. Energy is processed more efficiently, stores of fat are converted to lean body mass, and the structure of the body is repaired and rebuilt at a faster rate.

enact+ combines a proprietary Suma extract (Ekdisten) and Samambaia—two plants very high in natural ecdysterones—with stinging nettle root (Urtica dioica) extract (aqueous extract) to accelerate the body's natural, revitalizing anabolic drive.

Both formulations are the wonderful work of nutritional researcher, Brad King.

In Canada	In the United States
ehn inc. (greens+ Canada)	ehn inc. (greens+ Canada)
Toronto, Ontario	Toronto, Ontario
Toll-free: (877) 500-7888	Tel: (416) 977-3505
Web site: www.greenspluscanada.com	Web site: www.greenspluscanada.com

SPECIAL ACIDOPHILUS FERMENTED YOGURT

In Canada and in the United States

Bio-K+ International Inc.

Montreal, Quebec

Toll-free: (800) 593-2465

Web site: www.biokplus.com

THREE TOP-NOTCH PUBLICATIONS AND ONLINE RESOURCES

There is one newsletter that has the most up-to-date health information that I highly recommend everyone should subscribe to. It is *Health and Healing* by the brilliant and dedicated Dr. Julian Whitaker, M.D.

It is a vibrant publication, informative, practical and encouraging.

In Canada and in the United States

Health and Healing

Healthy Directions, Inc.

Potomac, Maryland

Toll-free: (800) 722-8008

Web site: www.drwhitaker.com

A must-read monthly magazine of exceptional quality, cutting-edge health information for health-care professionals and serious students of health and nutrition that I highly recommend is *Life Extension Magazine*.

In Canada and in the United States

Life Extension Magazine

The Life Extension Foundation

Hollywood, Florida

Toll-free: (800) 544-4440

Web site: www.LifeExtension.com

The most informative and well-written online resource worldwide is written monthly by Hans R. Larsen, M.Sc., of Victoria, British Columbia. Monthly he gives an overview of the latest, most practical, nutritional research. The online service, *International Health News*, is in its tenth year of publication.

In Canada and in the United States

International Health News

E-mail: health@pinc.com

REFERENCES

Abbas, Abul K., et al. *Cellular and Molecular Immunology*. Philadelphia, PA: W.B. Saunders Company, 1994.

Adachi, K, et al. "Suppression of the hydrazine-induced formation of megamitochondria in the rat liver by coenzyme Q10." *Toxicol Pathology*, 23 (1995): 667–676.

Adams, P.B., S. Lawson, A. Sanigorski, and A.J. Sinclair. "Arachidonic acid to eicosapentaenoic acid ratio in blood correlates positively with clinical symptoms of depression." *Lipids*, 31 (1996): 157–161.

American Heart Association. 1997 *Heart and Stroke Statistical Update*. Dallas, TX: American Heart Association, 1996.

American Journal of Clinical Nutrition, 1999: 69: 411–418. (Greenlanders study)

Ascherio, A., C.H. Hennekens, and W.C. Willett. "Trans-fatty acid intake and risk of myocardial infarction." *Circulation*, 89 (1994): 94–101.

Atkins, Robert C., M.D., and Sheila Buff. *Dr. Atkins' Age-Defying Diet*. New York: St. Martin's Press, 2001.

Austad, S.N. *Why We Age*. New York: John Wiley and Sons, 1997.

Balch, James F., M.D. *10 Natural Remedies That Can Save Your Life*. New York: Doubleday, 1999.

Balin, Arthur K. *Practical Handbook of Human Biological Age Determination*. Boca Raton, FL: CRC Press, 1994.

Bark, Joseph P., M.D. *Your Skin... An Owner's Guide*. New York: Prentice Hall, 2000.

Barnard, Neal, M.D. *Eat Right Live Longer*. New York: Harmony Books, 1997.

Barnard, Neal. M.D. *The Power on Your Plate*. Summerton, TN: Book Publishing Co., 1990.

Batmanghelidj, F. *Your Body's Many Cries for Water*. Falls Church, VA: Gobal Health Solutions, 1995.

Bierhaus, A., M.A. Hofmann, R. Ziegler, et al. "AGEs and their interaction with AGE-receptors in vascular disease and diabetes mellitus." *Cardiovascular Research*, 1998, 37(3): 586–600.

"Bioenergetic Therapy for Aging." *Life Extension Magazine*, February 2001: 24–32.

Blakeslee, Sandra. "The Surprising Theory on the Body Clock: Illuminate the Knee." *The New York Times,"* January 16, 1998.

Bland, Jeffrey S., Ph.D., and Sara Benum, M.A. *Genetic Nutritioneering*. Keats Lincolnwood, IL, 1999.

Bland, Jeffrey, S.Ph.D. "Dietary Fibers: Insoluble and Soluble." *Technical Bulletins*. Education/Technical Focus. GIG Harbor, WA: Health Communications International, Inc., 1995.

Blundell, J., and C. Halford. "Serotonin and appetite regulation." *CNS Drugs*, 9 (1998): 473–495.

Borek, Carmia. *Maximize Your Life Span with Antioxidants*. New Canaan, CT: Keats Publishings, 1995.

Brink, Susan. "Sleepless Society." *U.S. News and World Report*, October 16, 2000.

Broadway, J., et al. "Bright Light Phase Shifts the Human Melatonin Rhythm during the Antarctic Winter." *Neuroscience Letters*, 79 (1987): 185–189.

Brooke, Martin. "The Species Enigma: Disappearing Life Going Extinct." *New Scientist*, June 13, 1998.

Brownson, C., A.R. Hipkiss. "Carnosine reacts with a glycated protein." *Free Radical Biological Medicine*, 2000, 28(10): 1564–1570.

Burke, Edmund R., Ph.D. *Optimal Muscle Recovery*. Garden City Park, NY: Avery Publishing Group, 1999.

Burr, G.O., and M.M. Burr. "A new deficiency disease produced by the rigid exclusion of fat from the diet." *Journal of Biological Chem*istry, 82 (1929): 345–367.

"Cellular Nutrition for Vitality and Longevity." *Life Extension Magazine*, April 2000: 24–28.

Christensen, L. "The effect of carbohydrates on affect." *Nutrition*, 13 (1997): 503–514.

Colgan, Michael, Ph.D. *Essential Fats for Athletes*. Vancouver, BC: Apple Publishing Group, 1999.

Colgan, Michael, Ph.D. *The Right Protein For Muscle and Strength*. Vancouver, BC: Apple Publishing Co., 1998.

Conner, M. et al. "Primitive Diets of Our Ancestors." *New England Journal of Medicine*, 31 (January 1985): 4–8.

Cummings, S., B. Truong, and D. Gietzen. "Neuropeptide Y and somatostatin in the anterior piriform cortex alter intake of amino acid-deficient diets." *Peptides*, 1998.

D'Adamo, Peter, J., N.D., and Catherine Whitney. *Eat Right 4 Your Type*. New York: G.P. Putnam's Sons, 1996.

Dean, Ward, M.D. *Biological Aging Measurement Clinical Applications*. Los Angeles: The Center for Bio-Gerontology, 1988.

Di Pasquale Mauro, M.D. *The Anabolic Diet*. Toronto: Optimum Training Systems, 1995.

Di Pasquale, Mauro, M.D. "Dietary Protein: The Anabolic Edge." *Anabolic Research Review*, 1996, 1(3): 12–21.

Di Pasquale, Mauro, M.D. "High-Tech Supplementation." *Anabolic Research Review*, 1996, 1(5): 1–15.

Dilbert, M.S., et al. "Suicide Gene Therapy for Plasma Cell Tumor." *Blood*, September 15, 1996, 88 (6): 2192–2200.

Dineen, Sean. "Metabolic Effects of the Nocturnal Rise in Cortisol on Carbohydrate Metabolism in Normal Humans." *Journal of Clinical Investigation*, November 1993, 92(5): 2283–2290.

Drewnowski, A. "Why do we like fat?" *Journal of American Diet*, 1997, supplement: 558–562.

Dumas, M., et al. "Age related response of human dermal fibroblasts to L-ascorbic acid: study of type I and III collagen synthesis." *CR Academy of Science III*, Dec. 1996, 319 (12): 1127–1132.

Duncan, David Ewing. "Counting the Days." *New Scientist*, August 22, 1998.

Dunlap, Jay. "An End in the Beginning." *Science*, June 5, 1998.

Eaton, Boyd S., M.D., M. Shostak, and Melvin Konner, M.D., Ph.D. *The Paleolithic Prescription*. New York: Harper and Row, 1988.

Evans, W., and I.H. Rosenberg. *Biomarkers*. New York: Simon and Schuster, 1991.

Fauler, J., C. Neumann, D. Tsikas, and J. Frolich. "Enhanced synthesis of cysteinyl leukotrienes in psoriasis." *Journal of Investigative Dermatology*, 99 (1992): 8–11.

Felig, P., J.D. Baxter, and L.S. Frohman. *Endocrinology and Metabolism*, 3rd ed. New York: McGraw-Hill, 1995.

Fishman, Alfred P., M.D. "Hibernation in Animals." *Circulation*, August 1961: 433.

Fossel, Michael, M.D. *Reversing Human Aging*. New York: William Morrow, 1996.

Garcia-Closas R., A. Agudo, C.A. Gonzales, and R.E. Riboli. "Intake of specific carotenoids and flavonoids and the risk of lung cancer in women in Barcelona, Spain." *Nutritional Cancer*, 32 (1998): 154–158.

Gaziano, J.M., C.H. Hennekens, C.H. O'Donnell, J.L. Breslow, and J.E. Buring. "Fasting triglycerides, high-density lipoprotein, and risk of myocardial infarction." *Circulation*, 96 (1997): 2520–2525.

Georgakas, Dan. *The Methuselah Factors: Learning from the World's Longest Living People*. Chicago: Academy Chicago Publishers, 1995.

Giovannucci E. "Tomatoes, tomato-based products, phytonutrients, lycopene and cancer: review of the epidemiological literature." *Journal National Cancer Institute*, 91 (1999): 317–331.

Gould, K.L. "Very low-fat diets for coronary heart disease: Perhaps, but which one?" *Journal of the American Medical Association*, 275 (1996): 1402–1403.

Graci, Sam. *The Power of Superfoods*. Toronto: Prentice Hall, 1997.

Gulyaeva, N.S., A.M. Dupin, and I.P. Levshina. "Carnosine prevents activation of free-radical lipid oxidation during stress." *Exploratory Biological Medicine*, 1989, 107(2): 148–152.

Gulyaeva, N.V. "Superoxide-scavenging activity of carnosine in the presence of copper and zinc ions." *Biochemistry* (Moscow), 1987, 52 (7, Part 2): 1051–1054.

Haas, Robert. *Eat to Win for Permanent Weight Loss*. New York: Harmony Books, 2000.

Hag, I., M. Jamieson, and A. Ormerod. "Randomized trial of aromatherapy. Successful treatment for alopecia areata." *Archives of Dermatology*, 134 (1998): 1349–1352.

Hakkinen, S., et al. "Screening of selected flavonoids and phenolic acids in 19 berries." *Food Research International*, 32 (1999): 345–353.

Hayflick, L. *How and Why We Age*, 222–262. New York: Ballantine Books, 1994.

Heller, Richard, Ph.D., and Rachael F. Heller, Ph.D. *The Carbohydrate Addict's LifeSpan Program*. New York: Penguin Books, 1997.

Hipkiss, A.R., C. Brownson. "A possible new role for the anti-ageing peptide carnosine." *Cellular Molecular Life Sciences*, 2000, 57(5): 747–753.

Hirschberg, A. "Hormonal regulation of appetite and food intake." *Annals of Medicine*, 30 (1998):7–20.

Horning, M.S., L.J. Blakemore, and P.Q. Trombley. "Endogenous mechanisms of neuroprotection: role of zinc and copper and carnosine." *Brain Regulations*, 1 (2000): 56–61.

Horrobin, D.F., ed. *Omega 6 Essential Fatty Acids*. New York: Wiley-Liss, 1990.

Jazwinski, S. Michael. "Longevity, Genes, and Aging." *Science*, 273 (July 1996): 54–58.

Kagawa Y. "Impact of Westernization on the Nutrition of Japanese: Changes in Physique, Cancer, Longevity, and Centenarians." *Preventive Medicine*, 7 (1978).

Kagawa Y., M. Nishizawa, M. Suzuki, T. Miyatake, T. Hamamoto, K. Goto, E. Montaonga, H. Izumikawa, H. Hirata, and A. Eibhara. "Eicospolyenoic acids of serum lipids of Japanese islanders with low incidence of cardiovascular diseases." *Journal of Nutritional Science Vitaminology*, 28 (1982): 441–453.

Katahn, Martin, Ph.D. *The Tri-Colored Diet*. New York: W.W. Norton and Company Inc., 1996.

Khalsa, Dharma, S., M.D., with Cameron Stauth. *Brain Aging*. New York: Warner Books, 1997.

King, Brad. *Fat Wars: 45 Days to Transform Your Body*. Toronto: CDG Books Canada, Inc., 2000.

King, Brad, and Michael Schmidt, Ph.D. *BIO-AGE, Ten Steps to a Younger You*. Toronto: CDG Books, 2001.

Klatz, Ronald M., M.D. *Advances in Antiaging Medicine*, Vol. 1, New York: Mary Ann Liebert Inc., 1996.

Kleiner, Susan M., Ph.D., and Maggie Greenwood-Robinson. *Power Eating*. Champaign, IL: Human Kinetics, 1998.

Kniewald, Z., V. Zechner, and J. Kniewald. "Androgen hydroxysteroid dehydrogenases under the influence of pyridoxine derivatives." *Endocrine Regulations*, 26 (1992): 47–51.

Kronhausen, Eberhard, ED. D., and Phyllis Kronhausen, ED.D. *Formula for Life*. New York: Quill Books William Morrow and Co., 1999.

Lamb, M.J. *Biology of Aging*. New York: John Wiley and Sons, 1997.

Lamm, S. *The Virility Solution*. New York: Simon and Schuster, 1998.

Larsen, Hans R., M.A. *International Health News Yearbook 2001*. Victoria, BC: International Health News, 2000. (http://www.com/healthnews)

Larsen, Hans, R. Editorial. *International Health News*. September 2000: 105.

Lass, A., et al. "Comparisons of coenzyme Q bound to mitochondrial membrane proteins among different mammalian species." *Free Radical Biological Medicine*, 1999: 220–226.

Lass, A., et al. "Mitochondrial ubiquinone homoloues, superoxide radical generation, and longevity in different mammalian species." *Journal of Biological Chemistry*, 1997.

Lassus, A., and E. Eskeline. "A comparative study of a new food supplement, viviscal, with fish extract for the treatment of hereditary androgenic alopecia in young males." *Journal of International Medical Research,* 20 (1992): 445–453.

Laux, M., and C. Conrad. *Natural Women, Natural Menopause.* New York: HarperCollins, 1995.

Lee, T.H. "Beneficial Effects of a Mediterranean Diet: A Randomized Trial." *Journal Watch,* December 1996,16(23): 114–126.

Lichenstein, A.H., and L. Van Horn. "Very low fat diets." *Circulation,* 98 (1998): 935–939.

Linet, O.I., and F.G. Orginc. "Efficacy and safety of intracavernosal alprostadil in men." *New England Journal of Medicine,* 334 (1996): 1–7.

Linnane A.W., et al. "Mitochondrial DNA mutations as an important contributor to ageing and degenerative diseases." *Lancet,* 1989: 642–645.

Linnane, A.W., et al. "The universality of bioenergetic disease. Age-associated cellular bioenergetic degradation and amelioration therapy." *Ann NY Academy of Science,* 1998: 202–213.

Macieira-Coelho, Alvaro, ed. *Molecular Basis of Aging.* Boca Raton, FL: CRC Press, Inc., 1995.

Martin, S.J., et al. "Ordering the cytochrome c-initiated caspase cascade: Hierarchical activation of caspases-2, -3, -6, -7, -8, and -10 in a caspase-9-dependent manner." *Journal of Cell Biology,* 144 (Jan. 25, 1999): 281–292.

Mattes, R., Ph.D. "Physiologic responses to sensory stimulation by food: Nutritional Implications." *Journal of American Dietitians,* 97 (1997): 406–410.

Mazur, A. "Aging and endocrinology." *Science,* 279 (1998): 305–306.

McFarland, G.A., and R. Holliday. "Retardation of the senescence of cultured human diploid fibroblasts by carnosine." *Experimental Cell Regulations,* 1994, 212(2): 167–175.

Miller, Martin. "Ageless Quest for Fountain of Youth Is Alive and Well." *Los Angeles Times,* April 9, 1998.

Mimura, G. K. Murakami, and M. Gushiken. "Nutritional factors for longevity in Okinawa-present and future." *Nutritional Health,* 8 (1992): 159–163.

Mindell, Earl, Ph.D. *Earl Mindell's Anti-Aging Bible.* New York: Doubleday, 1999.

Moore, Thomas. *Life Span: Who Lives Longer and Why.* New York: Simon and Schuster, 1993.

Moss, Robert. "The Problem with Evolution: Where Have We Gone Wrong?" *The Scientist,* October 13, 1997.

Murray, Michael. *The Healing Power of Herbs.* Rocklin, CA: Prima Publishing, 1995.

Nissinen, A., and K. Stanley. "Unbalanced diets as a cause of chronic disease." *American Journal of Clinical Nutrition,* 49 (1999): 993–998.

Norman, A.W., and G. Litwack. *Hormones,* 2nd ed. New York: Academic Press, 1997.

Packer, L., Ph.D., and Carol Colman. *The Antioxidant Miracle.* New York: John Wiley and Sons, 1999.

Pelchat, M. "Food cravings in young and elderly adults." *Appetite,* 28 (1997): 103–113.

Pinnell, S. "Regulation of collagen biosynthesis of ascorbic acid: A review." *Yale Journal of Biological Medicine,* 58 (1985): 553–559.

Pirisi, Angela. "The Road to Lifelong Health." *Life Extension Magazine.* Holly, FL, January 2001.

Randall, V. "Role of 5-alpha-reductase in health and disease." *Baillieres Clinical Endocrinology and Metabolism,* 8 (1994): 405–431.

Reddy, A.C.P., and B.R. Lokesh. "Studies on spice principles as antioxidants in the inhibition of lipid peroxidation of rat liver microsomes." *Molecular Cellular Biochemistry,* 1992: 111–117.

Regelson, W., and C. Colman. *The Super-Hormone Promise.* New York: Simon and Schuster, 1996.

Rennie, John, Michelle Press, and Steve Mirsky. "The Quest to Beat Aging." *Scientific American,* September 6, 2000.

Ricklefs, Robert E., and Caleb E. Finch. *Aging: A Natural History.* New York: Scientific American Library, 1995.

Roth, J.S., M. Gluck, R.S. Yalow, and S.A. Berson. "The influence of blood glucose on the plasma concentration of growth hormone." *Diabetes,* 13 (1964): 335–361.

Rousseau, J.J. "Discourse on the Original of Social Inequality." *The Social Contract and Discourses.* Paris, 1755.

Schiffman, S., and C. Gatlin. "Clinical physiology of taste and smell." *Annals Registered Nutrition*, 13 (1993): 405–436.

Science News, 19, 151 (April 1997): 239.

Sears, Barry, Ph.D. *The Anti-Aging Zone*. New York: Regan Books HarperCollins, 1999.

Sears, Barry, Ph.D. *The Soy Zone*. New York: Regan Books HarperCollins, 2000.

Sears, Barry, Ph.D. *The Zone*. New York: Reagan Books, 1995.

Simopoulos, A.P., and J. Robinson. *The Omega Plan*. New York: HarperCollins, 1998.

Sinkovics, J., and J. Horvath. "Apoptosis by Genetic Engineering." *Leukemia*, April 1998 (8): 98–102.

Siple, Molly, M.S. *Healing Foods for Dummies*. Foster City, CA: IDG Books Worldwide, 1999.

Snodderly, D.M. "Evidence for protection against age-related macular degeneration by carotenoids and antioxidant vitamins." *American Journal of Clinical Nutrition*, 1995.

Somer, Elizabeth, M.A. *Food and Mood*. New York: An Owl Book, 1999.

Spirduso, Waneen W. *Physical Dimensions of Aging*. Champaign, IL: Human Kinetics, 1995.

Stamatiadis, D., M.C. Bulteau-Portios, and I. Mowszowicz. "Inhibition of 5 alpha-reductase activity in human skin by zinc and azelaic acid." *British Journal of Dermatology*, 119 (1988): 627–632.

Susan, S.A., et al. "Mitochondria as regulators of apoptosis: doubt no more." *Life Extension Magazine*, February 2001: 24–31.

Taub, Edward A., M.D. *Balance Your Body, Balance Your Life*. New York: Kensington Publishing Co., 1999.

"The Wonders of Whey Restoring Youthful Anabolic Metabolism at the Cellular Level," *Life Extension Magazine*, May 1999.

Timiras, P.S., ed. *Physiological Basis of Aging and Geriatrics*, 2nd ed. Boca Raton, FL: CRC Press, 1994.

Timiras, P.S., W.B. Quay, and A. Vernakdakis, eds. *Hormones and Aging*. Boca Raton, FL: CRC Press, 1995.

Tsai, L., et al. "Basal concentration of anabolic and catabolic hormones in relation to endurance exercise after short-term changes in diet." *European Journal of Applied Physiology and Occupational Physiology*, 1993, 66(4): 304–308.

Ullis, Karlis, M.D. *Age Right*. New York: Simon and Schuster, 1999.

Valentine, Tom. "Interview with Dr. Johanna Budwig, M.D., Ph.D." *Health Letter*, Jan/Feb. 1993.

Walford, Roy, M.D., and Lisa Walford. *The Anti-Aging Plan, Strategies and Recipes for Extending Your Healthy Years*. New York: Four Walls Eight Windows, 1994.

Wechsler, Pat. "A Short in the Dark." *New Yorker*, November 11, 1996.

Weil Andrew, M.D. *Eating Well for Optimum Health*. New York: Alfred A. Knopf Publishers, 2000.

Weindruch, Richard. "Calorie Restriction and Aging." *Scientific American*, 274 (January 1996): 46–52.

Weissberg, Steven M., M.D., and Joseph Christiano, A.P.P.T. *The Answer Is in Your Blood Type*. Lake Mary, FL: Personal Nutrition USA, Inc., 1999.

"What's Missing From Multi-Vitamin Supplements?" *Life Extension Magazine*. Wilton Manors, FL, November 2000: 19–38.

Whitaker, J., M.D., and Carol Colman. *Shed 10 Years in 10 Weeks*. New York: Simon and Schuster, 1999.

Wiley, T.S. and Bent Formby, Ph.D. *Lights Out*. New York: Pocket Books, 2000.

Wilson, J.D., and D.W. Foster, eds. *Williams Textbook of Endocrinology*, 8th ed. Philadelphia, PA: W.B. Saunders Co., 1992.

Yeager, Selene, and editors of Prevention Health Books. *New Foods for Healing*. New York: Bantam Books, 1999.

Yen, S.S., et al. "Replacement of DHEA in aging men and women: Potential remedial effects." *Ann NY Academy of Science* 774 (December 1995) : 128–142.

INDEX